cir 82
271 - Lunari

Nursing care of patients with
UROLOGIC DISEASES

Nursing care of patients with
UROLOGIC DISEASES

CHESTER C. WINTER, M.D., F.A.C.S.

Professor of Urology, The Ohio State University College of Medicine;
Director of Urology, University Hospital,
Columbus, Ohio

MARILYN ROEHM BARKER, R.N., M.S.

Instructor, The Ohio State University School of Nursing;
Assistant Director of Nursing Service and Systems Research, University Hospital,
Columbus, Ohio

THIRD EDITION

With 200 illustrations

THE C. V. MOSBY COMPANY

SAINT LOUIS   1972

Preface

The third edition of *Nursing Care of Patients with Urologic Diseases* follows the purpose and plan of the previous edition: a text designed for use by nurses and nurses' assistants who work on any type of urologic unit—outpatient clinic, inpatient service, cystoscopy suite, or urologic surgical area. Sections of the second edition are retained in original or rewritten form, but the major portion of the book represents revised and current concepts concerning urologic disorders and their nursing management. Many new illustrations are included to emphasize the visual method of teaching.

In the introduction to the book the origin of urology is traced back to 3000 B.C. A glossary of urologic terms is provided for the novice. The chapter on anatomy, anomalies, and physiology has been revised and enlarged to include diseases related to the urologic organs. Urologic equipment is described and illustrated in Chapter 3. The largest section in this text is devoted to the general principles of urologic nursing and brings special procedures and up-to-date concepts to the nurse's attention.

The physiologic and psychologic differences resulting from variations in age that affect urologic problems are emphasized in Chapter 5. Full descriptions of the nurse's role in urologic diagnostic procedures are given in Chapter 6; many of these tests are new. The principal categories of urologic diseases are discussed in separate chapters: renal parenchymal diseases, obstructive uropathy, infectious diseases, urinary calculi, genitourinary neoplasms, neurogenic disorders, urologic afflictions peculiar to women and men, and, finally, diseases of the adrenal glands amenable to surgery.

The chief audience for this text is the nurse in a hospital situation, but both office and public health nurses should find considerable information of value in this book, as should nurses in other medical specialties or those concerned with general duty. By the same token, the urologic nurse is encouraged to seek additional guidance from texts on general nursing and surgical nursing care.

A list of current and key references for more definitive reading concerning urologic problems is included at the end of each chapter and a few older but classic references have been retained.

A new addition to each chapter is a list of pertinent questions, the answers to which are found in the textual material for that chapter. This should be especially useful to the nursing student for review as well as applicable for use by teachers in testing retention of reading assignments.

Chester C. Winter

Marilyn Roehm Barker

Contents

CHAPTER 1

Introduction

Urology or genitourinary surgery is concerned with the prevention, diagnosis, and treatment of diseases of the urinary system in both sexes and of the reproductive system in the male. The development of urology as a surgical specialty began at the turn of the twentieth century but was forecast by the invention of the cystoscope by Nitze in 1876. Edison's invention of the incandescent lamp in 1888 and Roentgen's discovery of x-rays in 1895 made possible the direct visual examination of the lower urinary system as well as the indirect delineation of the upper urinary tracts. Radiopaque contrast materials were first injected into the upper urinary system in a retrograde fashion in 1907, making possible the outline of the renal pelvis and ureters. Intravenous pyelography was introduced in 1923 and furnished a means of estimating renal function in addition to outlining the urinary collecting system by the use of roentgenography. Urologists today can diagnose genitourinary diseases with greater accuracy utilizing the many instruments and diagnostic procedures made available through developments in radiologic procedures and nuclear medicine.

The basic diagnostic urologic tool is the hollow tube, or catheter, that is known to have been used as far back as 3000 B.C. by the Egyptians. Excavations from the ruins of Pompeii, a city buried during the volcanic eruptions of A.D. 79, have revealed sounds used to dilate the urethra. Woven silk catheters similar to those in use today were in evidence during the eighteenth century in Europe. Since then, latex, nylon, and silicone rubber tubes have been developed.

The earliest reported urologic operation was a lithotomy, the incision and removal of stones from the urinary system. Stone removal from the bladder was carried out as early as 600 B.C. The mortality rate was high. Special instruments were developed to insert through incisions in the perineum and into the urethra and bladder for crushing and removing stones. The marvel of these operations is greater when it is realized that they were performed without anesthesia or sterile techniques as used to-day. With the advent of general anesthesia in the 1840's, the first nephec-tomy was possible and was successfully carried out by Simon of Heidel-berg in 1869. Urology has made great strides in the last few decades due to the introduction of chemotherapy and the antibiotic agents, which have markedly reduced the morbidity and mortality rates. The most exciting developments in recent urologic history are the use of the artificial kidney and renal transplantation. When the renal transplant rejection phenomenon is finally solved, kidney transplantation and perhaps substitution of other organs in the urologic tract will become a specialty in itself.

The training of a urologist, in addition to 36 months of medical school, in-cludes a year of internship and 4 years of surgical-urologic residency. Nurses hoping to achieve full practical competence in the field of urology need spe-cial preparation and training in the care of patients with urologic diseases. The urology clinic provides a wealth of training in special diagnostic maneu-vers, in the use of urologic instruments, and in radiologic procedures. Since urologic disorders can occur at any age, the urology nurse must be properly prepared in the fields of pediatrics, obstetrics, gynecology, endocrinology, pharmacology, internal medicine, and geriatrics. A sound background in psychiatric disorders is paramount in understanding the emotional needs and disorders of the urologic patient. Urologic nursing therefore offers a wide experience with a diversity of disorders and patients to be encountered. Urology is not as limited a field as might be thought in view of the rather small number of organs of the body that are involved and their anatomic location. Preventive medical principles are also becoming more applicable in modern medical practice and concepts in epidemiology and in the pre-vention of diseases should be understood. The nurse who plans to enter clinical practice in urology will be a much greater asset to the physician if she has some knowledge of office procedures and organizational efficiency. Finally, a nurse must develop a pleasing and confident personality that will aid and comfort the sick patient, who frequently is fearful and has not even a rudimentary knowledge of the many mysteries of medicine.

A word of caution should be kept in mind by all nurses reading this book. Throughout the text, advice is offered on how the nurse can give psychologic and social aid to the patient. The nurse must be very certain that her ministrations are appropriate, tactful, constructive, and within the bounds of her professional background and experience. Especially im-portant is the knowledge that the therapeutic measures she uses conform to the desires of the physician in charge of the patient. She should try to keep informed as to the goals of the physician and consult with him rather than boldly striking out on her own.

GLOSSARY

agenesis Absent at birth.

anuria Less than 250 ml. urine output per 24 hours (technically, none).

azotemia Asymptomatic elevation of blood level of urea nitrogen and other metabolic products.

bougie à boule Straight rod with an olive or cone tip used for calibrating the urethra or ureter (Fig. 3-4).

caliectasis Enlarged renal calyces.

calycectomy Excision of renal calyx (segmental resection of kidney).

catheter Hollow tube for traversing the urethra or a hollow organ (Fig. 3-2).

    Councill catheter—Foley catheter with open end, allowing wire guide with screw on its tip to attach to a filiform.

    Foley catheter—Double-lumened retention catheter with an inflatable bag near its end (the large channel is for drainage and the smaller lumen is for inflation of the bag).

    Malecot catheter—Preformed retention catheter with two, three, or four collapsible wings near its tip.

    Pezzar catheter—Performed retention catheter with its collapsible end shaped like a mushroom.

    Robinson catheter—Straight, hollow tube with eyes near its end.

contrast material Material containing iodine or heavy metal and producing roentgenologic contrast.

coudé Curved tip of catheter or other instrument (Fig. 3-3).

Credé maneuver To press on the lower abdomen in order to empty the bladder.

cystocele Prolapse of bladder into vagina.

cystolitholapaxy Crushing and removal of calculi from bladder by means of instruments (Fig. 3-10).

cystolithotomy Removal of calculi by incision of bladder.

cystoscopy Indirect visualization of bladder by means of an instrument (Figs. 3-7 and 3-8).

cystostomy Percutaneously (or vaginally) placed tube in bladder.

cystotomy Incision made in bladder.

cystectomy Surgical removal of bladder.

diuria Frequency of micturition in daytime.

dysplasia Grossly abnormal tissue at birth.

dysuria Painful urination.

-ectomy To remove.

ectopic Congenital misplacement of an organ.

endogenous Source from within the human body.

endoscopy Indirect visualization of lower urinary tract by means of an instrument with a multiple lens system (Fig. 3-8).

enuresis Involuntary nocturnal micturition.

exogenous Source from outside the human body.

filiform Long, small-caliber, flexible rod for traversing urethral strictures or for catheterization (Fig. 3-4).

follower Solid or hollow tube attached to filiform for dilating urethral strictures or for catheterization (Fig. 3-4).

French (Fr.) Unit of measurement of a tube that equals 1 mm. in circumference.

frequency Increased incidence of voiding, day or night.

hematuria Blood in the urine; termed gross, micro-, initial, terminal, or complete.

hesitancy Difficulty in initiating micturition.

hydrocele Fluid-filled sac around testis or in spermatic cord.

hydronephrosis Abnormal enlargement of renal pelvis and calyces (Fig. 8-9).

incontinence Involuntary micturition.

    paradoxical incontinence Involuntary overflow voiding.

stress incontinence Involuntary micturition on pressure such as sneeze or cough.

urgency incontinence Involuntary micturition with strong urge to void.

intermittency Interrupted passage of urine while voiding.

-itis Inflammation.

litholapaxy Crushing and removal of urinary calculi.

lithotomy Incisional removal of intact calculi.

lithotomy position Supine, with hips and knees flexed and abducted (Fig. 6-1).

lithotripsy Crushing of urinary calculi with lithotrite.

lithotrite Instrument for crushing calculi internally (Fig. 3-10).

lithuria Passage of urinary stones or gravel.

micturition Voiding, or urination.

nephrectomy Surgical removal of kidney.

nephrogram Opacification of kidney parenchyma by contrast agent.

nephrolithotomy Incision of kidney and removal of calculus (Fig. 10-5, *B*).

nephropexy Fixation of kidney in its normal position.

nephrostomy Intubation of kidney.

nephrotomy Incision into kidney.

nocturia Frequency of micturition at night.

oliguria Between 250 and 500 ml. urine output per 24 hours.

orchiectomy Removal of testis.

orchiopexy Fixation of testis in normal location.

-ostomy To intubate or to open to the surface.

-otomy To cut.

paraphimosis An abnormally tight prepuce above the glans penis (Fig. 2-10, *B*).

-pexy To fix in position.

phimosis An unretractable foreskin (Fig. 2-10, *A*).

-plasty To repair.

pneumaturia Passage of urine containing gas.

prostatism Difficulty in micturition due to any cause in either sex (paradoxical in females and children).

pyelectasis Enlarged renal pelvis.

pyelogram Roentgenographic outline of internal architecture of kidney with contrast medium.

    excretory pyelogram (IVP) Made following intravenous injection of contrast agent (Fig. 6-14).

    retrograde pyelogram Made by introducing contrast material through ureteral catheters (Fig. (6-16).

pyelolithotomy Incision of renal pelvis and removal of calculus (Fig. 10-5, *A*).

pyeloplasty Operative reconstruction of renal pelvis and its ureteric junction (Fig. 8-13).

pyelotomy Incision of renal pelvis.

pyuria Abnormal number of white blood cells in urine.

reflux Backward flow of urine.

renogram Radioisotope test tracing obtained from kidney (Fig. 6-12).

resectoscope Endoscopic instrument for cutting and fulgurating tissue under indirect vision (Fig. 3-9).

residual urine Volume of urine in bladder immediately after micturition.

scintiscan Radioisotope test for outlining the kidneys (Fig. 6-13).

sound Metal rod used to calibrate or dilate the urethra (Fig. 3-4).

stranguria Painful and difficult passage of urine.

tenesmus Painful bladder spasms and painful straining to urinate.

transureteroureterostomy Implanting one ureter into the wall of the other.

uremia Symptomatic blood elevation of metabolic products usually found in urine.

ureterolithotomy Incision of ureter and removal of calculus (Fig. 10-5, *C*).

ureteroneocystostomy Reimplantation of ureter into bladder (Fig. 8-10).

urethroplasty Surgical reconstruction of urethral deformity (Fig. 8-3, *B*).

urethrotomy To cut the urethra.
urgency Intense desire to void.
uroflometry Graphic depiction of rate of urine flow.
urogram Roentgenologic appearance of urinary tract outlined with contrast medium.
uropathy Urinary tract disease.

QUESTIONS

1. What inventions made possible the development of urology as a specialty?
2. The foundation of urology rests upon what instruments?
3. What is the oldest urologic operation?
4. When was the first nephrectomy performed? By whom? Where?
5. Urology overlaps what other medical specialties and why?
6. In what manner may a nurse allay the fears and doubts of the urologic patient?
7. Why must a nurse be cautious in what she tells the patient?

REFERENCES

Immergut, M. A.: Classical articles in urology, Springfield, Ill., 1967, Charles C Thomas, Publisher.
Morel, A.: A unified urological nursing unit, RN 8:54, 1968.
Morel, A.: The urologic nurse specialist, Nurs. Clin. N. Amer. 4:475, 1969.

CHAPTER 2

Anatomy, anomalies, and physiology of male and female urinary tracts and the male reproductive system

Urinary system

Intelligent care of urologic patients is dependent upon an understanding of the subject's disorder and thus the nurse must have a thorough knowledge of the structure and function of the genitourinary system. Frequent reference to this chapter will be made throughout this book.

The urinary systems of the male and female differ in respect to their anatomic relationships with other organs of the body. The ureter and bladder in the female have a close relationship to the genital system. The male urethra is anatomically and physiologically different from that of the female. While these differences are clinically significant, in the following discussion the anatomy of the upper urinary system and its functioning in a normal person are treated as a common system for both sexes. Pertinent dissimilarities in the lower urinary tract are pointed out.

KIDNEYS

Renal function is essential to the maintenance of life and two and a half times the minimal functional requirement is provided for normal persons. Thus a human being can live in good health with only one normal kidney, allowing an individual to donate one kidney for renal transplantation to another individual. The remainder of the urinary system consists of two ureters, a bladder, and the urethra, which serve to transport, store, and discharge urine. The entire urinary system lies extraperitoneally, that is, behind and below the peritoneum that surrounds the organs in the abdominal cavity.

Anatomy

The adult kidneys (Latin, *renal;* Greek, *nephros*) are two bean-shaped organs about 4¼ inches long and 2½ inches wide; they are encapsulated by thin but tough, fibrous connective tissue. One lies on each side of the spinal column on the paraspinal muscles at the level of the lower thoracic and upper lumbar vertebrae (twelfth thoracic to the third lumbar). The right kidney is located slightly lower than the left because the liver lies above and anterior to it. It is also more mobile and in the female frequently descends when the subject is upright. The upper pole of each kidney is apposed to the diaphragm superiorly and about half of each kidney lies within the lower rib cage. The gallbladder lies directly anterior to the right kidney. This may cause difficulty in distinguishing x-ray shadows of renal and biliary calculi (kidney stones and gallstones). Frequently some confusion may occur regarding symptoms resulting from diseases of the biliary, digestive, and urologic organs. The adrenal glands (suprarenal glands) cap the medial upper pole of each kidney. The ascending colon and duodenum lie adjacent to the right kidney, while the left is abutted by the spleen above, the descending colon anteriorly, and the tail of the pancreas medially.

The kidneys are held in place by perirenal fat and connective tissue fascia (Gerota's), which is contiguous with the fascia of surrounding structures. The renal blood vessels and the ureters are important direct attachments.

Blood vessels, lymphatics, and nerves enter each kidney at the concave central portion on its medial aspect, which is known as the hilum. The renal pelvis, a funnel-shaped extension of the ureter, also is attached to the kidney at the hilum (Figs. 2-1 and 2-2). It lies posterior to the renal vascular pedicle and this relationship explains why the urologist uses a posterior flank surgical approach for operations on the renal pelvis as well as for some kidney operations. In contrast, operations upon the renal vessels and for removal of large tumors of the kidney are best approached anteriorly via the transabdominal route.

The kidneys are richly supplied with blood, receiving about one fourth of the cardiac output or about 1200 ml. per minute. The renal arteries are short vessels that branch directly off the abdominal aorta. The right renal artery is the longer of the two and passes behind the vena cava, making it difficult for the surgeon to approach. One out of five kidneys has an accessory artery. Within the kidneys the renal arteries divide into anterior and posterior branches that run to the boundary zone between the cortex and medulla and there subdivide into the arcuate arteries that radiate into all parts of the cortex of the kidney. Small afferent arterioles branch off the arcuate arteries along their course, and each afferent vessel joins to a small tuft of capillaries known as a glomerulus. These capillaries again join to

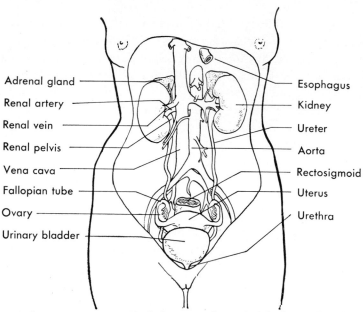

Fig. 2-1. Female urinary tract. Right kidney usually is slightly lower than left. Ureters pass anterior to iliac vessels and posterior to uterine arteries. Lower ureter is frequently injured in gynecologic operations or secondarily involved by diseases of female reproductive tract. (Adapted from unpublished illustration of Dr. B. G. Clarke and Dr. L. Del Guercio.)

form the smaller efferent arterioles. Each of the efferent vessels breaks up into peritubular capillaries, providing the sole blood supply to the renal tubules. The blood from the peritubular capillaries flows into the venules and thence into the renal vein, which empties directly into the inferior vena cava. The right renal vein is very short since the inferior vena cava is close to the right renal hilum. Only the longer left renal vein receives the left gonadal vein (ovarian or spermatic). Since the arteries do not intercommunicate, the kidney is really made up of four or five main units, each capable of being destroyed (infarction) if its segmental artery becomes occluded or severed.

It is the belief of some anatomists and physicians that there exists a shunt mechanism in the kidney that in time of acute body need allows blood to pass directly from the efferent arterioles into the venous system, bypassing the peritubular capillaries. This phenomenon is known as the juxtamedullary circulation of Trueta.

The renal lymphatics accompany the renal blood vessels, the renal tubules, and the renal capsules; they ultimately drain into lymph nodes at the junction of the renal vascular pedicles and aorta. The renal lymph glands communicate with other lymph channels along the abdominal aorta,

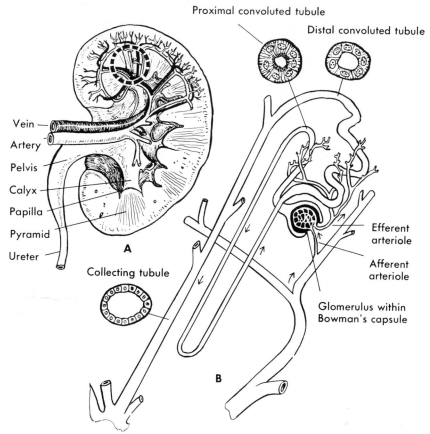

Fig. 2-2. Anatomy of kidney. **A,** Renal blood supply, pelvis, upper ureter, medulla, and cortex. **B,** Nephron unit. Note variations in lumenal caliber and cellular size in different parts of tubule. Blood supply of glomerulus and tubule is also shown. (Adapted from unpublished illustration of Dr. B. G. Clarke and Dr. L. Del Guercio.)

the inferior vena cava, and the periureteral sheath. They move renal products back into the circulation and serve as safety valves in case of blockage of the renal vein or ureter.

The kidneys are supplied with both sympathetic and parasympathetic nerve fibers. Both types of fibers pass with the branching blood vessels to the arterioles, the glomerular capillaries, and the renal tubules. These nerves have not been found to be essential for urine formation, but strong stimulation of the sympathetic nerves does diminish production of urine by constricting the afferent arterioles and thus decreasing the blood supply to the glomeruli, where the first process in urine production occurs. This has been demonstrated by the fact that the transplanted kidney functions well despite a severed nerve supply.

The renal parenchyma (solid portion of the kidney) is divided into two sections: the cortex and the medulla. The cortex, the thinner outer layer and the paler of the two, is situated between the renal capsule and the base of the renal pyramids and extends in fingerlike projections between the pyramids. The medulla is the segment of the kidney between the cortex and the renal pelvis. It is composed of the renal pyramids, which insert (as a papilla) into the calyces of the renal pelvis (Fig. 2-2). The renal pyramids consist of the collecting tubules and ducts and their supporting structures. The collecting ducts empty into the calyces (Greek word meaning "cups") of the renal pelvis. The normal kidney contains from seven to twelve of these cuplike structures. The calyces are joined by infundibula (Latin word meaning "funnels"), which in turn join to form the renal pelvis (Greek word meaning "basin"), which narrows as it joins the ureter; this junction is known as the ureteropelvic junction and is frequently a site of ureteral obstruction (Fig. 2-2).

The functioning unit of the kidney is called the nephron. Each kidney parenchyma contains approximately 1 million nephrons. Each nephron consists of a glomerulus (renal corpuscle or malpighian body) and a renal tubule. Bowman's capsule (dilated upper portion of renal tubule) snugly adheres to the tuft of glomerular capillaries. The glomerulus is located in the cortex of the kidney parenchyma. The renal tubule is an unbranched, tortuous duct, which on leaving the renal corpuscle is known as the proximal convoluted tubule. It then becomes straight and narrow and proceeds for a variable distance into the medulla, where it sharply bends and returns to the vicinity of the glomerulus. The straight portion is divided into three sections: the descending tubule, the loop of Henle, and the ascending tubule. At the level of the renal corpuscle the tubule again becomes convoluted and is called the distal convoluted tubule. It then empties into a collecting tubule; many of these tubules unite to form a collecting duct that courses back through the medulla to empty into one of the calyces of the renal pelvis (Fig. 2-2).

Anomalies

Normally the renal outline is symmetrical, but if an uneven outline is seen, it is labeled fetal lobulation and has no other significance. A small but otherwise normal kidney is known as a hypoplastic kidney and is not to be confused with a diseased kidney. Anomalies of the renal system are horseshoe kidney (two kidneys joined at the lower pole by a symphysis and very rarely at the upper pole), pancake-shaped kidney, abnormally rotated ectopic kidney that is located low in the body or even on the other side (crossed ectopia), and a divided kidney that has separate drainage systems. The latter are called supernumerary if they are completely separated or duplicated if they are contained under one capsule. The duplicated kidney is more common and usually enlarged. When only the renal pelvis is divided, the kidney is called bifid. Ectopia is related to improper upward migration of the kidneys in the embryo. Occasionally a person is born with only one kidney or has only a small amount of nonfunctioning nephrogenic tissue on one side (agenesis and dysplastic kidney, respectively). Congenital cystic disease will be considered in Chapter 11.

Physiology

The kidneys have two essential functions—homeostatic and excretory. The homeostatic function helps to maintain the constant composition of body fluids within limits essential to the maintenance of life. The excretory function, closely related to homeostatic function, is concerned with elimination from the body of the waste products of body metabolism such as urea, uric acid, creatinine, and excessive ketone bodies and elimination of excesses of normal fluid and electrolyte components of body cells and tissues. It also provides for removal of certain medications, poisons, and other foreign substances from the body.

The kidneys, by conserving or eliminating fluids and electrolytes present in the blood plasma that passes through them, continually adjust the osmotic pressure, volume, and ionic structure of the body fluids. It is estimated that the total blood volume (approximately 4000 to 5000 ml.) passes through and is acted upon by the kidneys about every half hour. This means that at least 190 liters of plasma are processed each day by the kidneys. The nephrons are the units responsible for the discriminatory function of the kidneys. The processes involved are glomerular filtration and tubular reabsorption, secretion, and excretion.

Glomerular filtration. The process of urine formation begins in the glomeruli. About 125 ml. of fluid (water filtrate) passes from the blood through the walls of the glomerular capillary system, through Bowman's membrane, and thence into the proximal convoluted tubules. The fluid is then known as glomerular filtrate. The glomeruli may be visualized as sieves through which the blood plasma, containing all its constituents except the proteins, is forced by the hydrostatic (push) pressure of the blood flowing into the glomeruli; this pressure is estimated to be about 70 mm. Hg. Only about one half of this pressure is effective, however, in driving the fluid through the membrane since it is counterbalanced by colloidal osmotic (pull) pressure exerted by the plasma proteins in the blood and a back pressure exerted by any of the fluid already in the tubule. The plasma proteins and the blood cells are too large to pass through the walls of the normal glomerular capillaries in any appreciable quantity. The glomerular filtrate is rich in creatinine, urea, and electrolytes.

Glomerular filtration is affected by the blood pressure and heart rate in normal individuals. The rate of filtration increases with rises in the blood pressure and pulse rate (coffee and tea increase urine output by increasing pulse rate and afferent arteriole pressure); it drops with decreases in blood pressure. When the arterial pressure remains between 80 and 200 mm. Hg, however, there is little change in the flow rate. Arterial pressures below 60 mm. Hg reduce glomerular filtration to zero. The effects of shock therefore can have serious consequences on the vital regulatory mechanisms of the body provided by renal function; that is, shock can cause body fluid and electrolyte imbalances that may be incompatible with life.

Tubular reabsorption. Both waste products and many constituents essential to normal body function pass from the glomeruli into the renal tubules indiscriminately, and a remarkable selective process occurs. The tubules eliminate substances in excess of normal body need and conserve those needed from the glomerular filtrate. The substances to be retained are reabsorbed through the tubular walls into the interstitial fluid (fluid in the tissue spaces) and thence into the bloodstream via the peritubular capillaries. Since quantities of substances necessary for life far in excess of body reserves are filtered each day, marked disturbance in the reabsorptive process of the kidney can rapidly lead to death.

It is fairly well known in which parts of the renal tubules absorption of various substances takes place or by what mechanisms absorption of certain substances are controlled. Two distinct mechanisms seem to play important roles—diffusion and active transport. Diffusion is a passive process by which a solution of low concentration (with low osmotic pressure) is pulled toward a region containing a solution having a higher osmotic pressure until such time as the two fluids become isotonic (equal in osmotic pressure). This is sometimes called obligatory movement of fluid. There is a gradual osmotic gradient extending from the renal capsule to the pelvis as well as within the tubule. The highest concentration of constituents of both urine and interstitial tissue fluid is found in the medulla. Active transport is a process requiring the expenditure of energy to move a substance from an area of low concentration to one of high concentration. Intracellular enzymatic reactions, as yet not well understood, are necessary for active transport to occur.

Most of the water, sodium, and chloride seem to be reabsorbed from the glomerular filtrate in the proximal convoluted tubules. This may occur by diffusion since the blood in the proximal peritubular capillaries has a high osmotic pressure as a result of a fifth of its fluid content being filtered off in the glomerulus. On the other hand, sodium may also be actively transported from the glomerular filtrate into the peritubular blood, and its (the sodium's) positive charge may attract the chlorides, which are negatively charged ions. The sodium chloride thus formed would then create an osmotic force that would in turn pull the water. Active reabsorption of other substances such as glucose, amino acids, phosphates, and sulfates also adds to the osmotic pressure of the blood in the peritubular capillaries and tends to pull water into them. Anything that causes abnormally large quantities of osmotically active substances such as glucose, urea, or proteins to be present in the renal tubular fluid, however, impedes the reabsorption of water by the tubules and acts as a diuretic, that is, increases the urinary output.

After the glomerular filtrate has passed through the proximal convoluted tubules, about 20% of its water content remains. Practically all of this water is normally absorbed in the distal convoluted tubules and collecting ducts. Vasopressin, the antidiuretic hormone (ADH) produced by the posterior pituitary gland, however, appears to control the amount of water eliminated or reabsorbed in the distal convoluted tubules and collecting ducts. If fluid is needed by the body, this hormone apparently makes the walls of the collecting tubules permeable so that water is readily reabsorbed. When the body needs less fluid, vasopressin production stops and the water is excreted rather than absorbed (diuresis). The collecting tubules and ducts descend through the medulla, which has a high osmotic pressure in its tissues; therefore the glomerular filtrate, although already concentrated, is hyposmotic to the medullary tissues. More water can thus be reabsorbed from it during its passage through these ducts when their walls are made permeable by vasopressin.

Hormones probably play a role in the reabsorption of other substances besides water. For example, when there are high concentrations of the adrenocortical hormone (aldosterone) in the blood, an excessive amount of sodium is reabsorbed and more potassium is excreted than normally. Low levels of this hormone cause sodium to be excreted regardless of the body's need. When the concentration of parathormone (parathyroid hormone) in the blood is high, calcium is reabsorbed in larger quantities than usual and less phosphorus is reabsorbed.

The kidneys contain many juxtaglomerular apparatuses, each composed of a portion of the afferent arteriole to the glomerulus and a portion of the distal convoluted tubule. Under conditions of hypotension or ischemia these structures will enlarge and secrete renin, a hormone capable of acting upon a polypeptide formed in the liver that eventually can be broken down into a powerful vasoconstrictor agent known as angiotensin II. Angiotensin, in addition to causing peripheral vasoconstriction and hypertension, also stimulates an increased production of aldosterone from the adrenal glands. Aldosterone in turn acts upon the distal tubules to cause reabsorption of fluid and sodium, which expands the vascular system. This feedback mechanism is thought to play an important role in the regulation of a normal person's blood pressure through a balancing of electrolytes and fluids. In the presence of a constricting lesion of the renal artery, however, overproduction of renin is not reduced by excessive aldosterone production and the blood pressure remains elevated and the electrolytes are often unbalanced (low serum potassium and elevated CO_2 and sodium).

From the 125 ml. of glomerular filtrate passing into the renal tubules each minute under usual conditions, all but about 1 ml. of the water content is reabsorbed for use by the body. The glucose and vitamin C in the filtrate are, under normal physiologic and dietary circumstances, almost completely reabsorbed and thus are not normally found in any substantial amount in urine. If, however, more of any of these substances is filtered than the tubule can completely reabsorb during the time required for the filtrate to pass through it, the substance will then be found in the urine. Excessively large amounts of substances such as glucose may be present in the filtrate as a result of high concentrations of the substances in the blood or an increase in the amount of blood filtered each minute. For example, patients with diabetes mellitus have abnormally high amounts of sugar in the blood and consequently have glycosuria (sugar in the urine). Sugar may also be present for several hours in the urine of a person who has eaten an excessive amount of candy or received intravenous dextrose. Glycosuria may also appear temporarily following any situation that causes a marked rise in blood pressure and a consequent increase in the glomerular filtration rate.

Following the filtration and reabsorption processes, urea is normally excreted as a waste product and is found in high concentrations in urine. However, it is a substance which, when highly concentrated in the glomerular filtrate, is readily reabsorbed. This causes the high blood urea level that commonly occurs in situations in which there is a small urine output, as in the severely dehydrated patient.

Tubular secretion. In addition to their role in selective reabsorption of water and other substances from the glomerular filtrate, the tubules have a direct secretory function. Some substances are secreted directly into the tubule from the blood through the tubular cells. While some of these substances are only secreted, others are partially filtered through the glomeruli and partially secreted directly into the tubules. Tubular secretion serves to transport unfiltered materials from areas of low concentration in the peritubular plasma to areas of high concentration in the glomerular filtrate. It favors rapid elimination of substances normally occurring in low concentration in the plasma, and it provides another means of exchanging useless or harmful substances in the plasma for desirable ones in the glomerular filtrate.

Phenolsulfonphthalein, penicillin, iodopyracet (Diodrast), sodium iodohippurate (Hippuran), para-aminohippuric acid, hippuric acid, and exogenous creatinine are secreted in the proximal convoluted tubules. Among these, hippuric acid is the only natural (endogenous) product. Because penicillin is so readily secreted, in order to maintain therapeutic blood levels, originally it was prepared with a chemical agent that aided in blocking its rapid secretion by the proximal tubules.

In the distal convoluted tubules, excess hydrogen and potassium ions circulating in the blood of the peritubular capillaries are exchanged for sodium ions in the urine. Since urine must not become too acid, the direct exchange of hydrogen ions (producing acidity) for sodium ions would be restricted without some compensatory mechanism to control the acidity. This compensation is accomplished by the tubular cells synthesizing ammonia, which diffuses into the glomerular filtrate in the tubules, neutralizing it and permitting the hydrogen ion exchange to continue. This process is essential to the kidneys' function of maintaining a normal blood pH by eliminating acid (hydrogen ions—H^+) from the plasma and maintaining the base reserves (bicarbonate ions—HCO_3^-). Since acid is a normal end product of many metabolic processes, there is a natural tendency for the hydrogen ion level to rise in the blood. Failure of the kidneys' ability to remove enough hydrogen ions from the blood is the reason acidosis frequently accompanies renal disease.

Renal excretion. By passing through the renal tubules, the glomerular filtrate changes from an isotonic to a hypertonic fluid known as urine that has a specific gravity up to 1.030, depending on the body's need for fluid and the amount of excretory products. Urine excreted during the hours of sleep is normally more concentrated since the fluid intake is nil and the urine volume excreted is less than that during the waking hours. The urine specific gravity rises also when a person perspires more heavily and less urine output is required. The specific gravity may drop below 1.010 when fluid intake is excessive and in disease states such as diabetes insipidus and renal failure. Urine is usually somewhat acid in reaction. The pH varies, however, with dietary intake and body needs; it may also be alkaline. About 1 to 2 ml. of urine per minute flows into the bladder. Under usual conditions the normal adult person has a urinary output of about 1200 to 1500 ml. per day, with about twice as much urine being excreted during the waking hours as during sleep. Table 1 shows the substances and the average amounts of each that may be found normally in each 1000 ml. of urine.

Proteins and glucose are not usually found in the urine of a normal person. Salt and ascorbic acid, although mostly reabsorbed, are present in small amounts because of the large amount of these substances commonly consumed in the United States.

An occasional white blood cell and a rare red cell seen in microscopic examination of the urine is not considered abnormal. Up to 1 million epithelial and white blood cells and approximately 330,000 red

Table 1. Chemical content of normal urine (gm./1000 ml or 24-hour excretion as noted)*

Electrolytes	
Calcium	0.1–0.3 (5 mEq.)
Chlorides, such as NaCl	10–15
Magnesium	0.05–0.2
Phosphorus, inorganic	0.9–1.1 (41 mEq.)
Potassium	1.5–2.5 (46 mEq.)
Sodium	4 (100 mEq.)
Other inorganic elements	
Arsenic	0.05 mg. or less
Iodine	50–250 μg
Iron	0.1–0.2
Lead	50 μg or less
Sulfur	1–2
Steroids	
17-Hydroxycorticosteroids	3–9 mg.
17-Ketosteroids	
Males	8–21 mg.
Females	4–14 mg.
Children (4-15 years)	0.8–11.3 mg.
Vitamins	
Ascorbic acid	15–50 mg.
Nicotinic acid	3–10 mg.
Riboflavin	0.5–0.8 mg.
Thiamine	0.03–0.3 mg.
Nitrogenous constituents	
Amino acids	0.4–1 gm./24 hours
Ammonia	0.3–1 (N 0.4)
Creatine	0–0.06
Creatinine	1.0–1.8
Hippuric acid	0.1–1
Nitrogen	12.5
Phenols	0.1–0.3
Proteins ("albumin")	0–0.1
Purines	0.05
Urea	25–35 (N 10–12)
Uric acid	0.2–2
Others	
Diastase	1.4–1.16
Ketones	0.3–1
Lactic acid	0.05–0.2
Porphyrins	0–30 μg
Urobilinogen	0–4 mg.

*From A pocketbook of normal laboratory values, rev. ed., Philadelphia, 1963, Smith, Kline & French Laboratories.

Table 2. Urine output per day in children*

Age	Amount (ml./24 hours)
First and second day of life	15–60
Third to tenth day of life	100–300
10 days–2 months	250–450
2 months–1 year	400–500
1–2 years	500–600
3–5 years	600–700
5–8 years	650–1000
8–14 years	800–1400

*From Campbell, M., editor: Urology, ed. 2, Philadelphia, 1963, W. B. Saunders Co.

cells may normally be present in a 12-hour collection of urine; this is less than one cell per cubic millimeter. An occasional cast (mold of the renal tubule) may also appear (up to 5000 per 12-hour urine specimen). These values represent the normal Addis count, which also includes less than 60 mg. of protein.

The average total output of urine per day in children varies with the age of the child and the fluid intake. Amounts shown in Table 2 may be considered average.

During the first few days of life, glomerular filtration and tubular resorptive powers are low; the urine is strongly acid and usually contains albumin, white blood cells, casts, mucus, and uric acid or urate crystals. It may also contain sugar. After the first few days of life (neonatal period) the urine is similar to that of an adult.

URETERS
Anatomy

The two ureters, distensible fibromuscular tubes lined with mucosa, connect the kidneys to the bladder and provide a passageway for urine. They vary in length from 25 to 30 cm. in the adult, the left ureter being slightly longer than the right because of the higher placement of the left kidney. Each ureter extends from the ureteropelvic junction of its respective kidney to the upper level of the vesical (bladder) trigone on its respective side (Fig. 2-3). The ureters pass obliquely through the bladder wall. They have no sphincters, but their oblique courses are somewhat sphincterlike in action and function as one-way flutter valves to prevent reflux (flow of urine back up the ureters from the bladder).

The lumen of the ureter varies in size along its course. There are three sites at which each ureter is normally narrower than elsewhere: (1) at the ureteropelvic junction, (2) where the ureter crosses the iliac vessels and passes into the bony pelvis, and (3) within the wall of the bladder. The narrow areas of the lumen have diameters of only about

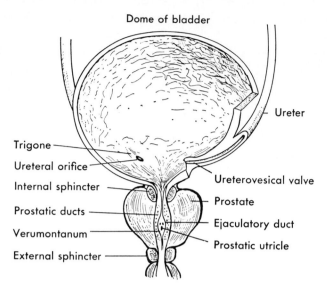

Fig. 2-3. Urinary bladder, prostate, and urinary sphincters. Each ureter enters bladder at upper outer corner of trigone. Intramural ureter acts as one-way valve. Ejaculatory ducts pass through prostate and empty at verumontanum in posterior urethra. External urinary sphincter controls urinary continence in male. Prostate surrounds posterior urethra like a doughnut. (Adapted from unpublished illustration of Dr. B. G. Clarke and Dr. L. Del Guercio.)

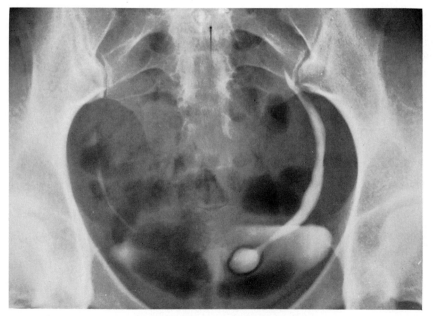

Fig. 2-4. Intramural ureter dilated and shaped like cobra head; represents a ureterocele seen during excretory urogram.

3 mm. and are thus of particular significance in the passage of renal calculi since only small stones can pass through these narrow passageways. Larger stones pass rarely due to the elastic quality of the ureter.

Along their course from the kidneys to the bladder the ureters lie close to the retroperitoneum and to many blood vessels. In the male each ureter enters the bladder in the vicinity of the upper end of the respective seminal vesicle (Fig. 2-9). In the female the ureters pass behind the reproductive organs (Fig. 2-1), and the enlargement of any of these organs may place them in close approximation to a ureter. Because of these relationships, inflammatory processes in structures such as the appendix or sigmoid colon in either sex, in the cervix, uterus, oviduct, ovary, or parametrium in the female, and in the seminal vesicles in the male may produce ureteral symptoms or the process may actually involve a ureter. In pelvic surgery there is danger of inadvertently ligating or lacerating a ureter. During pregnancy the enlarging uterus tends to obstruct the ureter and is an additional factor in the hydronephrosis that physiologically occurs during the last trimester of pregnancy. Progesterone is thought to be the main stimulus to such changes in pregnancy.

The ureters are richly supplied with blood; the ureteral vessels arise from the renal, lumbar, gonadal, and vesical arteries and empty into corresponding venous channels. The ureteral lymphatic vessels drain in various directions—those from the upper ureter flow toward the kidney; those from the lower ureter turn into the pelvic and lumbar lymph glands.

The nerve supply to the ureters is derived from the autonomic nervous system and probably is coordinated with the nerve supply to the renal pelves and that to the bladder. Although the neurogenic origin of the impulses that stimulate the motor functions of the ureters (peristalsis and tonus) is not positively known, it is suspected that ganglia located within the ureteral tissue itself are responsible.

Anomalies

Duplication of ureters may occur, and if complete, the distal most orifice may be located in the bladder or ectopically, causing incontinence if it ends beyond the urethral sphincter. It may end in a ureterocele, producing obstruction (Fig. 2-4). Triplication of the ureter is known to occur. The ureter may rarely cross behind the vena cava (retrocaval ureter) or cross to the other side of the bladder (crossed ectopia). If the kidney is absent at birth, there is also agenesis of the ureter. An attenuated ureter or fibrous cord accompanies renal dysplasia. The ureter is of normal length in the presence of ptosis of the kidney but is shortened when an ectopic kidney is found. The two entities can be differentiated roentgenographically on this basis.

Physiology

Although the mechanism by which urine is transported through the ureters from the kidneys to the bladder has not been fully determined, it is probable that peristaltic action plays the major role. The urine flow through the renal collecting ducts from the nephrons is still driven by a slight hydrostatic pressure. This pressure, however, has markedly decreased as the glomerular filtrate has passed through the renal tubules, and the remaining pressure is probably not great enough even to force the urine out of the ducts into the calyces of the renal pelves. All of the large collecting structures (collecting ducts, calyces, infundibula, renal pelves, ureters), however, have walls of smooth (nonstriated) muscle which, like the intestine, are the site of continuous coordinated peristaltic action. This peristaltic action exerts a detrusor (thrusting) action against the urine as it becomes pooled in a portion of the collecting system and transports the urine from segment to segment of the system until it is finally emptied in a small spurt into the bladder. The area above and below any section in which urine is momentarily pooled is always contracted. This accounts for the contracted and distended portions of the ureter seen in intravenous pyelograms. Urine is not moved to the next section until the section above the proximal contracted area is filled. Under normal conditions the flow is one way, bladderward, and the time taken for one jet of urine to pass from the calyces to the bladder is about 1½ seconds.

The muscle tone of the renal pelves and the ureters varies with the amount of urine flow. When the flow is large, the tonus decreases and the lumen is larger than when the flow is scant. The tonus apparently determines how much urine is allowed to empty into a section of the collecting system before the collecting stage switches to the detrusor stage. The renal pelvis of an adult or a child over 5 years of age will usually hold only 3 to 5 ml. of fluid. However, when manually filled during retrograde pyelography, the renal pelvis of an infant holds only about 1.5 ml. Larger amounts cause pain in the flank.

When the bladder becomes full enough, the ureters and kidneys receive neurologic signals and the ureteral tonus appears to decrease so that more urine is held in each sector, while the kidneys produce less urine. The ureter will continue to empty because muscle action against a heavy column of urine is more effective in acute situations. Under these circumstances urine will be ejected into the bladder less frequently but in larger amounts at each ejection. Any condition that causes the force needed to transport urine from one section of the collecting system to the next to be markedly above normal will cause the entire tract to become distended above the point of impasse. This situation may force urine back into the kidney pelvis, into the collecting ducts, or into the

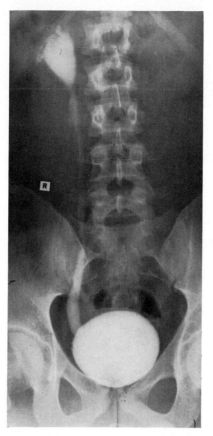

Fig. 2-5. Retrograde cystogram showing complete reflux of contrast material into right upper urinary system.

pyelolymphatic circulation. In *chronic* overdistention of the bladder the ureters lose tone and become tortuous. Their peristaltic activity is then feeble.

Vesicoureteral reflux, a common abnormality and an important cause of pyelonephritis, is the result of congenitally short intramural ureters or bladder inflammation and produces malfunction of the ureterovesical valve. It occurs most commonly in females and in children (Fig. 2-5).

BLADDER
Anatomy

The urinary bladder in the adult is a spherical, hollow muscular sac. It normally lies in the pelvic cavity, but when distended, it projects above the symphysis pubis. In the child whose pelvis is relatively small the bladder is a lower abdominal organ that is oval in shape when full. The bladder, similar to the rest of the urinary tract, is extraperitoneal; the peritoneum, however, is adherent to the dome of the bladder.

The base of the bladder is the only fixed portion of the organ. It is continuous with the prostate and urethra in the male and with the urethra in the female. The remainder of the bladder is freely movable and capable of considerable distention. Its normal capacity in the adult is 300 to 500 ml.; the child who has learned bladder control usually has a bladder capacity of 200 to 400 ml. The bladder can distend tremendously, however, and when its outflow is obstructed, the adult bladder may hold 1000 ml. of urine or more. This amount of distention may cause tissue damage and loss of tone.

Anterior to the bladder and posterior to the symphysis pubis there is a space filled with loose connective tissue (space of Retzius). This space is a potential area of infection in retropubic and suprapubic surgery and in traumatic rupture of the bladder neck. Posteriorly the bladder is separated by only a fascial sheath from the seminal vesicles and the rectum in the male and from the vagina and uterus in the female.

It consists of a vault or dome (superior portion), two lateral walls, a base, and a trigone. The trigone on the floor (base) of the bladder is the triangular area, the ureteral orifices forming its base angles and the urethral orifice forming its apex angle (Figs. 2-3 and 2-6).

The muscular wall of the bladder is made up of intertwining fibers of nonstriated or smooth muscle known as the detrusor muscle. The vesical (bladder) lining is a pale pink mucous membrane which, except for the smooth area over the trigone, falls into many folds when the bladder is empty. As the bladder distends, the mucous membrane smooths out. The connective tissue between the mucosa and muscle is known as the submucosal layer. There are two sphincters, an internal (involuntary) and an external (voluntary) one. The internal sphincter is located at the internal urethral orifice, which in the male lies just above the prostate gland. The external sphincter lies about 2 cm. beyond the internal sphincter—in the female it is near the middle of the urethra; in the male it is just beyond that portion of the urethra surrounded by the prostate gland (the prostatic urethra). The membranous urethra lies within the external urinary sphincter in the male and the entire structure is also known as the urogenital diaphragm and triangular ligament.

The bladder is well supplied with blood from the vesical arteries that originate from the hypogastric, hemorrhoidal, and uterine arteries. Its lymph drains into nodes along the obturator and internal, external, and common iliac vessels.

The nerve supply to the bladder muscle is from the autonomic (parasympathetic and sympathetic) nervous system. The parasympathetic afferent (sensory) fibers carry the impulses of practically all bladder sensation of desire to void to the spinal cord, and parasympathetic efferent (motor) fibers carry the motor impulses to the bladder. The reflex con-

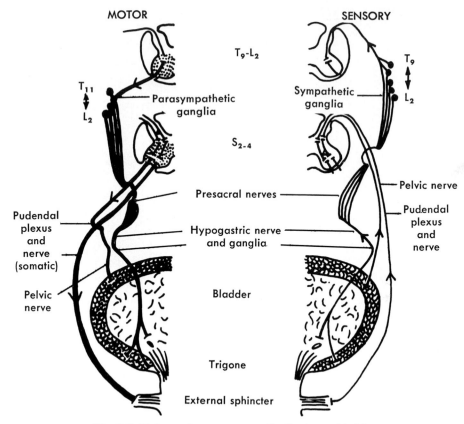

MOTOR   SENSORY

T_9-L_2

T_{11} — Parasympathetic ganglia   Sympathetic ganglia — T_9 / L_2

L_2

S_{2-4}

Presacral nerves ———   — Pelvic nerve

Pudendal plexus and nerve (somatic)   Hypogastric nerve and ganglia ———   Pudendal plexus and nerve

Pelvic nerve   Bladder

Trigone

External sphincter

Fig. 2-6. Motor and sensory nerve distribution to bladder.

nections of these afferent and efferent fibers are made in the second, third, and fourth sacral segments of the spinal cord. Both the afferent and efferent parasympathetic fibers are carried by the pelvic nerves (nervi erigentes). The sympathetic fibers supplying the bladder are chiefly sensory (pain) and arise from the twelfth dorsal to the second lumbar segments of the spinal cord passing via the presacral nerve and sacral sympathetic chain to the inferior hypogastric plexus. Sympathetic fibers seem to have little effect on micturition (act of urinating). Sympathetic efferent fibers carry the motor impulses necessary for ejaculatory mechanisms in the bladder neck and urethra. The somatic nervous system innervates the external sphincter of the bladder. The pudendal nerves arising in the third and fourth sacral segments of the spinal cord carry motor fibers to the external sphincter and perineal muscles. Sensory fibers from the perineum are also carried in these nerves. The somatic nerve elements help bring about voluntary control of micturition; the parasympathetic nervous system seems to regulate the involuntary factors of micturition (Fig. 2-6).

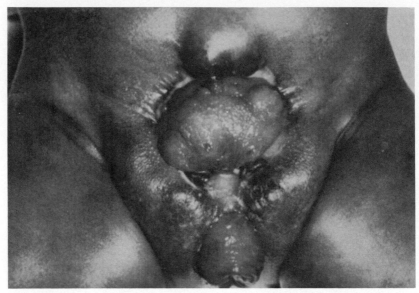

Fig. 2-7. Exstrophy of bladder shown with complete absence of lower abdominal musculature and anterior portion of bladder. Congenital prolapse of rectum is also seen in lower portion of photograph.

Anomalies

Embryonic vestiges of the umbilical artery may be seen as fibrous cords attached to the dome of the bladder. The obliterated urachus is likewise often encountered there. Cystic or patent urachal remnants extending from the bladder toward the umbilicus are occasionally found. The latter is recognized by leakage of urine from the umbilicus.

Failure of the midline to close in the embryo may result in absence of the anterior bladder, anterior abdominal wall, and symphysis pubis, a condition known as exstrophy (Fig. 2-7). Epispadias (absence of the dorsum of the urethra) is the usual accompaniment and other congenital anomalies of the gonads, anus, and extremities are frequently associated. There is a slight tendency for congenital disorders to be familial. The patient is always wet and the exposed mucosa is easily excoriated. The bladders are neither histologically nor physiologically normal; therefore the "turn-in" operation to close the bladder is rarely successful. The vesicoureteral valves are usually incompetent, allowing reflux when a bladder is formed. Operative reconstruction of the urinary sphincter rarely succeeds in making a person continent. More often, the bladder is removed and the upper urinary systems diverted to the skin or bowel. If ureterosigmoidostomy is performed, it is wise to wait until anal sphincter control is complete, since the anus is frequently abnormal in patients with exstrophy of the bladder.

Epispadias is repaired by urethroplasty, but if the sphincter is not intact, the patient may remain incontinent and require urinary diversion.

Children with this anomaly are subject to long and repeated hospitalization and frequently require a series of operations. The emotional stress upon patient and parents is great and calls for the utmost nursing and medical skill to cope with all aspects of the disease.

Other bladder anomalies include diverticulum, two to four separate bladder compartments with two urethras, an enlarged atonic bladder (megacystis), and fistula.

Physiology

Micturition is a reflex visceral function that the child learns to voluntarily control. Normal voluntary and involuntary muscle action coordinated by a normal urethrovesical reflex is essential for bladder control. Urine enters the bladder from the ureters in rhythmic jets. As the bladder fills, the pressure within it gradually increases. The detrusor muscle (bladder muscle) responds to this stretch by relaxing to accommodate a greater volume. As the urine continues to collect, a certain point of filling is reached when distention and the desire to void are recorded by the sensory parasympathetic endings in the detrusor muscle. In the child this usually occurs at about 200 ml.; in the adult, at 300 to 400 ml. The stimuli are transmitted to the reflex center for micturition in the spinal cord. In the normal person, if the time and place are not proper, completion of the reflex act can be interrupted and voiding postponed by release of a stream of inhibitory impulses from the cortical center and voluntary contraction of the external sphincter. When micturition is desired, the higher level inhibition is suppressed and reflex detrusor muscle contraction occurs smoothly and powerfully in tonic action. The internal sphincter, which is normally closed, now reciprocally opens, and urine enters the posterior urethra. Relaxation of the external sphincter and the perineal muscles follows, and expulsion of the bladder contents is accomplished. Contraction of the abdominal and diaphragmatic muscles may be used to help express the urine.

The infant is born with only the involuntary control of micturition intact; he will void as soon as distention of the bladder causes stimuli to reach the reflex center for micturition in the spinal cord. He must learn to respond to the sensory stimuli indicating a need to void and learn to use the muscles making voluntary control possible. The time this requires varies with individual children, but most children have complete control, both during the day and at night, by the age of 3 years.

The male bladder neck (internal sphincter) can be excised without causing incontinence. However, it may result in infertility due to retrograde ejaculation. Excision of the female bladder neck will occasionally produce incontinence.

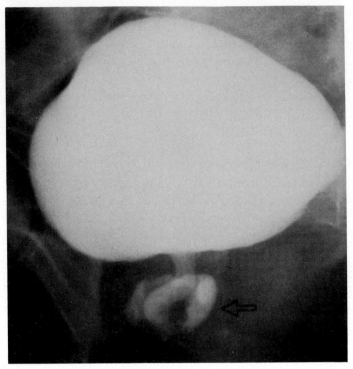

Fig. 2-8. Oblique view of voiding cystourethrogram shows two diverticula of urethra (arrow).

URETHRA
Anatomy

Male urethra. The urethra of the male is a long, curved narrow tube about 20 cm. in length leading from the bladder through the penis to the urethral meatus at the tip of the glans penis. The muscles of the perineum surround the posterior portion (proximal) of the urethra; the anterior portion extends beyond the pubic bones. Urine is discharged from the bladder in a stream through the urethral (external urinary) meatus. The male urethra is divided into four sections: prostatic (posterior), membranous, bulbous, and pendulous (anterior). The prostatic urethra is about 2 to 4 cm. long and is encircled by the prostate gland; the internal sphincter at the bladder neck surrounds the proximal end of this section and just beyond the prostate the external sphincter surrounds it. The ejaculatory ducts carrying spermatic fluid (sperm) from the testicles and seminal vesicles open into the prostatic urethra through a small elevation on its posterior wall called the verumontanum (Fig. 2-3). The membranous urethra is about 1 cm. long and lies between the prostatic and bulbous sections of the urethra. The bulbous urethra, about

5 cm. long, runs from the membranous urethra to the penile-scrotal junction. The pendulous urethra makes up the remainder and has a thin wall surrounded by part of the penile erectile tissue (see Fig. 8-3).

Numerous glands empty into the male urethra. Cowper's glands (bulbourethral), which secrete an alkaline fluid favorable to the life and motility of sperm, enter it at the junction of the bulb and the external sphincter. Scattered along its course are the tiny glands of Littre that lubricate the urethral membrane and occasionally become the sites of infection (gonorrhea and nonspecific urethritis).

Female urethra. The female urethra, a short straight tube, is about 3 to 5 cm. long. The external meatus, opening between the labia minora, is anterior to the vaginal orifice. It is relatively close to both the vaginal and anal openings. The external sphincter lies in the midurethra. Numerous small glands (paraurethral glands and the paired Skene glands) open into the female urethra. No portion of the female urethra is external to the body proper as in the male. It is subject to strictures, diverticula (Fig. 2-8), fistulas, infections, and tumors. The external meatus is the most common site of stricture.

The arterial supply comes from the inferior vesical and vaginal arteries. The veins join Santorini's plexus and vaginal veins. The meatal lymphatics pass to the superficial inguinal nodes, but the majority drain into the hypogastric lymph system, joining those of the bladder.

Anomalies

The urethra is subject to anomalies, the most common in the male being hypospadias. This anomaly is a deficiency of a portion of the ventral aspect of the urethra and its skin covering in which the meatus may be located at any site between the perineum and the glans penis. Mild degrees of this disorder require no correction. It can be recognized also by the absent ventral prepuce and the ventral curvature of the erect penis due to a chordee restriction.

Fortunately the patient's continence is not affected by hypospadias. Moderate to severe degrees should be repaired by urethroplasty. This may be a one- to three-stage operation. Circumcision should never be performed since the dorsal hood of the prepuce is generally used in the repair. The chordee is corrected in the first stage after 1 year of age, and urethroplasty may be postponed for another year until all tissues are soft and pliable. In all stages the urine is diverted by a perineal urethrostomy or suprapubic cystostomy. Pressure dressings are not usually removed for 7 days. Fistula formation is a common complication, but eventual successful outcome is the rule. Operative repair should be complete by school age.

Epispadias is partial or complete absence of the dorsal urethra and its coverings and is most often encountered with exstrophy of the bladder. In intersexual patients the urethra may open into a sinus that is a vaginal remnant. Intersex anomalies should be suspected in all urethral anomalies.

Other anomalies include stricture, fistula, and two urethras.

Physiology

The primary function of the urethra is to serve as a passageway through which urine can be expelled from the bladder and to act with the sphincter as a valve to control continence. In the male the urethra has another function—it serves as a passageway for semen containing sperm (male reproductive cells). The function of the urethral sphincters is discussed under physiology of the bladder.

Male reproductive system

Anatomy

The penis and scrotum constitute the external genitalia of the male. The testes from which sperm (spermatozoa) originate lie in the scrotum. Sperm form within the spermatogenic tubules of the testis; these tubules drain through the rete testis and ductuli efferentes carrying the sperm into the epididymis. (The combined testicular-tubular systems made up of the spermatogenic tubules, rete testis, and ductuli efferentes are called the seminiferous tubules.) Then the sperm traverse the long vas deferens and join with the seminal vesicles, from whence they enter the prostatic urethra via the ejaculatory duct (Fig. 2-9).

Penis. The penis is an erectile organ made up of three tissue masses richly supplied with blood vessels having sympathetic innervation. The three masses are the paired corpora cavernosa, which run parallel to and above the urethra, and the smaller corpus spongiosum, which surrounds the urethra. At the distal end of the penis is a cone-shaped structure known as the glans penis, at the apex of which the urethral meatus opens as a vertical slit. The glans is covered by a thin semimucous membrane containing many sebaceous glands and nerve endings.

The pudendal arteries supply the penis with blood that normally (in the flaccid state) is shunted into the venous plexuses and passes through the veins of Santorini back into the general circulation. Psychogenic or local stimulation causes the venous valves to shut during an erection and the shunts between the arterioles and venules are closed so that blood is trapped within the corpora cavernosa. When the pudendal nerves are unable to transmit nerve impulses in certain neurologic diseases, the penis may be unable to respond and become erect. This is notable in lower motor neuron disease. However, in upper motor neuron disease the penis is capable of abnormally sustained erections. In pathologic conditions such as priapism the venous blood cannot escape and the penis may have

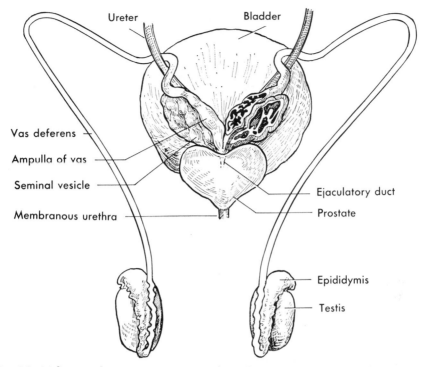

Fig. 2-9. Male reproductive system. Sperm formed in testes pass into epididymides and thence through vasa deferentia, join with the seminal vesicles, and finally empty into prostatic urethra through ejaculatory ducts. These systems do not intercommunicate. Note relationship of vas deferens and ureters.

an abnormally prolonged and painful erection unassociated with sexual desire. The corpus spongiosum is not involved in this condition, nor is the glans penis, which is part of the corpus spongiosum system.

In the act of ejaculation (male sexual climax), semen is expressed from the urethra in rhythmic spurts.

The skin of the penis is very thin and loose which, when the corpora becomes engorged with blood, allows for distention. In the normal newborn infant the penile skin forms a redundant fold over the glans; this is known as the prepuce, or foreskin, and can be retracted behind the glans. The foreskin is often removed soon after birth by an operation known as circumcision. After circumcision the foreskin is either greatly shortened or absent. This is a near perfect prophylaxis against carcinoma of the penis when performed at birth. The lymphatics of the prepuce and glans penis drain into the superficial inguinal lymph nodes. The lymphatics of the shaft and proximal penis drain into the pelvic lymph nodes.

The sympathetic nervous system supplies the innervation of the erectile muscles in the penis; the internal pudendal nerve supplies sensory fibers to the organ.

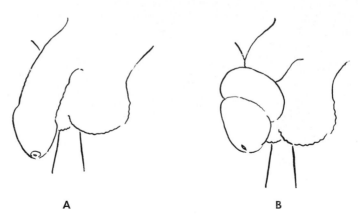

A   B

Fig. 2-10. A, Phimosis. Prepuce is tightly drawn over glans penis and cannot be re-tracted. **B,** Paraphimosis. Prepuce has been retracted behind glans penis and because of edema cannot be easily drawn over glans penis. (Courtesy Dr. B. G. Clarke and Dr. L. Del Guercio.)

PHIMOSIS AND PARAPHIMOSIS. Phimosis (Fig. 2-10, A) is a condition in which the opening of the prepuce is too small to allow it to be retracted over the glans penis. It may be congenital or acquired. In the adult it is frequently associated with edema and inflammation caused by balanitis, an infection of the glans penis. It is treated by circumcision (surgical excision of the prepuce) or a dorsal slit. Nowadays most male babies are circumcised soon after birth since the procedure markedly decreases the incidence of infections of the glans penis as well as carcinoma of the penis. This may be performed quite simply by use of a Gomco clamp. No anesthesia is required if it is done within a few days of birth.

A petrolatum gauze dressing is usually placed over the glans penis following circumcision at any age. Some patients are hospitalized for only a few hours after this operation. Before being discharged, the older children and adults or the mothers of infants must be taught to change the dressing and must be alerted to watch for bleeding. If severe bleeding occurs, a firm bandage should be applied to the penis, and the patient should return at once to the doctor or to a hospital emergency room. When bleeding occurs, the doctor usually applies a pressure dressing. This dressing is bulky, but the patient is usually still able to void. On discharge from the hospital the adult patient or older child should be given a tube of an antibiotic ointment and dressings to use at home until the wound is well healed. The infant rarely needs a dressing after a day or two. Prepucial adhesions are usually present at birth and must be severed at the time of circumcision; they have a tendency to recur. Frequently an estrogen preparation is prescribed for adult patients to take for several days preoperatively and postoperatively to prevent penile erection, which might disrupt the sutures or cause hemorrhage.

In patients with paraphimosis (Fig. 2-10, *B*) the foreskin cannot be reduced after it has been retracted behind the glans and the penis is constricted. This causes severe pain, and there is danger of necrosis and sloughing of penile tissue unless paraphimosis is treated early. Paraphimosis is frequently associated with an infection of the glans or follows urethral instrumentation. After such operations the penis should be checked to make sure the foreskin in uncircumcised males has been reduced. The prepuce can sometimes be gently reduced. In others, however, a circumcision is done as an emergency treatment to prevent recurrence and to provide for easier eradication of the infection in the glans penis. A dorsal slit of the prepuce is the easiest and quickest solution to the problem.

Scrotum. The scrotum is a sac of loosely folded skin and smooth muscle that contains the testes and the epididymides; one of the latter is attached to each testis. The wall contains smooth muscle fibers known as the dartos that cause it to undergo involuntary rhythmic contractions. The scrotum is divided by a septum of connective tissue into two noncommunicating compartments, each of which contains a testis, its attached epididymis, and the beginnings of one vas deferens. The scrotum is posterior to the penis, anterior to the anal opening, and dependent to the perineum. Its lymph drains into the femoral, inguinal, and then the iliac nodes. The scrotum is believed to have a thermoregulatory function. Its temperature of a few degrees below that of the body is thought to aid spermatogenesis. A varicocele may increase the intrascrotal temperature and reduce spermatogenesis.

Spermatic cords. A spermatic cord suspends each testicle in the scrotum. The cords originate at the right and left internal abdominal (inguinal) rings and course through the respective inguinal canals to emerge at the external abdominal (inguinal) rings and proceed into the scrotum (Fig. 2-11). Each spermatic cord is composed of the vas deferens and the spermatic blood vessels and nerves of the testicle suspended from it. Surrounding the vessels of the cord and the vas deferens is the cremaster muscle, which regulates the length of the spermatic cord and the distance of the testis from the body. Torsion of the cord is painful and may cause loss of testicular function by strangling the blood supply (Fig. 2-12).

Testicles. The testes are oval-shaped structures weighing between 20 and 30 grams each; they are about the size of a walnut. One is suspended by its spermatic cord in each scrotal compartment.

The testes are composed of closely packed tubules, microscopic in size (seminiferous tubules), and enclosed in a dense fibrous sheath (tunica albuginea). A closed serous sac (tunica vaginalis) adheres to the anterior and lateral surfaces of each testis and then extends outward to line the scrotal compartment. When an excessive amount of fluid is con-

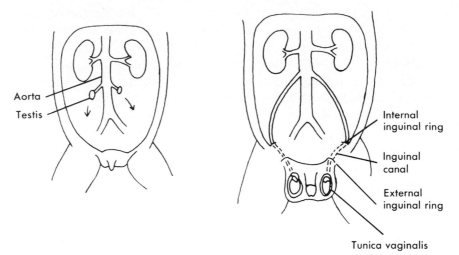

Fig. 2-11. Descent of testicles from embryonic origin in abdominal cavity to scrotum. Note that spermatic arteries arise from aorta. This explains why pain in lateral abdominal and flank regions is referred to testis.

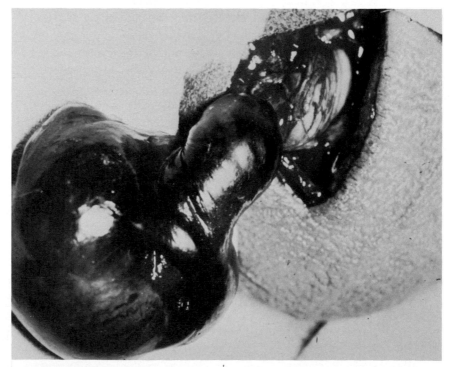

Fig. 2-12. Torsion of spermatic cord is demonstrated at surgery through a scrotal incision; the testicle and its twisted cord are shown. Note dark or cyanotic appearance of the testicle due to its blocked blood flow.

tained in the tunica vaginalis, a hydrocele is formed (see Fig. 11-12). This is the most common mass to be found in the scrotum and is to be distinguished from solid masses by its ability to be transilluminated.

The blood supply for the testicles arises in the abdominal cavity (spermatic and vas deferens arteries) and the lymph drains into the periaortic nodes. The nerve supply arises at the lumbar level. The abdominal origin of the vessels and nerves of the testes is the result of the testes developing intra-abdominally in the fetus and explains why lower ureteral pain is transferred to the testis (Fig. 2-11).

Epididymides. The epididymides are long, narrow, coiled collecting tubules packed together to form structures that are apposed to the posterior wall of each testis. The seminiferous tubules of each testicle empty into their own epididymis, which in turn empties into the respective vas deferens (Fig. 2-9). They are highly susceptible to inflammation (epididymitis), abscess formation, and occlusion (Chapter 9).

Vasa deferentia. There is a right and a left vas deferens; they are thick-walled, fine-lumened, fibromuscular tubes. The vas deferens arises from the epididymis and passes as part of the spermatic cord through the internal abdominal ring, where it runs behind the bladder to form the ejaculatory duct, which is joined by the duct from the seminal vesicle. Each vas deferens is about 46 cm. long (Fig. 2-9). Their obliteration or ligation causes infertility.

Seminal vesicles. The seminal vesicles are twin structures that lie behind the base of the bladder, above the prostate, and in front of the rectum. Each is made up of a single, long-winding, and narrow saccular tube (Fig. 2-9). Near the base of the prostate the duct from the seminal vesicle joins the respective vas deferens to become the ejaculatory duct, which empties into the verumontanum of the prostatic urethra.

Prostate gland. The prostate gland is a multilobular gland located at the base of the bladder and encircling the urethra (Figs. 2-3 and 2-6). It is about 4 cm. long and weighs between 10 and 20 grams. It drains into the urethra. Glandular tissue makes up most of the lateral and central portions of the gland; the posterior portion is primarily fibromuscular connective tissue. The prostate gland is encapsulated by fibrous connective tissue. In hyperplastic glands the fibrous capsule is augmented by a shell of normal prostate tissue compressed outward by the hypertrophied prostate tissue; this shell of normal tissue is called the surgical capsule. The prostate gland is well supplied with blood from the inferior vesicle and pudendal arteries. Its venous channels empty into the venous plexus of Santorini. It is innervated by the pudendal nerves. It is an accessory sex gland but not essential for life. Like the appendix, it is frequently removed. It is highly susceptible to inflammation, stone formation, hypertrophy, and cancerous degeneration.

Anomalies

Maldescent of the testis is a common birth defect (cryptorchid if in the normal path of descent, ectopic if outside). The malformation may be bilateral, but it is a little more common on the right than on the left. Cryptorchidism in its extreme form consists of unilateral agenesis of the testicle. The cryptorchid testis is found in the abdomen in 15% of the cases and at inguinal, femoral, or perineal sites in the remainder. Indirect inguinal hernia, an embryologically related malformation, occurs in a great proportion of patients with testicular maldescent.

When the testis remains undescended after puberty, the tubules degenerate and spermatogenesis does not occur, although androgen secretion is maintained. A testis transplanted to the scrotum no later than at 6 years of age has the best chances of achieving normal sperm production. Prospects of normal spermatogenesis lessen progressively until puberty is complete. After this, spermatogenesis does not occur in maldescended testes. The incidence of cancer in undescended testes is reported to be twenty times greater than it is in normal testes. This is true even after successful surgical placement of the testes within the scrotum.

The child may be given gonadotropic hormones to stimulate testicular descent. Successful use of this therapy is reported, but it is difficult to prove in these instances that descent would not have occurred had normal maturation been allowed. If the cryptorchid testicle does not descend into the scrotum spontaneously, orchiopexy (surgical placement and fixation of the testicle in the scrotal sac) is necessary. If the patient also has a congenital inguinal hernia, operative repair of the hernia is done at the time orchiopexy is carried out.

If a single testicle remains in an ectopic position after puberty has ended and if the other testicle is normal, it is often recommended that the ectopic testicle be surgically removed because of the increased incidence of cancer in such an organ. Bilateral ectopic testes are not removed but are surgically fixed in the scrotum because, even though they produce no sperm and are susceptible to cancer, they supply the androgens essential for normal development and maintenance of male sex characteristics.

Since orchiopexy is usually performed on youngsters who are normally very active, the major concern in caring for them may be to restrict their physical activity. The surgeon may wish the child to be kept on bed rest for several days or to be allowed up in a chair only. Often the scrotum, with the testicle sutured into it, is temporarily fixed to the thigh with sutures to give additional traction. The child then needs frequent reminding not to actively move his leg. Interesting activities should be provided to help keep the child quietly occupied. It is often helpful for a member of the family to stay in the hospital with the child during his waking hours.

The doctor usually will not want the child to participate in active sports or to ride a bicycle for about 6 weeks postoperatively. He may, however, return to school and other normal activity. The child, or his parents, depending upon his age, should examine the testis monthly so that if cancer of the testis should develop it will be detected early. Annual examinations should be continued throughout the patient's lifetime.

Intersexuality

Recent advances in child psychiatry, cytology, and endocrinology as well as in medicine, surgery, and the basic sciences have yielded important new information concerning intersexuality. A true hermaphrodite is defined as a person possessing gonadal tissue of each sex, ordinarily with intermediate body manifestations. Other intersexual individuals are referred to as pseudohermaphrodites. In these individuals, genital structures, endocrinologic makeup, or the character of the chromosomes do not conform to those usually associated with their gonadal sex. Buccal smears, steroid determinations, roentgenologic examinations, and surgical exploration and gonadal biopsies are the usual diagnostic tests.

During the past decade, long-term follow-up studies have been completed on a large number of intersexual individuals, and the following plan has been proposed:

1. Very early in life make the best decision possible on the basis of the available evidence in assigning a gender to the individual.
2. Rear the child accordingly.
3. As the child develops, carry out any reconstructive surgery or endocrine replacement therapy that may be necessary to simulate the characteristics of the assigned sex.
4. Do not worry about the individual's social and psychologic adjustment. It will almost always be good regardless of whether the assigned sex conforms to the biologic sex provided the child has been permitted to grow up under normal conditions associated with the assigned sex.

Infertility

The problem of infertility among married couples is of major medical and social concern. Goldzieher states that one out of every seven couples in the United States is unwillingly childless. The problem rests with the wife 45% of the time, with the husband 20% of the time, and with both partners 35% of the time. It was many years before the husband was considered a possible cause of sterility. However, it is now recognized that over half a million men in the United States are responsible for barren marriages. Thus both the husband and wife should be urged to seek medical attention.

Some doctors prefer to carry out a complete examination of the husband first since it is more easily accomplished. Following a thorough physical examination, the first special test will be repeated semen examinations to determine the presence, number, morphology, and motility of the sperm. The husband should produce the specimen in the doctor's office by masturbation or bring the specimen of semen immediately from home to the doctor. The date of the previous sexual activity and the hour of collection of the present specimen should be accurately recorded. If sperm are not present in the semen, it may indicate strictures along the vasa deferentia or it may indicate absence of sperm production. Rarely, both vasa deferentia are congenitally absent.

A *biopsy of the testicle* will show sperm production if the absence of sperm (azoospermia) is due to stricture of the tubal systems above the testes. Occasionally, strictures may be repaired by a plastic surgery procedure (vasoepididymal or vasovasal anastomosis), but this may not be successful in many patients. Bilateral cryptorchidism, or undescended testicles, even though corrected, may be the cause of sterility because of failure of the testicles to develop their sperm-producing function. This is particularly true if the correction is not done before puberty. Men sometimes will have no further sperm production following bilateral orchitis (especially with mumps) and following irradiation exposure of the testicles. Rarely, hypothyroidism is found to be the cause.

When the husband is completely aspermatic or when the wife has an irremediable structural defect, conception is impossible and the couple should consider adoption of children if they desire a family. However, if sperm are present but the count and the motility rate of the sperm cells are low, the doctor may encourage the patient to eat a well-balanced diet, to maintain normal weight, to obtain adequate rest, and to participate in moderate exercise (preferably outdoors). The doctor may suggest that the couple have frequent intercourse during the fertile period (14 to 16 days after the beginning of the menstrual period); several days of abstinence should be practiced just prior to this period. If these methods are unsuccessful, the injection of the husband's semen (which may be concentrated by combining the first portions of several semen samples) into the upper portion of the cervical canal may produce a pregnancy or artificial insemination may be elected.

If the examination indicates that the man is fertile, examination of his wife is undertaken. (For a discussion of female infertility evaluation, consult a nursing textbook on gynecology.)

The testicular cells secrete testosterone and are under the influence of the anterior pituitary gland, which in turn secretes a gonadotropic hormone. A feedback mechanism exists and an excessive production of testosterone will suppress the anterior pituitary hormone. Testosterone stimulates the development of the phallus and the secondary sexual organs and characteristics. It has some influence upon the size of the prostate gland. In a male castrated prior to puberty or with inadequate development of the testes prior to this stage, the prostate will not mature. The secretion of the male hormone reaches its maximal peak at the period between puberty and the age of 25 years, after which it begins to wane, but this varies considerably among men.

Spermatogenesis, the production of sperm from germ cells, takes place in the testicle. The secretion of androgen in adequate amounts is essential to this process. With the approach of puberty there is an increase in the amount of circulating male hormones and, unless interrupted by some extraneous circumstance, this continues until death. The production of sperm may continue, therefore, from puberty until death.

Growth and development, general health, and nutritional state all influence spermatogenesis. Inadequacies in any of these may either structurally alter sperm, reduce their numbers, or abolish their formation. To impregnate an ovum, sperm must be sufficiently numerous, perfectly formed, and active. Although only one sperm fertilizes an ovum, millions of sperm must be present in the ejaculated semen for fertilization to occur. The reason for this is still not known. Endocrine disorders, especially those involving the anterior pituitary gland, may inhibit spermatogenesis.

Once formed, the sperm, suspended in fluid, are moved along the tubules to the ejaculatory duct by the muscular activity of the duct system and the action of cilia lining the ducts. Some of the fluid in which the sperm are suspended is secreted by the testicles, but most of it is supplied by the epididymides, seminal vesicles, prostate gland, and Cowper's glands. The seminal vesicles and prostate gland add nutrients to the fluid. When the fluid with its suspended sperm moves down the urethra, it is known as semen. For the semen to be ejaculated into the female reproductive tract, the engorgement of the penile corpora and the action of the erectile muscles of the penis are essential. The life of the sperm in the female reproductive tract is influenced by the vaginal pH; hyperacidity of vaginal secretions may kill them. Under optimum conditions, sperm stay motile in the vagina for 12 to 36 hours.

QUESTIONS

1. What comprises the genitourinary system?
2. How does the urinary tract differ in the two sexes?
3. Describe the anatomy of the kidney.
4. What is the relationship of the adrenal glands and the kidneys?
5. What other organs are adjacent to the kidneys?
6. How does the arterial system of the kidney differ from that of the venous system?

7. What is the role of the renal lymphatics?
8. Is the nerve supply essential to the functioning of the kidneys?
9. Name three anatomic sections of the kidney.
10. What is a nephron?
11. List several anomalies of the kidney.
12. What is the function of the glomerulus?
13. What is the function of the renal tubule?
14. Name some hormones that either originate in the kidney or act upon that organ.
15. What is an Addis count?
16. What is the role of the ureter?
17. What is the significance of vesicoureteral reflux?
18. How many urinary sphincters are there and where are they located?
19. Discuss the nerve supply of the bladder.
20. What is exstrophy of the bladder?
21. What is the difference between hypospadias and epispadias?
22. Describe the difference in the male and female urethras.
23. What is the relationship of the prostate to the urinary tract?
24. List the segments composing the male reproductive system.
25. What is the difference between phimosis and paraphimosis?
26. What is the difference between cryptorchidism and an ectopic testis?
27. Orchiopexy is usually performed at what age?
28. Outline a plan for the management of a patient with an intersex problem.
29. Semen or seminal fluid is composed of what elements?

REFERENCES

Amelar, R. D.: Infertility in men, Philadelphia, 1966, F. A. Davis Co.

Anthony, C. P.: Textbook of anatomy and physiology, ed. 8, St. Louis, 1971, The C. V. Mosby Co.

Barsocchini, L. M., and Smith, D. R.: Diaper phenolsulphonphthalein test in the newborn infant, J. Urol. **91:**195, 1964.

Bergman, H.: The ureter, New York, 1967, Harper & Row, Publishers.

Boatwright, D. C., and Moore, V.: Suburethral diverticula in the female, J. Urol. **89:** 581, 1963.

Davis, B. L., and Robinson, D. G.: Diverticula of female urethra: assay of 120 cases, J. Urol. **104:**850, 1970.

Ehrlich, R. M., Dougherty, L. J., Tomashefsky, P. T., and Lattimer, J. K.: Effect of gonadotropin in cryptorchism, J. Urol. **102:**783, 1969.

Garduno, A., and Mehan, D. J.: Testicular biopsy findings in patients with impaired fertility, J. Urol. **104:**871, 1970.

Harrow, B. A., Sloane, J. A., and Salhanick, L.: Clinical evaluation of renal function test, J. Urol. **87:**527, 1962.

Hodgson, N. B.: One-stage hypospadias repair, J. Urol. **104:**281, 1970.

Lung, J. A., Painter, M. R., and Lewis, E. L.: Urethral prolapse, J. Urol. **102:**361, 1969.

MacKay, M., and Edey, H.: Law concerning voluntary sterilization as it affects doctors, J. Urol. **103:**482, 1970.

MacLeod, J.: Semen analysis for infertility, Clin. Abst. Gynec. **8:**115, 1965.

Marshall, V. F., and Muecke, E. C.: Functional closure of typical exstrophy of bladder, J. Urol. **104:**205, 1970.

Mountcastle, V. B., editor: Medical physiology, ed. 12, St. Louis, 1968, The C. V. Mosby Co.

Newman, H. F., Northup, J. D., and Devlin, J.: Mechanism of human penile erection, Invest. Urol. **1:**351, 1964.

Ney, C., and Friedenberg, R. M., editors: Radiographic atlas of the genitourinary system, Philadelphia, 1966, J. B. Lippincott Co.

Prior, J. A., and Silberstein, J. S.: Physical diagnosis, St. Louis, 1969, The C. V. Mosby Co.

Scott, W. W.: The role of the urologist in the diagnosis and treatment of pseudo-hermaphroditism, Postgrad. Med. **29**:481, 1961.

Skoglund, R. W., McRoberts, J. W., and Raade, J.: Torsion of spermatic cord: review of literature and analysis of 70 new cases, J. Urol. **104**:604, 1970.

Smith, D. R.: Estimation of the amount of residual urine by means of phenolsulfon-phthalein test, J. Urol. **83**:188, 1960.

Stewart, B. L.: Impotency in the male, Lancet **83**:2, 1963.

Winter, C. C.: Kidney function tests in children, Calif. Med. **94**:127, 1961.

Winter, C. C.: Exstrophy of the bladder: a re-evaluation of the treatment, J. Urol. **93**: 700, 1965.

Winter, C. C.: Excretory urography as a renal function test. In Ney, C., and Frieden-berg, R. M., editors: Radioisotope atlas of the genitourinary system, Philadelphia, 1966, J. B. Lippincott Co., pp. 719-721.

Winter, C. C.: Practical urology, St. Louis, 1969, The C. V. Mosby Co.

Winter, C. C.: Vesicoureteral reflux and its treatment, New York, 1969, Appleton-Century-Crofts.

3

Urologic equipment

Urology is distinguished from the other surgical specialties by the special instruments used. Some equipment is commonly used in both bedside and office management of patients, while other special equipment is used in surgery. The urologic clinic and surgical nurses should become thoroughly familiar with the various instruments and equipment. This chapter is designed to acquaint the nurse with the various types, use, and care of urologic equipment.

CATHETERS

The catheter is a hollow tube that may be rigid if made of metal, plastic, or glass or flexible if made of material such as rubber, nylon, silk, or plastic. Both the rigid and flexible catheters may be preformed into specific shapes. The size of the catheter is designated in French units. One French unit is equal to 1 mm. in circumference or 0.33 mm. in diameter. The circumference measurement is used to designate the size of the catheter. In the adult female the most widely used urethral catheters range in size from 14 to 20 Fr., while in the adult male, sizes 16 to 22 Fr. are generally used. Correspondingly smaller catheters are used in children and infants. The adult ureters are intubated with sizes 4 to 6 Fr.; 4 or 5 Fr. is used in the pediatric age group. The ejaculatory ducts are catheterized with special size 3 Fr. catheters. The size of the catheter to be used depends upon the purpose to which it is being applied. If the patient is being catheterized to obtain a urine specimen, a small catheter is sufficient and less likely to cause trauma. However, if the tube is being placed in the bladder or kidney for temporary drainage, a catheter of larger size is more efficient. A catheter placed in the kidney is called a nephrostomy tube, while one placed in the bladder is called a cystostomy tube. The operations performed for placement of these catheters are called nephrostomy and cystostomy, respectively. Catheters

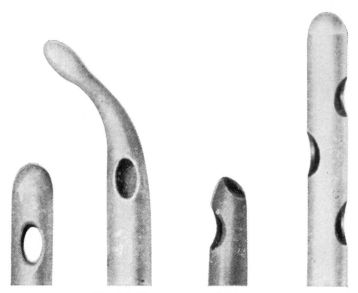

Fig. 3-1. Variations in catheter tips.

have additional descriptive names relating to their shape, number of openings near the tip (eyes), and the construction of the tip, which may be solid or hollow (Fig. 3-1).

Straight catheter

The Robinson catheter is made of rubber or plastic material and has a rounded hollow tip. If the tip is solid and has only one eye, it is known as a Nelaton catheter. The Robinson catheter generally has two or more eyes. It is the catheter used most often for obtaining a urine specimen or for temporarily relieving the patient of acute bladder retention. It is moderately flexible and has a better ratio of internal to external diameter than the Foley retention catheter. It may be strapped to the male penis with strips of adhesive and used as an indwelling catheter. Modifications of this type of catheter include a whistle tip, which has an oblique open end, a coudé tip, which is curved and has a rounded or bulbous tip (Tiemann catheter) that facilitates passage in the tortuous male urethra, and a hole-in-tip catheter (similar to the Councill catheter) (Figs. 3-2 and 3-3).

Self-retaining catheters

The Foley catheter is the most popular self-retaining catheter. It has a double lumen, and the additional lumen leads to an inflatable balloon near its tip, permitting it to be retained in the bladder or kidney (Fig. 3-2). The balloon generally comes in a 5 or 30 ml. capacity. Like-

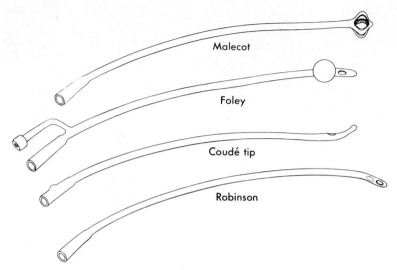

Fig. 3-2. Commonly used catheters; top two are retention catheters.

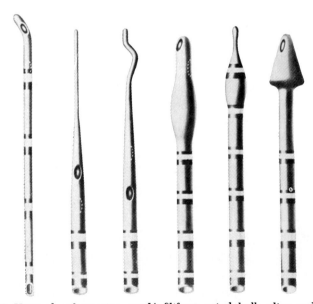

Fig. 3-3. Ureteral catheter tips: coudé, filiform, spiral, bulb, olive, and acorn.

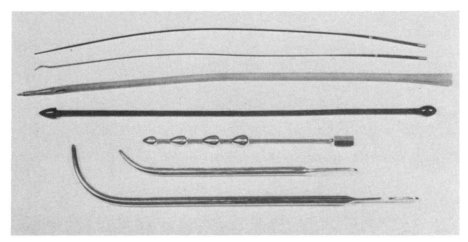

Fig. 3-4. From bottom: solid steel male sound, solid steel female sound, Thaxton urethral bougie, bougie à boule with olive and acorn tips used for urethral calibration, Phillips catheter (follower), and two filiforms.

wise, the tip of the catheter may have one or two eyes, may be straight or coudé shaped, and may have a short or long tip. After an operation on the bladder neck or prostate a Foley catheter with a large bag (hemostatic catheter) may be used to compress the vessels in the operative site by having traction placed upon the catheter. The balloon is filled with sterile water using a syringe. Some of the channels to the balloon have valves to which the syringe or a needle may be attached, while others are merely hollow rubber tubes that require an adapter connecting the syringe. A three-way Foley catheter is one in which a third lumen is used for the inflow of irrigating fluids. The larger channel is used as an outflow tract and this arrangement permits continuous irrigation. This type is particularly useful when the operative site is bleeding and continuous irrigation is necessary to dilute the blood and keep it from forming clots that might obstruct the catheter, especially if it is attached to dependent drainage. The chief disadvantage of the Foley catheter is the small lumen of its outlet channel compared to its external diameter. The Councill catheter is a Foley catheter with an open tip. This allows intubation of the catheter with a stylet having a screw on its end for attachment to a threaded filiform (Fig. 3-4). This filiform is useful for negotiating strictures, and the Councill catheter is to be left indwelling by removing only the stylet and attached filiform.

The Malecot catheter has a large single channel and its tip is in the shape of two or four wings that collapse into the shape of the tube when traction is applied (Fig. 3-2). It is very useful for temporary or permanent indwelling drainage of the bladder or kidney. It is made of rubber or plastic. Either material becomes soft in the presence of body heat,

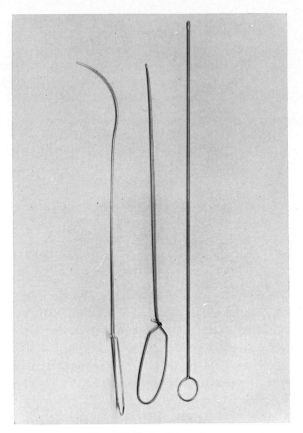

Fig. 3-5. Catheter guides.

allowing the wings to straighten readily upon traction without trauma when the catheter is removed.

The Pezzer or mushroom catheter is similar to the Malecot catheter except that its preformed tip is in the shape of a mushroom and it does not collapse into the shape of a tube when it is released from the body, making its removal more traumatic. Some Pezzer tips have open ends.

Ureteral catheters

Ureteral catheters are smaller and longer than urethral tubes. They are passed through a cystoscope, by which means the urologist is able to intubate the ureters. They are made of nylon, polyethylene, Teflon, dacron, silicone rubber, woven silk, or rubber. Each type has a special use to which it is adapted (Fig. 3-3).

The mandarin is a catheter guide, or metal stylet, that is straight or curved (Fig. 3-5). It is inserted in the catheter to make it rigid. It allows for greater ease in catheterizing the male, for maneuvering past false urethral passages, and for replacing cystostomy or nephrostomy tubes.

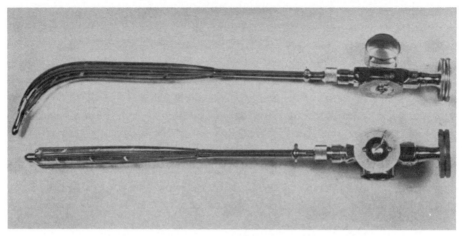

Fig. 3-6. Straight and curved Kollman urethral dilators.

The stylet should be well lubricated with jelly or mineral oil so that it may be removed without dislodging the catheter. Its use is potentially hazardous and should be employed only by the urologic specialist.

Urologic dilatation. When the urethra or sinus tracts to the bladder and kidney become constricted, the passageway may be dilated with special instruments or catheters (Fig. 3-4). The simplest method of dilatation is to pass a small rubber catheter, which tends to swell after a few hours and therefore enlarges the channels gradually. By inserting a larger catheter every day, the channel may be dilated gradually in a nontraumatic and nonpainful fashion. However, if one wishes to dilate the channel abruptly, local or general anesthesia should be used. The most popular local anesthetic for this use is 2% lidocaine jelly or liquid. It is instilled for 10 minutes. The following instruments are used for dilatations.

SOUNDS. A sound is a smooth, solid, cylindrical rod of stainless steel. The female sound has a short, straight shaft that tapers to a rounded end. The male sound often has a sweeping curve at one end and its tip is also rounded (Fig. 3-4). They are made in even sizes—8 to 36 Fr. The male urethra is generally stretched to a caliber no higher than 30 Fr., while the female urethral circumference may be made as large as 45 Fr. In order to achieve the latter size a special instrument called the Kollman dilator is used. It has four metal wings that expand to dilate the urethra when a wheel on the outer end is turned (Fig. 3-6).

BOUGIES. The bougie is similar to a sound except that its tip may have either an acorn or olive shape (Fig. 3-4). The acorn tip is more useful in calibrating the urethra or ureter and locating the site of stricture since the narrowest caliber will cause it to "hang up" when pulled out. The olive end is more applicable for dilatation of a channel since it will slip forward and backward more readily than the acorn tip. Bougies are generally constructed of nylon or woven silk and impregnated with gum or wax. The latter allows it to develop a softer consistency when it is heated by the body temperature or soaked in warm water. Some bougies are made of metal (Thaxton bougie) and these are especially valuable in calibrating the female urethra and its meatus.

The Phillips dilator (follower) is also made of nylon or silk with wax or gum impregnation and has a screw on its tip that attaches to a long, fine, flexible threadlike tip (filiform) (Fig. 3-4). The filiform is about 12 inches in length and is passed through the urethra into the bladder. It is most useful when dealing with strictures. The Phillips followers are attached and may be passed into the bladder by stretching the stricture. Progressively larger followers may be attached and used without removing the filiform from the urethra completely so that the continuity with the bladder is maintained.

In preparing catheters for use, sterilization methods suitable to their composition are followed. Most urologic tubes, sounds, or bougies may be autoclaved and prewrapped for use. The instruments that cannot withstand heat are soaked in germicidal solutions. All parts should be separated for cleansing and sterilization.

The Le Fort catheter (follower) is similar to the Phillips type but differs in that the follower is made of metal and is hollow with an eye near its end so that the bladder may be drained after the urethra is negotiated. It is not intended to be left indwelling. However, the hollow Phillips follower may be left in the bladder temporarily and is strapped into place with adhesive.

The Councill catheter is a Foley catheter with a small hole in its tip. This allows a stylet with a screw in its tip to be inserted and connected to a filiform. After the catheter is passed and its balloon inflated, the stylet and attached filiform are withdrawn.

CYSTOSCOPIC EQUIPMENT
The cystoscope

The cystoscope is an instrument used for indirect visualization of the inside of the bladder, urethra, and occasionally the interior of other parts of the body such as the kidney. Its outer cover is called a sheath and the solid portion placed in the sheath to aid its passage is called an obturator. The obturator comes with an optional flexible or inflexible end. The former is called a Timberlake obturator. Various types of observation lenses are available. These include one that allows visibility straight ahead, a for-oblique angle of 15 degrees, a right-angle view, and a retrospective examination. The first lens is most useful in examining the urethra, the bladder

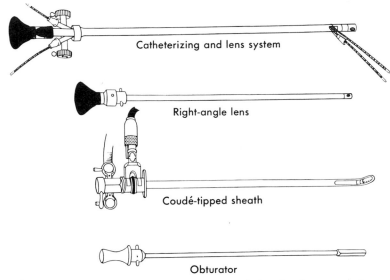

Catheterizing and lens system

Right-angle lens

Coudé-tipped sheath

Obturator

Fig. 3-7. Brown-Buerger cystoscope. Parts consist of sheath, obturator, right-angle lens, and working element that has retractable lid used to deflect catheters in order to pass them into ureters. Note coudé beak of sheath.

neck, and the interior of the prostate, while the latter is used to inspect the bladder just proximal to the bladder neck. With the use of these combinations of lenses, there is no area of the bladder that cannot be observed. To pass ureteral catheters or to perform transurethral surgery, the observation lens is replaced by a catheterizing unit with a smaller lens or with a surgical device. Some units have a fin, so that when two catheters are passed they will remain separated in their respective channels. A lid on the end of the unit may be tilted to deflect the catheter so that it may be passed into a ureteral orifice. The right-angle lens of the Brown-Buerger cystoscope (one with a coudé tip sheath for easier passage in the male, Fig. 3-7) is larger than the similar lens of the McCarthy cystoscope (one with a straight sheath) (Fig. 3-8). Cystoscopes vary in size from 11 (infant) to 28 Fr. The largest cystoscopes permit use of stone extractors, forceps, scissors, biopsy and fulguration instruments.

The resectoscope is a modification of the cystoscope in that its working element contains a movable part. This is generally a wire loop connected to an electric current that enables it to cut or burn tissue. There are various methods of moving the loops, such as springs or a movable handle for manual manipulation by the urologic surgeon (Fig. 3-9).

The Thompson punch resectoscope uses a guillotine blade to cut out bits of tissue without the use of electric current. Fulguration is accomplished by inserting an electrode.

The lithotrite is another instrument closely allied to the cystoscope.

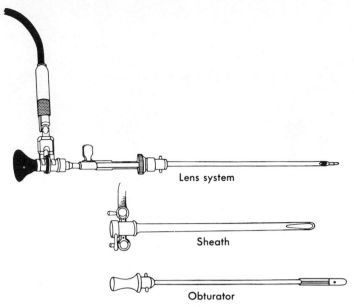

Fig. 3-8. McCarthy cystoscope or panendoscope. Its parts consist of sheath, variety of telescopic lenses, and an obturator.

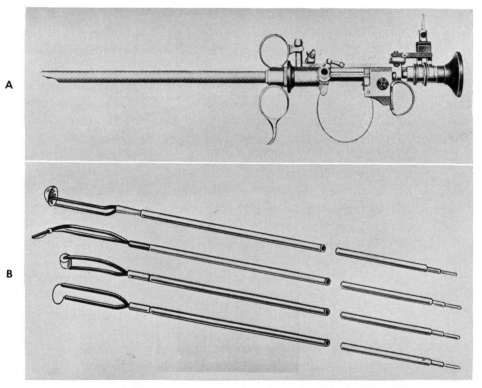

Fig. 3-9. A, Resectoscope, which contains movable wire loop that will cut through tissue or fulgurate bleeding points when electrically energized and projected. B, Four types of cautery attachments for resectoscope.

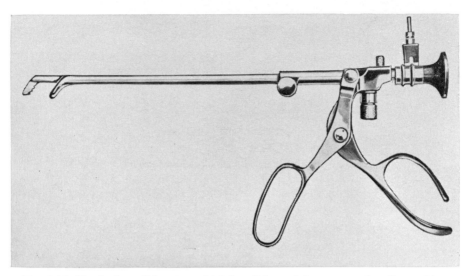

Fig. 3-10. Hendrickson lithotrite, which has light and lens system for direct vision.

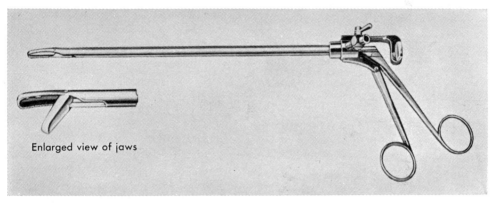

Enlarged view of jaws

Fig. 3-11. Lowsley forceps, which is useful for grasping small foreign objects or stones within bladder.

The Bigelow lithotrite is a large instrument with rounded, movable jaws on its tip that are closed when passed into the full bladder but are then opened to engage and crush large stones. This is a blindly manipulated instrument and is more hazardous to use than smaller lithotrites containing a lens system for direct vision. A small percentage of bladders are ruptured by using these instruments. Few urologists have mastered the ability of using the Bigelow lithotrite and it is becoming a lost skill. Litholapaxy for smaller stones is safer and the Hendrickson lithotrite (Fig. 3-10) is a popular instrument for such use. It contains a foroblique lens system with a light, allowing a stone to be engaged and crushed under direct vision. Other instruments used transurethrally or through cystostomy or nephrostomy openings are the Lowsley forceps (Fig. 3-11)

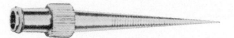

Metal catheter connector to fit Luer syringe — for use with all small-caliber funnel-end woven catheters

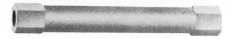

Rubber ureteral catheter adapter — red and green for differentiation of right and left kidneys

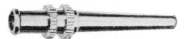

Metal ureteral catheter adapter

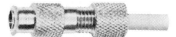

Tuohy Luer-Lok catheter adapter — replaceable rubber internal washer locks adapter firmly to catheters, sizes 3½ through 7

Fig. 3-12. Catheter adapters.

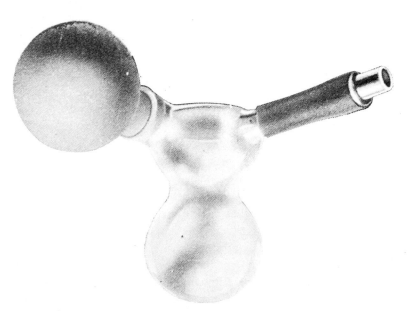

Fig. 3-13. Ellik evacuator used for removal of tissue or blood clots from bladder by attaching to resectoscope or cystoscope sheath.

that can grasp bits of tissue or stones for crushing and removal and flexible needles, scissors, meatotomy knives, and electrodes that can be inserted through the instruments and used under direct vision. Scissors and cold or electrode blades are useful for cutting the ureteral orifice in performing a ureteral meatotomy. Flexible cup biopsy instruments may also be employed through a cystoscope. It is obvious that these instruments must have battery or rheostat attachments for a light source, and the resectoscopes must have power units for cutting and fulgurating. Fiberoptic units are now available for improving the intensity of the lighting systems of cystoscopes, lithotrites, and resectoscopes.

ANCILLARY EQUIPMENT

Special catheter adapters made of metal or plastic material are available so that tubes of a variety of sizes may be connected to catheters (Fig. 3-12). The Asepto syringe, which is made of glass with a tapered end and a rubber bulb attachment for intermittent pressure and suction, is useful for most irrigations. The Ellik evacuator (Fig. 3-13) is used to remove tissue, stone fragments, or clots from the bladder through a cystoscope or resectoscope sheath. The Toomey syringe is a 2-ounce, piston-type syringe made of glass or plastic and has a large-caliber nozzle. It allows greater suction to be applied in irrigation and is most useful for removing clots from the bladder, particularly after surgery. Ureteral syringes are ordinary 5 or 10 ml. glass or plastic syringes. Adapters are necessary for connecting their ends to different types of catheters and are made of rubber or metal. However, ordinary hypodermic needles may be used. Urethral syringes are smaller, usually ½ to 1 ounce in capacity, and have tapered blunt tips so that they will fit into the end of the urethra. Today these are used primarily for the instillation of local anesthetics, while in the past they were commonly used for the introduction of medications.

Special clamps are available for holding solutions in the male urethra or for closing catheters or tubing (Fig. 3-14).

Stone extraction baskets are made of flexible metal, nylon, or woven silk and near their ends they contain strands of wire, nylon, or catgut that act to snare stones within the ureter (Fig. 3-15). The Dormia extractor is a popular basket in use today. It has a spiral wire end that expands when it is brought out of its sheath after it has been pushed past the stone. The Ellik loop catheter has a wire or catgut strand attached to the end of a 5 Fr. nylon ureteral catheter (Fig. 3-16). This strand is brought into the catheter lumen about 5 cm. from the tip. After the catheter has been passed into the renal pelvis, a loop is formed at the tip by pulling on the wire or catgut. The looped catheter is then pulled down the ureter to a level just above the stone. During the subsequent hours or days the loop engages the stone, aiding in its removal.

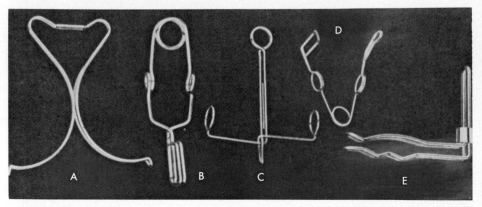

Fig. 3-14. Male penile clamps. Useful for holding anesthetic materials within male urethra.

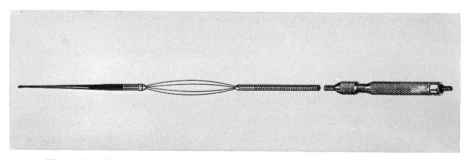

Fig. 3-15. Johnson stone basket used for extracting stones from lower ureter.

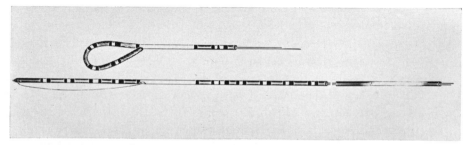

Fig. 3-16. Ellik loop catheter. Catheter is passed into renal pelvis where loop is formed, and loop is then pulled down the ureter in order to engage and extract ureteral calculus. Catheter is shown in open and closed positions.

DRAINAGE EQUIPMENT

The nurse plays a major role in the management of the drainage system of the patient with an indwelling catheter or tube in the bladder or kidney. The tube or catheter is connected to a long plastic tube that carries the drainage into a bottle or bag reservoir made of glass or plastic material. These collectors usually have capacity markers, making it convenient to chart the output. Most of the current drainage units in use are closed systems. These systems are not to be taken apart, nor do they have openings that will allow the entrance of bacteria. One such type has a drip area so that an air space is incorporated to prevent bacteria from entering the body. Another type of drainage system employs a Y tube connector so that an elevated bottle of irrigating solution may be introduced through the elevated arm while the dependent arm of the Y is attached to the drainage collector. Clamps are placed on the inlet and outlet tubes so that they may be turned off and on as the system is used. Other types of drainage tubes have outlets for collecting urine specimens for analysis or to attach syringes for manual irrigation.

The Y tube connector is also adaptable for decompression-type drainage. It is elevated above the bladder level to any height desired so that urine will accumulate in the bladder before it is drained by intermittent syphonage (Fig. 3-17). Some urologic surgeons prefer this type of drainage because the bladder is not always completely empty. This allows the blood to be diluted in the postoperative state, with less opportunity to form clots and obstruct the drainage tubes. Various types of suction machines may be applied to any of the drainage systems to keep the tubes open and the bladder or kidney empty. Making an air vent with a hypodermic needle somewhere along the line will keep the suction from being too great and thereby avoiding the blockage of the openings of the catheters with bladder mucosa.

When the urologist performs a transthoracic-transdiaphragmatic approach to the adrenal or kidney, he closes the diaphragm and chest wall but often leaves an indwelling catheter in the pleural space. The drainage tube passes beneath a water level in a bottle on the floor. Each time the patient inspires, some air is forced from the pleural space beneath the water level and it will bubble out. This type of water trap prevents air from returning into the pleural space. Within a few hours the lung will become fully expanded with this type of air evacuation.

CLEANSING AND DISINFECTION OF UROLOGIC EQUIPMENT

All urologic equipment must be carefully cleaned following its use. All parts should be disassembled. Difficulty is encountered in cleaning the inside of tubes, hollow instruments, and stopcocks. These must be thoroughly cleaned to remove all solid and infected material using mild

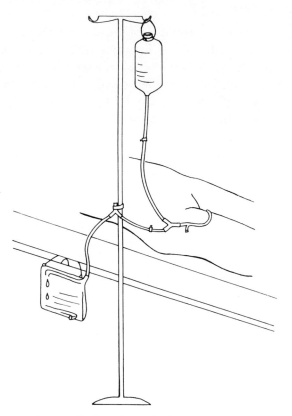

Fig. 3-17. Decompression urethral catheter drainage system. Note Y tube, which may be elevated to any desired level to maintain intermittent partial filling of bladder. An irrigation system is also connected to catheter and controlled by inlet and outlet clamps. This system is commonly used after transurethral prostatic surgery.

solvents, soaps, or detergents. When the instruments have been carefully cleaned, they are sterilized by autoclaving, gas sterilization, or liquid bactericidal solutions. In general, most metal and rubber instruments can be autoclaved. Many plastic materials are not heat resistant, however, and this must be ascertained before placing them in an autoclave. Silicone rubber goods may be autoclaved. Autoclaving is the most desirable type of sterilization because it is rapid and at high temperatures all bacteria, including *Mycobacterium tuberculosis*, microbacteria, and spores, are killed. Gas sterilization is a lengthy process but is less injurious to the lens systems of cystoscopes. Many instruments and catheters are sterilized in solutions such a Detergicide or Cidex. They have been found to be quite reliable when the directions for their use are carefully followed. One of the most commonly used but least reliable bactericidal agents is Zephiran chloride. If vapor gets inside the lens system of a cystoscope, it will become "foggy." It must then be returned to the factory for removal of the entrapped vapor.

QUESTIONS

1. List four different types of catheters and indicate what unit of measurement is used to depict their size.
2. What is the most commonly used retention catheter?
3. What is the most commonly used catheter for obtaining a urine specimen only?
4. What is a sound used for?
5. What are bougies used for?
6. Describe two different types of cystoscopes.
7. Describe two different types of resectoscopes.
8. What is the difference between a stone basket and an Ellik loop catheter?
9. Describe three types of catheter drainage systems.
10. Describe three methods of sterilizing urologic equipment.

REFERENCES

Baumrucker, G. O.: TUR—transurethral prostatectomy, techniques, hazards and pitfalls, Baltimore, 1968, The Williams & Wilkins Co.

Dreyer, C. V., and Winter, C. C.: Applications of the Dermo-Jet in urology, J. Urol. **104**:586, 1970.

Rogers, C.: Lists key points in care of endoscopic instruments, Hosp. Top. **43**:109, 1965.

Thompson, L. R.: Evaluating disinfectants, Amer. J. Nurs. **62**: 82, 1962.

Tyler, V. R.: Gas sterilization, Amer. J. Nurs. **60**:1596, 1960.

CHAPTER 4

General principles and procedures of urologic nursing

The material discussed in this chapter is common to the care of patients with urologic disorders and to avoid continuous repetition is presented before the discussion of care of patients with specific disorders. Since certain adaptations are necessary relative to the age of the patient, Chapter 5 should be read in conjunction with this chapter to better understand the various methods used.

Nurses' notes

The progress notes recorded in the patient's chart by the nurse serve an important function. The purpose of recording the type and frequency of fluid and dietary intake, the times, amount, or frequency of passage of excreta, and notations of mental status, patient verbalizations, symptoms, or signs is to aid the physician in the management of the patient and his disease and to guide the nursing personnel toward continuity of nursing care of the patient. It is obvious that if these documentations are accurate and thorough, a high quality of medical and nursing care will be achieved. One of the most difficult aspects of nursing duties seems to be the task of writing nurses' notes. It is insufficient to say, "the patient had a good day," and it reveals an incomplete appraisal of the patient and his problem to say, "the patient spent a restless night." Yet these trite remarks are of the usual caliber of records kept in many charts. Such notes are a waste of time for both the nurse and the physician and do not present a very accurate report. If the nurse really is interested and dedicated in helping the patient, she will follow a plan similar to the one that follows to accomplish her purpose. First, she must be thoroughly familiar with all aspects of the patient's problem. The patient may have a single disease with secondary or minor additional problems or a number of disorders.

The problem may be a symptom of unknown origin. The nurse's first note in the chart should therefore attempt to define this by her personal assessment of patient needs. When evaluating the patient, the nurse should be able to define his immediate needs using the patient, his family, health team members, and records as resource material. Her initial findings should be reflected in the admission note of a urologic patient such as the following.

Mr. John Adams was admitted on 6 East at 5 A.M. via the emergency room per cart. He states he received medication for severe pain in the right lower back thought to be due to a kidney stone. The pain still remains; however, the severity has decreased considerably. He is experiencing some nausea. His clean-voided, two-glass specimen of urine has been sent to the laboratory for analysis and culture. The urine was smoky in color. He states he is allergic to penicillin and commented about being frightened but willing to cooperate. The patient is oriented in all spheres. Pending laboratory tests, x-ray examinations and the procedure for straining all urine have been explained to the patient.

This example indicates clearly the patient's chief problem and the immediate course of management. It also alerts all nurses or doctors as to the line of treatment. Subsequent notes should be pertinent to the patient's illness; the following are examples.

9 A.M.—Mr. Adams' urine and blood specimens were sent to the laboratory for analysis. His urine is still coffee-colored. He had good results from his purgative and was sent to the radiology department for chest and urinary tract x-ray films. He has had only a mild right flank ache radiating to his right groin since admission and no longer requires pain medication. His electrocardiogram has been postponed, pending the outcome of these x-ray films. He does not now complain of nausea.

9 P.M.—Mr. Adams had a severe pain in the right genital region at 8 P.M. and subsequently voided a small white stone with relief of pain. The stone has been saved for Dr. Johnson. The patient seems quite relieved of his previous anxiety and is joking with the ward personnel.

These brief but fact-filled notes indicate a clear picture of the patient's problem and subsequent course of action. They show that some thought and analysis have gone into their preparation. The notes paint a vivid picture for other nurses and the attending physician. Valuable time can be saved, and more intelligent and efficient care can be given the patient. With patience and disciplined practice, the nurse can become a skilled writer of chart notes and assume a more important role in the management of the patient. She will obtain much greater satisfaction from this type of participation in the professional medical management of her patients and from the dependability, reliance, and judgment the physician will discover she possesses.

FLUID INTAKE AND URINARY OUTPUT

A primary concern in the medical treatment of patients is to maintain the urinary output within normal limits. Since the urinary system plays a primary role in the homeostatic functions of the body, failure to maintain an adequate urinary output can lead to serious illness. Deficiency in the urinary output reflects either inadequate intake of fluids or a faulty mechanism for excretion.

Measurement of fluid intake and output

Important nursing functions include careful observation and accurate recording of fluid intake and urinary output. During the acute stages of the urologic illness every patient should have a fluid chart. This record should be accurately kept and critically studied to determine if there is the expected ratio of intake to output. Any marked change in this ratio should be reported to the physician. Progressive reduction in daily urinary output despite adequate intake is a danger sign, heralding either urinary obstruction or renal failure due to nonobstructive disease. It should be definitely determined, however, that decreased urinary output is not caused by inadequate fluid intake or by retention of urine in the bladder. Conversely, it is well to be aware at this point that an occasional patient with partial urinary obstruction will be able to maintain a normal output of urine. Therefore an adequate output of urine should not be taken as reassurance that the patient has no obstructive uropathy.

A well-hydrated person who is not abnormally losing fluid by other routes such as through the skin (diaphoresis) or the gastrointestinal tract (vomiting or diarrhea) will excrete amounts of urine slightly more than his "liquid" intake. Almost equal amounts of fluid are usually taken in liquid and solid foods—about 1100 ml. a day in solids and 1200 ml. a day in liquids. (See Chapter 2 for discussion of urinary output of infants and children.) Postoperatively a patient tends to retain sodium and fluids for 24 hours, during which time his output will be less. He also loses slightly larger amounts of fluid than normal as "insensible water loss" (respiration and perspiration), and he usually eats less solid food. He will therefore need a higher "liquid" intake than normal to supply the body's fluid needs, and although he may have a liquid intake of 2000 to 3000 ml., he still may have a urinary output of only 1000 to 1500 ml.

Fluid chart

The fluid chart should provide an accurate *record of fluid intake and output.* The intake record should indicate the type and amount of all fluids received and the route by which they were administered (Figs. 4-1 to 4-4). Usually only the quantity of fluid taken by mouth is recorded. But, if a careful check of electrolytes such as sodium, potassium, and chlorides is needed, the type as well as the amount of fluids drunk must be noted. Notation of solid food intake may also be requested since dietary intake is an important way to replace essential electrolytes as

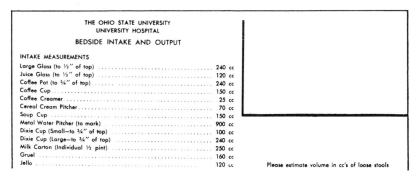

THE OHIO STATE UNIVERSITY
UNIVERSITY HOSPITAL

BEDSIDE INTAKE AND OUTPUT

INTAKE MEASUREMENTS

Large Glass (to ½" of top)	240 cc
Juice Glass (to ½" of top)	120 cc
Coffee Pot (to ¾" of top)	240 cc
Coffee Cup	150 cc
Coffee Creamer	25 cc
Cereal Cream Pitcher	70 cc
Soup Cup	150 cc
Metal Water Pitcher (to mark)	900 cc
Dixie Cup (Small—to ¾" of top)	100 cc
Dixie Cup (Large—to ¾" of top)	240 cc
Milk Carton (Individual ½ pint)	250 cc
Gruel	160 cc
Jello	120 cc

Please estimate volume in cc's of loose stools

Fig. 4-1. Intake measurement reference chart.

well as other nutrients. Space should be provided on the fluid chart for *recording urine output and for identifying other less common fluid losses such as wound drainage or vomitus.* Often a *daily weight record* is requested because this gives a good indication of changes in body fluid content. Daily weights of infants and postoperative patients are commonly obtained for this purpose.

Daily weights. To be useful as a measurement of body fluid content, the weight must be taken on the same scale and at the same hour each day with the patient wearing the same amount of clothing. Circumstances that might affect the weight must be kept as nearly identical as possible from day to day. Usually weights are taken in the early morning before the patient has eaten or defecated; it is preferable for the bladder to be empty.

Urinary output. Urinary output should be carefully recorded as to the time and amount of each voiding. If urine drains from more than one orifice, the output from each site should be recorded separately. Conspicuous signs posted on the patient's chart, at the bedside, and in the utility room help to prevent the inadvertent discarding of urine before it is measured or collected for special laboratory examinations.

Wound drainage. If there is excessive wound drainage, it is often necessary to measure this. When the drainage is from a fistula (opening) into the urinary tract, *catheters or collection bags may be used* so that more accurate recording of fluid loss is possible. A karaya gum ring plastic bag is quite useful over a drain site. At other times *it may be necessary to weigh the dressings and any wet linen at each change.* This may be done accurately by weighing the linen and dressings on a small gram scale prior to use; this is recorded as dry weight. Upon removal, the dressings and linen are again weighed and the dry weight is subtracted from the wet weight to give a record of fluid loss (1 gram = 1 ml. or 1 cc.).

Other output. Vomitus should be measured as accurately as possible and should be described as to color, contents, and odor. Electrolytes are

THE OHIO STATE UNIVERSITY HOSPITALS
INTRAVENOUS THERAPY
INTAKE WORKSHEET

DATE:

ROOM NO.	PATIENT'S NAME	SOLUTION ORDERS	11-7 GIVEN	11-7 LEFT	7-3 GIVEN	7-3 LEFT	3-11 GIVEN	LE
608	Michael Bernstein	#1000cc 5% Dextrose/Water	300	700	700			
		#1000cc 5% Dextrose/Saline			900	100	100	
		#1000cc 5% Dextrose/Water					1000	
		# ACCUMULATIVE TOTAL	300		1900		3000	
		#						
610	John Markham	#500 cc WHOLE BLOOD	500					
		#1000cc 5% Dextrose/Saline	100	900	900			
		#1000cc 5% Dextrose/Water			200	800	800	
		# ACCUMULATIVE TOTAL	600		1700		2500	
		#						
611	William Newberry	#200cc 3% NACL			200			
		#1000cc 5% Dextrose/Saline			450	550	550	
		# ACCUMULATIVE TOTAL			650		1200	
		#						
		#						
		#						
		#						
		#						
		#						
		#						
		#						
		#						
		#						
		#						
		#						

Form 5909—Rev. 3/70 (460102)

Fig. 4-2. Example of intravenous fluid intake worksheet for several patients in a nursing section. The day is divided into three 8-hour periods corresponding to the nursing work shifts.

THE OHIO STATE UNIVERSITY HOSPITALS

BEDSIDE INTAKE AND OUTPUT

ke Measurements Are to Be Recorded In Cubic Centimeters (cc's)

se Reference Card Posted in Patient Room To Obtain Exact "CC's"
For Each Container

KE	Measurements in cc's		TUBE FEEDING			OUTPUT			Measurements in cc's			
E	ORAL	OTHER	FORMULA	WATER		TIME	URINE	GASTRIC	EMESIS	STOOL	MISC.	
An.						12						
						1						
						2						
						3						
						4						
						5						
					8 Hr. Total	6						8 Hr. Total
						7						
											DRAINAGE	
	WATER 150					8²⁰	300					
	MILK 220					9⁴⁵	200					
	COFFEE 150					10						
	WATER 150					11³⁰	150					
h	JUICE 140											
	COFFEE 150					12						
						1					75	
	WATER 150				8 Hr. Total	2	175					8 Hr. Total
						3						
					1110							900
						4						
er						5						
						6						
						7						
						8						
						9						
						10						
					8 Hr. Total	11						8 Hr. Total
AL						TOTAL						
r.						24 Hr.						

6911—Rev. 2/71 (460118)

Fig. 4-3. Example of record for listing fluid intake and output. The day is divided into 8-hour periods.

Form 5006—Rev. 12/67
(460108)

THE OHIO STATE UNIVERSITY HOSPITALS

INTAKE AND OUTPUT RECORD

DATE	TIME	INTAKE			OUTPUT					
		ORAL	PARENTERAL	TOTAL	URINE	DRAINAGE	EMESIS	OTHER	STOOL	TOTAL
3/30/71	11- 7	200		200	400	90				490
	7- 3	910	500	1410	825	75				900
	3-11	1120		1120	1100	125				122.
	24 Hr. Total	2230	500	2730	2325	290				261.
	11- 7									
	7- 3									
	3-11									
	24 Hr. Total									
	11- 7									
	7- 3									
	3-11									
	24 Hr. Total									
	11- 7									
	7- 3									
	3-11									
	24 Hr. Total									
	11- 7									
	7- 3									
	3-11									
	24 Hr. Total									

4-1   INTAKE AND OUTPUT

Fig. 4-4. Example of fluid intake and output record covering a 5-day period.

lost in large amounts with excessive vomiting, and accurate measurement and description of losses are essential for the doctor in determining the type as well as the amount of fluid replacement needed. Gastric juices are watery, usually pale yellowish green, and have a sour odor. Excessive loss of gastric juices upsets the acid-base balance of the body and the vomitus may then smell "fruity" because of the presence of acetone. Bile is somewhat thicker than gastric juice and may vary from bright yellow to dark green in color. It has a bitter taste and acrid odor. Intestinal contents vary from dark green to brown in color, are likely to be quite thick, and have a fecal odor. Fluids from various parts of the gastrointestinal tract contain varying amounts of electrolytes. Gastric juices contain a great deal of sodium, chloride, and hydrogen ions; bile contains mainly sodium but also an important amount of potassium; and intestinal fluid contains primarily bicarbonate, chloride, calcium, sodium, and phosphate. Any *gastric* and *intestinal drainage* should also be measured; any irrigation fluid included in it should be carefully subtracted from the total drainage so that an accurate output of body fluids is recorded.

Fluid may also be lost in large amounts *in the stool.* If the patient has diarrhea, it is important that the number of stools, the color, and the approximate amount of each be recorded. Since infants are prone to losing large amounts of fluid in the stool, daily records of their stools are kept routinely.

Blood losses from any route should be carefully estimated and measured if possible. Since blood is often mixed with other fluid, the color and consistency of the fluid in which it is found should be recorded. This gives a basis for judging the amount of bleeding. Viscid, bright red drainage with clots is primarily blood.

Diaphoresis is difficult to measure, but when a careful check of fluid output is considered necessary by the doctor, it should be recorded. Although sweat volume cannot be measured except with special research facilities, note should be made of heavy perspiration and its approximate duration. Since fever speeds up metabolism and increases loss of fluid through the lungs and the skin (insensible fluid loss), careful checking and *recording of body temperature* helps the doctor to determine how much fluid the patient needs.

Fluid intake. Fluid is essential for all body processes, and large amounts of it are used each day. Without an adequate daily fluid intake, body functions are disturbed. In noncritical situations the best way to restore water to the body is by mouth. Electrolytes and nutrients are also best supplied by this route. Fortunately, most patients with urologic disorders are able to take food and fluids by mouth.

FORCING FLUIDS BY MOUTH. Because disease not only may aggravate fluid losses but also may increase the water requirement by speeding up some of the body processes, extra fluids are often needed. Therefore, unless the patient's cardiac or renal status contraindicates forcing fluids, patients with urologic disorders are often ordered to force fluids. Adults should then drink between 2000 and 3000 ml. of fluid a day. Larger amounts should not be given without a doctor's order. Infants and children, since they have less body fluids (although more proportionately) than do adults, should be given smaller amounts; the quantity varies with the age and size of the child. Infants under 12 months of age normally require a daily intake of up to 125 ml. per kilogram of body weight. When infants must have fluids forced, the normal intake must be exceeded, but the amount to be given should be specifically prescribed by the physician. Most children under 5 years of age can safely receive at least 75 ml. per kilogram of body weight a day. For children 5 to 10 years of age, 50 ml. per kilogram of body weight is usually adequate. This means that a 2-year-old sick child should usually be given 1000 ml. of liquids a day; a 12-year-old, 2000 ml. a day. The physician should be consulted, however, as to the desirable amount.

Many persons, especially when they are ill, find it difficult to drink large quantities of water. It is often very difficult to encourage children and elderly patients to drink fluids. There are many ways, however, that the nurse can help the patient take adequate fluids by mouth and thus avoid the need for parenteral fluids. Fruit ades, ginger ale, or other soft drinks may be substituted for part of the water. Juicy fruits or other solid foods with a high fluid content such as custards, ice cream, or gelatin may be more palatable than liquids for some patients. The amount of fluid thus given must be estimated and recorded. A juicy orange, for example, contains about 50 ml. of fluid. Soups, bouillon, milk, cocoa, tea, and coffee also provide fluid.

Care must be taken, of course, that any substitutions for water are acceptable on the diet prescribed for the patient. A patient whose salt intake is restricted, for instance, should not be given salty broths or milk drinks. The patient on a low potassium diet should not take fruit juices, tea, coffee, or chocolate drinks. A dietitian can help the nurse determine the approximate amount of fluid provided by various foods and will indicate to her those foods and fluids acceptable for patients on restricted diets.

The techniques used in presenting fluids to patients may influence the intake. Often small amounts of fluid given at frequent intervals are more easily taken than a large amount presented less often. Carbonated beverages or hot liquids may be better tolerated by patients who are nauseated. Attractively prepared food or fluids served in a pleasant atmosphere also help to improve the intake of most patients.

Fluids should always be spaced throughout the 24-hour period. Not only does this serve to maintain normal body fluid levels but it also helps the urinary system irrigate itself and prevents waste materials from passing through the system in concentrated form, predisposing to the formation of calculi. Fluid spacing also prevents overhydration.

Patients with urologic disease should take generous amounts of fluids not only during the acute stage of illness but also as a general health practice. They should be warned, however, not to take excessive amounts of fluid since this may cause *water intoxication,* a condition in which the kidneys are unable to excrete the fluid as fast as it is absorbed into the bloodstream. This causes the blood volume to increase and dilutes the normal salt content of the blood, causing symptoms of sodium depletion.

If patients can tolerate food and fluids by mouth but for some reason are unable to swallow them or refuse to take them, a feeding tube may be inserted through the nose into the stomach and *tube feedings* given. By this method, 250 to 500 ml. of a therapeutic feeding may be given to adults at spaced intervals. The feeding may also be given as a slow continuous drip. Infants and children are given a prescribed formula equivalent in amount to their usual feedings. The procedure for passing the tube for feeding (gavage) is described in medical-surgical nursing textbooks and pediatric nursing textbooks. The nurse should be alert for signs of aspiration of the fluid into the lungs. Coughing, choking, and cyanosis indicate aspiration, and if any of these symptoms occur, the feeding should be immediately discontinued. A small amount of water should always be given before the feeding itself because, if the tube is displaced, aspirated water is less likely to cause serious trouble. Following the feeding, water should also be given to flush out the tube.

PARENTERAL FLUIDS. When food and fluid cannot be taken by mouth, parenteral fluids are given. By far the most common method used to give parenteral fluids to all age groups is intravenous infusion (venoclysis). Hypodermoclysis (infiltration of subcutaneous tissues with fluids) is sometimes used, and infants and young children may be given fluids intraperitoneally. If continuous administration of fluids is desirable, a Rochester needle or an incision may be made into the vein to be used and the polyethylene catheter threaded into the vessel. The latter is called a *cutdown.* This catheter is usually left in place for several days, and at least a very slow drip of some infusion fluid must constantly run into it to prevent clogging of the lumen.

Amino acids and electrolytes as well as glucose are frequently given intravenously. When hemorrhage has markedly decreased the blood proteins, it may be necessary to give whole blood, plasma, albumin, or plasma expanders such as dextran to replace the protein loss before other fluid therapy is effective. Unless the patient has lost a large amount of blood, fluids to replace blood proteins must be given slowly because they tend to pull tissue fluids into the bloodstream. This may cause a sudden increase in the circulating blood volume and push fluid into the lungs, producing pulmonary edema (drowning in pulmonary secretions).

If any intravenous fluids are being given rapidly, the patient should be watched closely for signs of bounding pulse, engorged peripheral veins, hoarseness, dyspnea, cough, or pulmonary rales. At the first signs of any of these indications of increased blood volume, the rate of flow of the infusion should be greatly reduced and the doctor notified. Particular care must be taken with patients who are known to have cardiac disease, with infants, and with aged persons. Unless otherwise ordered, intravenous fluids should never be given faster than 3 ml. per minute. Moreover, when the patient is not dehydrated, infusions should be run at a rate roughly equal to the rate of fluid losses from all routes per minute. If run rapidly in this instance, the fluid will act as a diuretic (cause an increased output of urine) and will not be utilized.

Intravenous fluids containing electrolytes (sodium chloride, potassium, amino acids, molar lactate, calcium) need to be run slowly to allow the body to regulate their use. The patient should be carefully watched for signs of intoxication (excess of fluids or electrolytes). Many doctors do not write intravenous therapy orders until daily chemical analyses of blood have been reported.

Techniques for administering parenteral fluids are discussed in textbooks on fundamentals of nursing. Special techniques used for children are discussed in pediatric nursing textbooks.

CATHETERIZATION AND MANAGEMENT OF URINARY OUTPUT

To rid the body of its waste products, urine, once formed, must be excreted from the kidney and drained from the body. Failure to provide drainage of urine causes distention and back pressure in the urinary tract proximal to the portion not emptied. This predisposes to renal damage. In addition, whenever there is urinary stasis, infection of the urinary tract is a common sequel. Acute urinary retention is quite painful and predisposes to ileus.

Use of catheters

There are times when it is essential to insert one or more catheters into the urinary tract to provide urinary drainage. The usual indications for catheterization are anatomic obstructions of the tract, inability to voluntarily empty the tract, or the need to inactivate the tract to promote healing or to avoid forcing urine into adjacent tissues (extravasation). The catheter is placed so that it drains urine from the tract above the site of obstruction or the site desired to be inactivated.

Catheters should always be used with discrimination since there are many serious disadvantages to their use. When a catheter is being in-

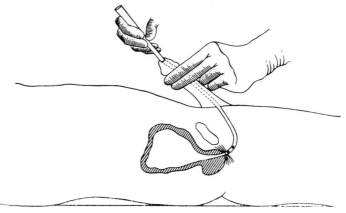

Fig. 4-5. Male catheterization. Note that urethra is straightened perpendicular to body, leaving only one bend to be negotiated. Resistance to catheter is often met at external urinary sphincter.

serted, there is always danger of introducing infectious organisms into the urinary tract of the male or female and into the male reproductive system. Aseptic and atraumatic techniques must therefore be carefully observed (Fig. 4-5). Following urethral catheterization, males are likely to develop epididymitis. Because the ejaculatory ducts open into the prostatic urethra, organisms easily enter at this point and proceed along the vas deferens to the epididymides. Epididymitis is not only a painful infection but one frequently complicated by vasoepididymal strictures which, if bilateral, cause sterility. Therefore, when possible, urethral catheterization of a male is avoided. In addition, a catheter left in the urethra and bladder for any length of time acts as a foreign body and causes irritation of the mucosal walls of the portion of the tract through which it passes. This in turn predisposes to inflammation of the mucosa and of the glands opening along the tract. Indwelling catheters, especially those not attached to a closed drainage system, have also proved to be a source of staphylococcal and other types of infection in the urinary tract. Of course, unless the drainage system itself is kept uncontaminated and is replaced periodically, it too may be a source of infection. Prolonged use of a catheter can lead to formation of urinary tract calculi because the urine, instead of maintaining its usual acidity, becomes alkaline as a result of urinary tract infection. Inorganic matter present in urine, especially calcium and phosphates, tends to precipitate in alkaline urine.

With a few exceptions, which will be mentioned under specific disorders, all catheters except urethral catheters are inserted by the doctor. On a urologic service many urethral catheterizations may also need to be done by the doctor. If in carrying out an order for catheterization the nurse finds it difficult to pass a urethral catheter, the procedure should be discontinued and the doctor notified. Traumatic catheterizations predispose to urinary tract infections and urethral strictures. It is not uncommon to be unable to pass a standard catheter in patients with urologic disease, especially in males with urethral and bladder neck obstructions. Catheterizations requiring the use of special equipment such as stylets, filiforms and Phillips catheters (followers), or sounds *are not nursing procedures.* A nurse should never introduce any hard or inflexible equipment through the urethra because there is danger of severe trauma such as perforation of the urethra or bladder. The nurse should, moreover, never catheterize a patient in the early postoperative period following urethral or bladder surgery.

The purpose of using a catheter in any patient with urologic disease is to provide better drainage of the urinary system. Unless the doctor specifically orders it, *catheters should never be left clamped.* A catheter that is draining a kidney directly must never be clamped for even a very short period since the normal renal pelvis in an adult has a capacity of only 4 to 8 ml. Special care must be taken that a catheter draining a kidney is not allowed to become completely or partially plugged. In case of accidental removal of any catheter inserted through a surgical opening, prompt reinsertion (within 30 minutes) is essential; these openings rapidly diminish in size.

If the ureter is obstructed or partially obstructed, a catheter may need to be placed into the renal pelvis to ensure adequate drainage. Where the catheter is placed depends on the location of the obstruction and the condition of the patient. If there is complete obstruction of the ureter, a catheter may be introduced directly into the kidney. A nephrostomy tube, usually a Foley, Pezzer (mushroom), or Malecot (batwinged) catheter (see Fig. 3-2), may be inserted through the substance (cortex and medulla) of the kidney into the renal pelvis from a surgical wound made laterally in the flank. A *pyelostomy tube,* usually a Foley, Pezzer, or Malecot catheter, is placed directly into the renal pelvis—it is not passed through the cortex and medulla of the kidney. The surgical opening for a pyelostomy is also made in the flank. It is not used as often since it is harder to replace than a nephrostomy tube. The kidney may be drained by a *ureterostomy tube* (a whistle-tipped or many-eyed Robinson catheter or a T tube), which is passed through a surgical opening into the ureter. This opening is made through an incision in the anterior flank. The catheter is passed up the ureter to the renal pelvis. If the ureter is unobstructed or only partially obstructed, the renal pelvis may be drained by a *ureteral catheter,* which is passed by means of a cystoscope into the bladder and up the ureter to the renal pelvis.

If there is obstruction below the bladder, constant drainage is necessary to preserve renal function because the back pressure produced by inadequate emptying of the lower urinary system may ultimately damage the nephrons. The most common means of draining the bladder is through the *urethral* catheter. Usually a self-retaining type of catheter (for example, a Foley) is used. Sometimes a coudé-tipped Tiemann, a many-eyed Robinson, or a filiform and Phillips catheter will be used as an indwelling catheter for male patients since a straight catheter can be adequately anchored to the penis. (See discussion on anchoring of catheters.) Occasionally a male patient may have a *perineal urethrostomy* (a new opening into the urethra from the perineum made to bypass an obstruction or surgery performed in the anterior urethra). In this instance the urethral catheter may be brought through the perineum. When the urethra is completely obstructed or when there is danger of infection of the male genital system because of prolonged use of a catheter, a *cystostomy tube* (usually a Foley, Malecot, or Pezzer) may be placed into the bladder through a suprapubic incision. Sometimes after bladder, prostatic, or urethral operations the bladder will be drained by both a cystostomy tube and a urethral catheter.

One kidney may be drained by a catheter while the other empties into the bladder as usual. The urinary output in this instance will be both voided and drained by a catheter. Each collection must be recorded separately. Actually this provides only an estimate of the output of each kidney. Since the drained kidney is still connected with the bladder, some urine from this intubated kidney may drain around the catheter into the bladder and be voided. This is especially common when ureteral catheters are passed up the ureter retrogradely through a cystoscope and left to drain. Although both kidneys may be intubated, some urine is forced down the ureters around the small catheters and the patient will void this as the bladder fills. If, in addition to the *ureteral* catheter, a *urethral* catheter drains the bladder, some drainage may return through both catheters.

Care of tissues surrounding a catheter. The skin surrounding an indwelling catheter needs to be carefully inspected at least once daily for dryness and cleanliness. It is a good practice, however, to routinely note the condition of the skin each time the catheter is checked for patency. It is especially important to check the area around the urinary meatus following a urethral catheterization because it may be edematous. Edema of the foreskin in a male patient is extremely painful and may limit circulation to the urethral tip. If edema is noted, it should be reported to the doctor immediately. He usually orders sitz baths or cold applications and special attention to local cleanliness. If paraphimosis is present, it must be reduced.

Cleansing of the urethral meatus and the adjacent catheter every 2 to 4 hours results in a diminished incidence of infection in patients with indwelling catheters. Sponges soaked with hydrogen peroxide or benzalkonium chloride are desirable for this cleansing. The reliable patient may be instructed to carry out this procedure himself. The importance of frequent cleansing to remove all crusts and mucus from around the catheter should be emphasized.

Inspection of the catheter and genital area will be less upsetting to the patient if it is done in a matter-of-fact, efficient manner and without undue exposure. The patient should be told why the inspection is being made. If a male nurse is available, it is usually preferable that he cleanse the genital area of a male patient.

Equipment needed for catheterization

Many different types of catheters are used. The kind selected for use will depend on the cavity being intubated, the size and shape of the passage through which the tube must be passed, and whether or not the catheter is to be left in place. Before setting up for a catheterization, the nurse should therefore ascertain the type of catheter to be used.

A size 14 to 20 Fr. catheter is commonly used for *uncomplicated urethral catheterizations* in the female and a size 16 to 22 Fr. in the male. A much smaller catheter, often size 8 or 10 Fr. or smaller, is used to catheterize the urethra of a child. A coudé or curve-tipped catheter (Tiemann) is often used for intermittent male urethral catheterizations because it is more easily passed through the curved male urethra. However, a whistle-tipped or a many-eyed Robinson catheter may also be used. A straight, soft, red-rubber catheter with a solid round tip is usually used for intermittent urethral catheterizations in the female. Should the doctor suspect that a patient has a large amount of residual urine in the bladder, he may want catheterization done with a self-retaining catheter (Foley; see Fig. 3-2), which can be left in place for drainage if necessary.

If the passage through which the urethral catheter must be passed is partially obstructed, a coudé-tipped catheter with an olive tip may be used. Sometimes the doctor may use a stylet (metal catheter director) in conjunction with the catheter. At times it is necessary for him to dilate the urethra with bougies or metal sounds before a catheter can be passed. At other times a filiform and Phillips catheter may be the only tube that he can insert into the urethra. When the urethra is partially obstructed, catheters of various sizes are usually needed. The doctor should be consulted about this.

Although any type of catheter may be left in the bladder (indwelling) for drainage, usually some type of self-retaining catheter such as a Foley or Malecot is used; a stylet must be used with the Malecot type.

Pezzer (mushroom) and Malecot (batwinged) catheters (see Fig.

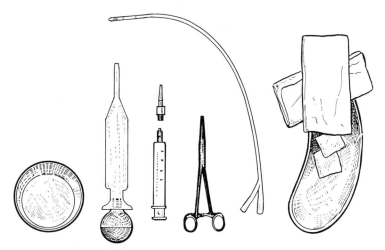

Fig. 4-6. Usual equipment necessary for inserting Foley catheter. Left to right: basin for irrigating fluid, Asepto bulb syringe, syringe for inflation of catheter balloon, hemostat to be used as forceps, Foley catheter, and waste basin with surgical towel and sponges for cleansing urethral meatus.

3-2) are most commonly used *to intubate the bladder through a cytostomy* (suprapubic surgical opening into the bladder) (see Fig. 8-3, *B*) *or to intubate the kidney through a nephrostomy* (surgical opening into the kidney) (see Fig. 8-13). The catheter used may be either straight or right-angled, according to the doctor's preference. The doctor should be consulted as to the type and size of the catheter. When inserting these tubes, a catheter director is needed.

A many-eyed Robinson catheter or a whistle-tipped catheter is usually used to *catheterize the renal pelvis through a ureterostomy* (surgical opening of the ureter onto the flank). The size needed will vary from patient to patient and may be as small as a 6 Fr. or as large as an 18 Fr.

The following equipment is needed for all catheterizations: a good light (preferably an adjustable lamp), sponges and solution for cleansing the local area, a sterile lubricant such as K-Y jelly, and a sterile field including a sterile drape, sterile gloves, forceps, and two catheters of the type to be used; two clean basins in which to collect the urine and a receptacle for used sponges; and a culture tube and specimen bottles. For a *routine female urethral catheterization* this basic setup is adequate. A 4 by 8 inch sponge for handling the penis should be added to the equipment when preparing for a *male urethral catheterization.*

If a self-retaining catheter with an inflatable balloon (Foley) is to be inserted, extra equipment will need to be added to the basic catheterization setup (Fig. 4-6). To determine if the catheter is correctly placed, equipment to irrigate the catheter will be needed. This includes a bulb syringe (Asepto), a basin, and irrigating solution such as sterile physiologic solution of sodium chloride. *Equipment is also needed to inflate the balloon* (this varies according to the type of catheter used). A syringe (5 to 30 ml., depending on the size of the balloon) is needed to inflate the balloon of a Foley catheter. Fortunately, more hospitals and offices are using disposable catheter and drainage sets. (These are available commercially.)

Whenever a catheter is to be left indwelling in the bladder or kidney, equipment for irrigating the catheter must be added to the basic catheterization setup. Although irrigation should be avoided whenever possible, studies have shown that the incidence of infection can be reduced by the use of a three-way catheter when an indwelling catheter is to be left in the bladder. The three-way catheter is connected to sterile irrigation and drainage equipment that eliminates the need for frequent disconnection of the system at the end of the catheter, thus preventing introduction of bacteria at this point. Unfortunately the drainage lumen in a three-way catheter is quite small and easily obstructed by clots or debris.

If a Pezzer or Malecot catheter is to be inserted, a stylet will need to be added to the routine urethral catheterization equipment. Extra lubricant should be available because the catheter director must be copiously lubricated so that it will slip out easily from within the catheter following insertion of both into the bladder or renal pelvis.

Principles of urethral catheterization

Preparation of patient for catheterization. Before beginning any physical preparation for catheterization, *the procedure should be explained to the patient,* even if the doctor is to do the catheterization.

Privacy should always be maintained, and patients should be properly positioned and draped for catheterization. This maintains their dignity and helps them to be less embarrassed and tense. Tenseness makes it difficult to pass a catheter. Teaching the patient to breathe deeply also helps to relax the vesical sphincters and makes the procedure less traumatic and uncomfortable.

A woman should be placed in a dorsal recumbent position for a urethral catheterization and draped as for a pelvic examination. A firm support under the hips makes visualization of the urethral meatus easier. Placing the patient on a treatment table rather than in bed allows for better support, position, and visualization. If the doctor catheterizes a woman, a female nurse should be present during the procedure.

As an alternative to the dorsal position for the female patient, the nurse may find placing the patient in a lateral position more advantageous both for herself and the patient. Particularly if the nurse is short in stature, the lateral position makes possible better visualization of the genital area,

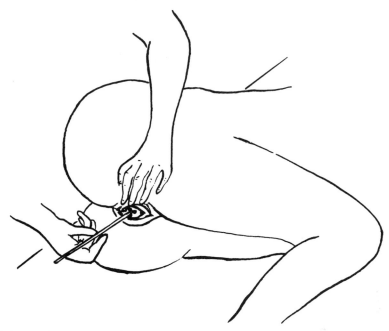

Fig. 4-7. Female patient in lateral or Sims' position. Labia are separated for urethral catheterization.

eliminates the need to work under the strain of an awkward position, and provides a greater area for the placement of equipment. If the patient has contractures of the hips and/or knees, the lateral position is more comfortable as well as less embarrassing. The patient is placed on her right or left side, depending on whether the nurse is right- or left-handed. The knees are drawn toward the chest, the buttocks placed on the edge of the bed, and the shoulders drawn toward the opposite side of the bed. The nurse need only lift up the labia for the urethral orifice to be made visible (Fig. 4-7).

For a male urethral catheterization the subject should be flat in bed and should lie upon a bath blanket placed from the chest to the knees and have the bed covers fan-folded back to the knees. After explaining the procedure, draping the male patient, and preparing the equipment, the female nurse should, after ascertaining from the doctor that her assistance is no longer needed, leave the patient with the doctor. When the catheterization is finished, she returns to see that the patient is comfortable and to take care of any specimens and the equipment. A male nurse may remain during the procedure.

A second person must always be present to hold and to talk with a child during a catheterization. Most young children will need both their arms and legs securely held to prevent sudden movement. One person

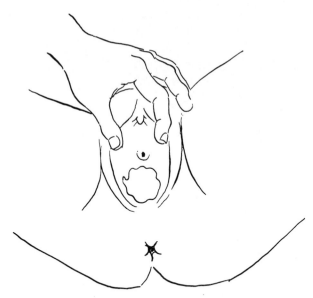

Fig. 4-8. Exposure of female urethral meatus. Note location between vaginal opening below and clitoris above. This area should be thoroughly cleansed prior to insertion of catheter. When voided urine specimen is collected for culture, labia should be separated in this manner and area cleansed with antiseptic solution.

can usually do this by standing at the child's head and holding each leg and by placing an arm over each arm of the child. The position for a child is the same as for an adult.

CLEANSING THE GENITALIA. Cleansing of the genitalia with soap and water may be necessary. Before catheterizing the urethra, the area about the meatus should be thoroughly cleansed with a disinfectant such as benzalkonium chloride (1:750 aqueous solution). The cleansed area should be kept uncontaminated until the catheter has been passed. In a woman this means that the labia should be kept well separated (Fig. 4-8). If gloves are used to pass the catheter in a female, they must be put on prior to cleansing and the area must be cleansed with use of a forceps to maintain the sterility of the gloved hand to be used in handling the catheter. In the male the foreskin should be retracted to cleanse the meatus and should be left retracted; the cleansed penis is placed on a sterile towel.

Passing the catheter. Insertion of a catheter should be done under aseptic conditions and without trauma. The catheter should be sterile, well lubricated with a water-soluble jelly, and handled and inserted with sterile gloves or a sterile instrument. Gloves should always be used with children or extremely nervous patients to avoid accidental trauma with an instrument. There should always be a sterile field beneath the catheter to prevent accidental contamination while passing it.

In catheterizing a female the thumb and first or second finger should be inserted well into the labia minora and then pulled upward toward the symphysis pubis to smooth out the area and make the meatus visible (Fig. 4-8). Asking the patient to breathe deeply will often make the meatus dilate slightly. A good light is also needed to adequately visualize the urethral meatus in the female.

The male urethral meatus should be readily visible at the tip of the penis. For catheter insertion the penis should be held upward, perpendicular to the body. This minimizes the urethral curvature and straightens the channel.

When passing a catheter, resistance is usually encountered at the urethral sphincter. The catheter should not be forced but a brief pause is allowed until the sphincter relaxes and then the catheter should pass through. In the female the catheter will need to be inserted 2 or 3 inches; in the male, from 7 to 10 inches.

Placing an indwelling catheter. If a catheter is to be left in the bladder, it should be inserted about 1 inch farther than the point at which urine first flows. When a balloon at the tip of the catheter is inflated to retain the catheter in the bladder, the patient should not experience pain. If he does, the balloon should be emptied and the catheter inserted farther. An indwelling catheter should be pulled gently outward for a moment following anchorage to ascertain if it is secure. It should also be irrigated to ensure proper placement for drainage. Irrigation fluid will return freely from a well-placed catheter.

Anchoring catheters. It is important that catheters be adequately anchored to prevent accidental dislodgment. *Self-retaining urethral catheters* are tethered with tape to the thigh. The *method of anchoring a straight catheter in the urethra* is as follows: Cut two strips of 1-inch adhesive tape 5 inches long. Cut four pieces of ½-inch tape 7 inches long. Apply tincture of benzoin to the penile skin. Place one end of each piece of the longer strips on each side of the penis and apply the shorter strips of adhesive to hold the long strips in place. Wind the four pieces of long tape in alternate directions around the catheter (Fig. 4-9).

Cystostomy, nephrostomy, and ureterostomy tubes should have two points of anchorage since the openings made for the insertion of these tubes are essentially fistulas that rapidly decrease in size upon removal of the catheter. In even a half hour after removal of a catheter it is often impossible to reinsert a catheter of the same size. If the catheter is inserted during an operation, it usually is sutured in place. If so, only a two-flap adhesive anchorage is necessary. If the tube is not sutured in place, a piece of adhesive tape should be placed around the catheter, leaving a tab to pin to the dressing, and a two-flap adhesive anchorage should also be used. When the patient has no dressing, the catheter can be gently curved

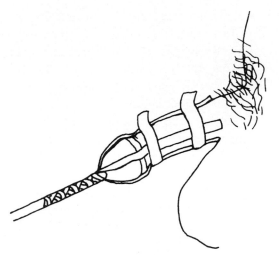

Fig. 4-9. Nonretention catheter may be strapped to penis with four strips of adhesive in fashion shown here. Two additional strips of adhesive are wrapped around penis to hold catheter attachments in place.

(taking care not to kink it) and attached to the abdomen at two points by two-flap adhesive anchorage.

Checking for patency of catheter. Catheters must be checked frequently to assure they are open (patent). The interval between each check varies depending on circumstances. A newly placed catheter or a catheter inserted to provide drainage postoperatively should be checked every 15 minutes until the nurse is sure that there is free drainage. If there is frank bleeding through a catheter, it should be constantly watched. The catheter of a patient who has hematuria but not frank bleeding or that of a patient who is restless and tends to kink the tubing should be checked at least hourly. Even catheters that are apparently draining well should be checked for patency three or four times a day.

In checking the patency of a catheter, disconnection of the catheter from the drainage tubing should be avoided because of the possibility of introducing bacteria during the procedure. Careful notation of urinary output or use of the recently developed fine measurement devices that can be attached between the drainage tubing and the drainage bag is preferred. However, if this is not possible, disconnect the drainage tubing at the catheter and allow the urine in the tubing to drain. Thoroughly cleanse the end of the catheter and the glass connector with a gauze saturated with 70% alcohol,* reconnect the catheter to the tubing, and

---

*The bottle of alcohol should not be left at the bedside to prevent any possibility that it may be inadvertently mistaken for the irrigating solution. Individually wrapped cotton pledgets saturated with alcohol are commercially available and are preferable in this situation.

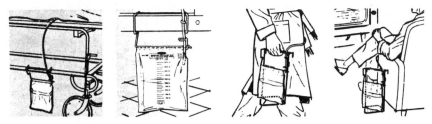

Fig. 4-10. Plastic bag for collecting and measuring urine output may be attached to bedside or carried by patient when ambulatory.

hold the glass connector at a slight elevation so that the urine is draining against gravity to fill the glass connector. If under these conditions urine appears in the connector within 1 or 2 minutes, the catheter is draining adequately. If there is little drainage, the nurse should make sure that the patient is not dehydrated. Drainage often will start within half an hour after the patient is given two or three glasses of water.

If drainage is not adequate, the drainage system, starting with the drainage bottle and working back to the catheter, should be systematically checked to make sure that it is not obstructed at any point. A catheter or the drainage tubing may be blocked by a blood clot or a plug of mucus. These obstructions may sometimes be dislodged by gently "milking" the tubing. If drainage remains poor, the catheter should be irrigated. The doctor often leaves an order to irrigate the catheter if it is necessary. If there is no order or if irrigation is not successful, the doctor should be called. No catheter should be allowed to drain inadequately for more than 1 hour.

Connection to various drainage systems. Proper maintenance of the drainage system to which a catheter is connected is an essential nursing function. The system must be properly set up initially and properly maintained. The lumen of the connectors and the tubing used should always be comparable to that of the catheter to which it is connected. The inner bore of any tube draining urine should be at least 8 mm. in diameter. When a white sediment begins to encrust a glass connector, or when a drainage tube rubbed between the fingers feels sandy, the drainage equipment should be changed. Usually the catheter will also need changing at this time. Ordinarily, tubing will need to be changed only once a week. If the drainage bottles are cleansed and boiled daily, there will be less odor. However, disposable calibrated plastic drainage bags are available commercially and obviate this problem (Fig. 4-10). Methods for cleaning and sterilizing urologic equipment are discussed in Chapter 3.

Care must be taken that neither the catheter nor the drainage tube is kinked or squeezed shut. If thick-walled latex tubing is used, obstruction of drainage caused by kinking of the tubing can be reduced. Care should be taken not to obstruct the lumen of the tube in attaching the drainage tubing to the bed. A large paper clamp is convenient to use and is unlikely to squeeze or kink the tubing. Tubes are frequently clamped off by the weight of a patient lying on them. To prevent this and also to lessen the danger of decubiti, it is best to run drainage tubing over the thigh. However, this may cause kinking of the catheter, and if so, the tubing should be run under the knee or directly to the foot of the bed, where it will not be under any part of the body. Special care must be taken that nephrostomy and ureterostomy tubes are not kinked by the patient lying on his side. (See Fig. 8-13 for location of nephrostomy tubes.)

GRAVITY DRAINAGE. Catheters are usually attached to *straight drainage* so that they will drain by gravity. *A kidney is always drained by this method.* To drain a closed cavity by gravity, air must be accessible in the drainage system. Since there is less danger of infection and since better drainage is provided when the tubing is not immersed in the urine collecting in a bottle, it is preferable to use a system in which a large tube is attached to a capped bottle or bag that has an air outlet as well as an adequate inlet for the urine or to one of the new disposable drainage bags. There seems to be less incidence of staphylococcal or other infections when a closed system of drainage such as this is used. This system also decreases odor.

To provide complete drainage of a cavity (renal pelvis or bladder) by gravity, the tubing must run directly from the level of the cavity to the drainage receptacle with no loops of tubing below the level of the drainage bottle. Clipping the tubing to the bed and coiling the excess length of tube on the bed help to prevent back pressure and incomplete emptying of the intubated cavity.

Use of a plastic leg bag provides a system of straight drainage for the ambulatory patient (Fig. 4-11). Patients should be cautioned not to fasten the bag so high that the catheter or tubing is kinked or must drain against gravity. Leg bags usually do not provide adequate drainage for the patient in bed because of lack of gravity. Moreover, drainage equipment for bed use does not provide convenient emptying of the urinary tract when the patient is out of bed. It is not only inconvenient but the tubing tends to loop below the level of the drainage bottle or bag and prevents complete emptying of the intubated cavity.

The patient usually can be taught to change from one drainage system to the other. He should cleanse the end of the catheter and the connectors with 70% alcohol or benzalkonium chloride (1:750) on changing from one type of drainage apparatus to the other. The connecting tube not in use should be left wrapped in a dry sterile gauze sponge saturated with benzalkonium chloride (1:750), a bacteriostatic agent, or covered with a commercially made protector. Individually wrapped benzalkonium

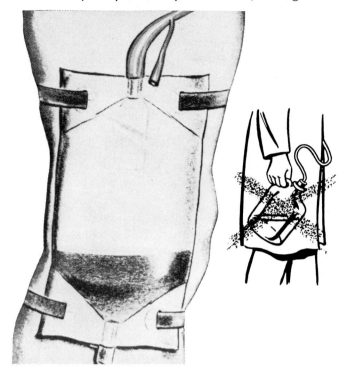

Fig. 4-11. Plastic bag attached to thigh and connected to indwelling urethral catheter so patient may be ambulatory. One-way flutter valve keeps urine in bag from returning into catheter. Bag is easily emptied through outlet at bottom.

chloride or alcohol sponges can be left at the bedside. A piece of aluminum foil, plastic, or waxed paper can be used to cover the container to prevent contamination and evaporation.

STERILE CLOSED DRAINAGE SYSTEMS. The closed drainage system is preferable whenever possible. With a closed system the possibility of bacteriuria can be reduced since no disconnections are made between catheter and drainage tubing, drainage tubing and collection receptacle, or at the time of irrigation. Manufacturers have improved the equipment in the last few years. Factors to be considered in purchasing such equipment include lumen size of tubing, length of tubing, airways in collection bags that do not foster the entrance of bacteria, drip chambers that prevent backflow and contamination, accurate measurements, ease in assembly and use with a patient reclining, sitting, or walking, and ease in emptying the bag without danger of contamination. A well-illustrated publication is now available for health workers and patients that describes closed drainage systems, positioning of equipment and the patient, plus methods of collecting specimens.* Various studies using closed drainage

---

*Seggreen, M.: The closed urinary drainage system, New York, 1970, The American Journal of Nursing Co., Educational Services Division.

systems are listed in the references at the end of the chapter; most of them give evidence that supports the use of such systems.

OTHER DRAINAGE SYSTEMS. Although the bladder is usually drained by gravity (straight drainage), occasionally the doctor may wish it to be drained by some other method. A catheter from the bladder may be attached to suction drainage to ensure that the bladder is kept completely empty. Weak suction must be used to avoid injury to the mucous membrane of the bladder. The patient with suction drainage may be allowed out of bed, but he must remain within range of the suction. Gomco intermittent suction may be used. The addition of an air outlet should be provided by inserting a 20-gauge needle into the catheter and taping it in place.

The desired negative pressure may also be obtained by attaching a small electric (Stedman) pump to tubing connected to one arm of the drainage bottle cap. The drainage tubing from the catheter is attached to the other arm and no air is allowed in this system.

Sometimes when the bladder is greatly distended or when there is bleeding from the prostatic fossa, the doctor may want to prevent total emptying of the bladder. This is accomplished by *decompression drainage* (see Fig. 3-17).

The color of urinary drainage should be checked and recorded. An accurate check of the color can be made only at the glass connector next to the catheter because the urine in the drainage bottle is a collection of several hours. Checking the color of drainage in this way is especially important in any situation in which there is bleeding from the urinary system. The total drainage returned from any catheter should also be noted and described because some changes are more easily noted in urine that has collected over a period of several hours and might not be apparent at the connector. In observing the collected urine, the nurse should be especially alert for urine that appears purulent or dirty (infection), cloudy (albuminuria), or smoky (hemoglobinuria); shreds of mucus and small pieces of tissue may also be noted.

Catheter irrigation. The purpose of catheter irrigation is to maintain the patency of the tube and to prevent obstruction to urinary drainage, *not to lavage the organ that the tube drains.* Vigorous irrigation of the kidney and bladder will tend to irritate these structures and spread infection, resulting in pain, hematuria, chills, and fever. Gentleness is mandatory. If adequate fluids are being given and if there is no hematuria with clots, it is unusual for a catheter to need irrigation. The safest and most effective means of irrigating the *urinary system* is by "internal irrigation"—maintaining a large fluid output by forcing fluids either by mouth or parenterally.

If a catheter is to be irrigated, the size of the cavity into which the fluid is being instilled must be considered. The renal pelvis of an adult should never be irrigated with more than 4 to 6 ml. of fluid, that of an infant (birth to 2 years of age) with no more than 1 ml., that of a child under 5 years of age with no more than 2 ml., and that of a child under 8 years of age with no more than 3 ml. The fluid should be instilled gently and allowed to drain back by gravity. Most adult patients will tolerate 75 to 100 ml. of fluid in the bladder, but no more fluid than a patient can tolerate without pain should ever be used. No more than 25 ml. should be used for an infant and 50 to 75 ml. for children under 8 years of age. Under usual conditions irrigations are carried out until the returns are clear. It is advisable to obtain a specific order from the doctor as to the quantity, frequency, and type of irrigation.

If in irrigating, fluid flows in readily but fails to return, there probably is a blood clot or mucus acting as a valve over the eye of the catheter. In this situation, do not continue to add fluid but try to dislodge the obstruction by "milking" the tubing. If this is unsuccessful, the doctor should be called. He may use a suction syringe to remove the obstruction. The Toomey syringe (50 ml. metal-tipped catheter syringe) or its disposable counterpart is the type often used. Only nurses who are specifically trained in the use of this syringe should irrigate or aspirate with it. If too much pressure is exerted, the mucous membrane lining of the bladder can be damaged.

Sterile physiologic saline solution is ordinarily used to irrigate catheters because its clearness makes observation of the return flow easy. Also, it is isotonic to the body fluids. Other solutions occasionally ordered for irrigating are dilute acetic acid (0.25% to 0.5%) and Renacidin. When acetic acid is being used, the doctor should be notified if burning sensations occur. Antibiotic solutions such as those containing 1% neomycin may be ordered. These should be instilled into the cavity and the catheter clamped for a few minutes or for as long as ordered. For patients with atonic bladders, who may require indwelling catheters for an indefinite period of time, 30 ml. of 5% or 10% Renacidin is instilled into the bladder and allowed to remain for 15 minutes. It is followed by repeated irrigation of 30 ml. of sterile physiologic saline solution until the return fluid is clear. The procedure is repeated twice daily. With this procedure, changing of the catheter is recommended every 4 weeks—sooner only if necessary.

INTERMITTENT IRRIGATION. If a urethral catheter needs frequent irrigation, it may be practical to set up intermittent irrigation. This is simply an adaptation of the method of irrigation in which a sterile syringe and a basin of sterile solution are used. A sterile closed reservoir flask holds the irrigating solution, and sterile tubing from the flask to the catheter allows the solution to flow into the bladder upon release of the clamp on this tubing; the drainage tubing from the catheter must be clamped until the specified amount of solution has entered the bladder. The inflow tubing from the reservoir is then clamped and the clamp is released from the drainage tubing. This method obviates the danger of contamination of the catheter during irrigation and makes using a new set for each irrigation unnecessary. This method of irrigation is not safe for irrigations of the renal pelvis because the inflow cannot be regulated carefully enough to allow only 8 to 10 ml. or less of fluid to be instilled at one time.

With intermittent irrigation, an accurate record of the amount of fluid used for irrigation must be kept because the solution returns into the drainage bottle. The amount of irrigating fluid used must be subtracted from the total drainage each time the drainage bottle is emptied so the urinary output may be accurately recorded.

CONSTANT IRRIGATION. If the catheter provides for both inflow or irrigating fluid and outflow of drainage (three-way Foley catheter) or if the patient has both a cystostomy tube and a urethral catheter in the bladder, the doctor may order constant irrigation. The equipment is identical to that used for intermittent irrigation, except that a drip-o-meter is placed below the reservoir flask. The rate of the drip may be increased or decreased as necessary to keep the catheter draining well. When this method of irrigation is employed, an accurate record of the amount of irrigating solution used must be kept and this must be subtracted from the measurement of total drainage.

Urine output after removal of indwelling catheter

Much has been said about providing for urinary output in patients with indwelling urethral catheters, but the nurse also needs to be aware of the urinary output of patients from whom indwelling catheters have been recently removed. The patient who has recently had a catheter removed may be asked to record the *time and amount of each voiding* for several days because this gives an idea of the adequacy of bladder function. The nurse should instruct the patient in the method to be used. If the patient is confined to bed, the nurse may do the recording herself. Regardless of whether the nurse or the patient records the output, the nurse should note the results at least every 4 to 8 hours.

No person who has an adequate fluid intake should go longer than 8 hours without voiding. After operations on the prostate gland or bladder, however, patients should void at least every 3 or 4 hours. Failure of these patients to void for as long as 8 hours probably signifies urinary retention and should be reported to the physician. This type of retention often results from edema at the bladder outlet, and it is not unusual for these patients to need a catheter replaced. It is impossible to know how much edema is present until after the catheter is initially removed. The output of these patients should therefore be checked with special care.

The color and consistency of the urine voided following removal of a catheter should be noted. Some patients develop cystitis (infection of the bladder). This may be caused by incomplete emptying of the bladder. The urine in this instance may appear cloudy or even purulent. (As mentioned before, it is normal for urine to be alkaline and cloudy after meals.) It is not unusual for some hematuria to occur following removal of a catheter used for drainage after bladder or prostatic operations. This is especially common if bleeding has been controlled during surgery by fulguration (electric desiccation). Eight to fourteen days postoperatively the dead tissue sloughs from the healing wound and bleeding may then result. The doctor should be informed about this because it is sometimes necessary to take additional steps such as using some method of hemostasis to prevent serious secondary hemorrhage.

For a few hours after a catheter is removed, the patient may have some dribbling when he voids. This usually is self-limiting or can be controlled by teaching the patient to do perineal exercises. (See instructions in discussion on incontinence caused by damage to the bladder sphincters.) Continued dribbling should be reported to the doctor since it may indicate that a vesical sphincter has been damaged or it may imply urinary retention and overflow incontinence. It is important to find out if the incontinence is complete (constant dribbling) or if it is only "on urgency" since such information guides planning for the patient's further treatment. Another pertinent observation is whether the patient is incontinent in all positions (lying, sitting, standing). If the major problem is muscular weakness, he will probably have the least difficulty with control when in a supine (lying) position and the most difficulty while walking. A patient who is having difficulty regaining normal urinary control should limit his fluids after 6 P.M. so that sleep will not be disturbed unduly.

Home care of patient with catheter drainage

Some patients must be sent home with catheters in place in the bladder or kidneys. This may be only a temporary arrangement (for a short period postoperatively or preparatory to further surgery) or it may be a permanent arrangement. The doctor usually wants the patient or a member of his family to be taught to care for the catheter. The nurse in the hospital should plan the teaching program so that the patient, under supervision and using his own equipment, will be able to assume complete care of the catheter before discharge. It is wise to ask a public health nurse to visit the patient at home to supervise his technique at least once more and to answer any questions he may have. The patient who knows he will have at least one visit from the nurse is usually less apprehensive about going home. The referral to the public health nurse, in addition to identifying information regarding the patient, should include the doctor's report, the nurse's report, and reports applicable from other services such as social service, dietary service, and occupational therapy. The nurse should give a detailed description of nursing problems and treatment, the patient's attitude, and response to care. She should include what was taught the patient and/or family, that is, the extent of self-care accomplished, individual understanding, and amount of help needed. Any other family health problems that affect the care of the patient should also be related. A call from the nurse caring for the patient in the hospital directly to the public health nurse will facilitate a smoother transition for the patient and provide an opportunity for the public health nurse to ask questions and/or share information. Written instruction for care of catheters should also be given to the patient and/or his family. They should include basic principles of cleanliness, methods of sterilization, equipment resources available, the step-by-step procedure, and care of the equipment. Solutions, equipment, and techniques will vary with the doctor, institution, and community resources. Therefore by planning with the doctor, the patient, and the public health nurse cooperatively, an individual plan that meets the patient's special needs can be established. The following general suggestions may be adapted for use by the patient with any type of indwelling catheter:

1. Follow the rules of good hygiene and cleanliness, which are essential for prevention of infection and odor. Frequent cleansing of the meatus with mild soap and water or benzalkonium chloride at the point where the catheter is inserted will, in addition, promote comfort.
2. Keep equipment other than presterilized disposable types clean with soap and water after use; just prior to use, boil for 10 minutes after water starts to bubble in order to sterilize it.
3. Wash permanent collecting bottles, leg bags, and tubing daily with soap and water, soak for 15 minutes in vinegar solution, and rinse with cold water containing a deodorant. Tubing should be boiled twice a week.
4. When disconnecting or prior to reconnecting the catheter to the drainage systems, protect ends of the catheter and tubing with sterile gauze or ready-made protector or preferably wipe with 70% alcohol.
5. When irrigating, press fluid gently into catheter. Allow fluid to drain via gravity unless otherwise ordered by the doctor. Repeat until fluid returns clear.
6. When using a leg urinal, secure it with leg straps. To give better support, the bag can be suspended from a belt placed around the waist.
7. Drink 2 to 3 quarts of fluid a day since this will provide continuous irrigation. If heavy sweating occurs, you should drink more fluid.
8. You may take a shower with your tubes in place unless you have a dressing. Simply plan to replace adhesive tape as soon as you are dry.
9. Change location of tapes frequently to prevent irritation of your skin. If your skin becomes sore, lie under a heat lamp with a 60-watt bulb. Place it 2 feet above your abdomen. *Do not use a sun lamp!*
10. If leakage occurs around the tube or if the tube stops draining:
    a. Check to see that all tubing and connections are clean. Crystals should not form in the tubing or connections if you care for them as outlined each day.
    b. Check to see that no part of tubing or bag is kinked.
    c. Be sure that you always have your drainage container at a level lower than opening from which tube comes.

    d. Be sure leg bag is closed tightly. You may need a new washer in bottom.

    e. Irrigate catheter.

    f. If you have checked all possible causes and still have trouble, return to clinic or your private doctor.

11. If catheter accidentally comes out, you should make arrangements to have it reinserted as soon as possible. The catheter should be changed at least every month or as directed by the doctor.

12. If you are going away on a trip, you will need to remember to pack equipment for caring for your tube and night drainage equipment. If you will not have access to a stove, you will need to take along a small electric hot plate or several cans of Sterno.

13. In some instances it may be easier for you to boil equipment at night. If you leave equipment tightly covered, you may use it in the morning, but do not leave it more than 12 hours.

14. If you follow directions for caring for equipment, there should be no problems of odor.

15. If you have back pain, fever, or any other unusual symptoms, contact your doctor.

16. To protect your mattress in case of leakage, plastic material such as a shower curtain, pillowcase, or oilcloth used only for this purpose may be placed under your sheet. Occasionally, if you are restless, you may kink a tube by lying on it and this might cause a slight leak. Some persons prefer to use plastic-lined pants, which can be obtained in any large department store.

17. Where to obtain your equipment: (*This information mu t be collected and listed for each individual patient, depending on the locality where he lives, his ability to pay for equipment, the community resources available to him, etc.*)

MANAGEMENT OF URINARY INCONTINENCE

Because of the contraindications to intubating the urinary tract, catheterization is avoided in situations that can be safely managed by other means. Indwelling catheters are usually ordered only as a last resort for patients who are incontinent of urine (unable to control voluntarily the discharge of urine) but who, nevertheless, completely empty their bladders. Indwelling catheters are also usually avoided if complete emptying of the bladder can be accomplished by the use of manual techniques.

Causes and techniques for managing

A person must have urethral sphincter control to be continent of urine. The lack of urethral sphincter control has many causes. Sometimes as a result of operative or traumatic openings (fistulas) into the urinary tract, the urine may be deflected temporarily or permanently through an opening in the tract somewhere above the urethral sphincters. This will permit constant, uncontrolled drainage of the urine. It is important that the sponge count be correct at the time of surgery and that no foreign body be left that could promote a fistula (Fig. 4-12).

Disorders involving the central nervous system pathways may result in loss of voluntary control of the bladder. Perception of the urge to void may be impaired or motor impulses may fail to reach the muscles that con-

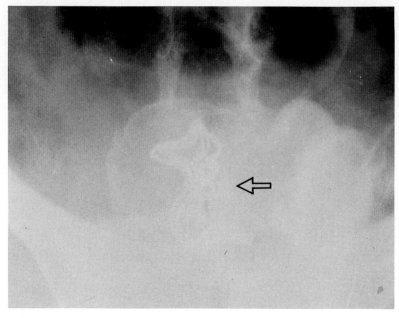

Fig. 4-12. Anteroposterior roentgenographic view of bladder or pelvic area. Note radiopaque markings in midbladder region. This represents the markings of a sponge retained in bladder after surgery (arrow).

trol micturition. Injury of the pudendal nerves or the hypogastric ganglia from which they arise also causes loss of voluntary control of micturition.

Damage to the spinal cord results in impairment of the nervous reflex mechanisms of the bladder. Infection at any point in the urinary tract may cause irritation of the bladder and produce heightened stimulation of the bladder reflex mechanism with resulting urgency in the need to void and incontinence of urine. Pressure of distended abdominal organs, tumor masses, or the gravid uterus on the bladder may also produce this effect.

Damage of the urethral sphincters or relaxation of the perineal supportive tissues may cause incontinence. A physiologic relaxation of the urethral sphincters and the perineal structures is quite common in older women. Urethral sphincters are frequently damaged during prostatic surgery. Finally, total incontinence from the time of birth suggests an ectopic ureteral orifice located distal to the external urethral sphincter.

To solve the problems presented by incontinent patients, the nurse needs to know the pathologic causes of incontinence. This helps her to determine with the physician whether functional rehabilitation of the bladder is possible or desirable. If not, she should try to make the patient as comfortable as possible by improvising equipment and by using commercial appliances at her disposal.

The patient who is unaware of the need to void and empties his bladder involuntarily may be treated in several ways.

Voiding schedule. A voiding schedule similar to that used in "toilet training" for children is often successful in treating neurogenic incontinence. The patient is encouraged to void at regularly scheduled intervals that are slightly shorter than the intervals between involuntary emptying of the bladder. People ordinarily void on awakening, before retiring, and before or after meals. If a diuretic such as coffee, tea, or cola has been taken, it is usually necessary to void about a half hour later. With this as a basic schedule, a record of the time of involuntary voiding and the kind and amount of fluids taken during the intervals between voidings should be kept for a few days. From this it is usually possible to determine the individual patient's normal voiding pattern. His toilet schedule can then be set accordingly. Each day similar kinds and amounts of fluids should be taken during the intervals between toileting to prevent unusual rapidity in filling of the bladder.

It is important to note the amount the patient voids at each urination and to see that the bladder is not still distended after he has voided. Frequent voiding of small amounts of urine may indicate that the bladder is not being adequately emptied. Exertion of manual pressure over the bladder may produce complete emptying; this is known as the *Credé maneuver.* With both hands, a continuous gentle but firm pressure is applied backward and downward over the lower abdomen. This may be done by the patient or the nurse. The patient with an upper motor neuron bladder will know of a variety of ways to stimulate his bladder to contract.

Increased frequency of urination may occasionally be caused by pressure of a distended bowel and, if so, may be relieved by the insertion of a rectal tube to release flatus or by giving an enema. The nurse must have a doctor's order for this. If increased frequency persists, the doctor should be notified since urinary tract infection may be the cause.

External drainage. It may be impossible to keep the patient on a well-regulated voiding schedule. If this is so, other means must be sought. A form of external drainage can ordinarily be used for a man because a watertight apparatus can easily be applied over the penis.

For the male patient a condom catheter may be applied. The procedure for improvising this type of external drainage is as follows: Attach the closed end of a condom (penile sheath) to drainage tubing either with a plastic catheter adapter or piece of hard or firm plastic or rubber tubing 2 to 5 inches long and two ⅛-inch pieces of rubber tubing (Fig. 4-13). Puncture a hole in the closed end of the condom with an applicator stick to allow drainage. Carefully cleanse and dry the penis and note any abnormalities such as edema, discoloration, or break in the skin before

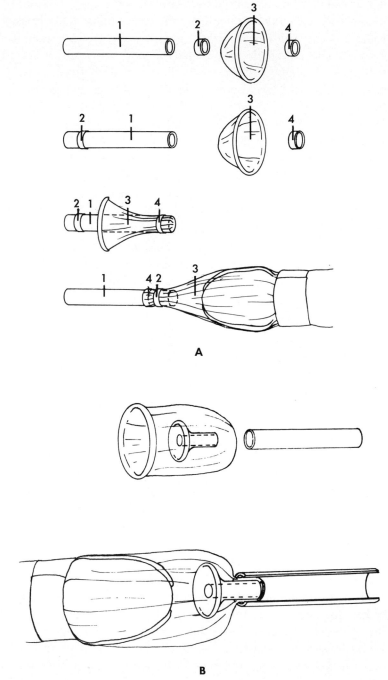

Fig. 4-13. A, Method for making external condom drainage attachment to penis. B, Alternate method for making external condom catheter attachment to penis. Note hollow button used to pierce and hold end of condom.

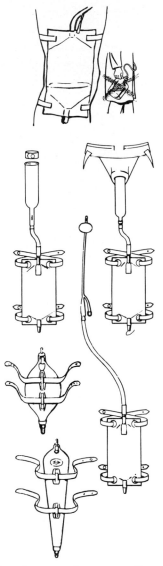

Fig. 4-14. Several types of male external urinary collecting devices for incontinence.

application of tincture of benzoin. Invert the condom and roll it onto the penis, leaving only about 1 inch between the meatus and the connection tube. Apply Elastoplast over the condom and around the penis. When applying, allow for some expansion. A commercially made penile sheath is available and has the advantage of being more rigid and less likely to twist and obstruct. This appliance can be attached interchangeably to a leg bag or bedside urinary drainage bag or bottle. To drain properly, the collecting apparatus must always be placed below the level of the bladder and the sheath and tubing should be straight and without kinks. The system should be checked frequently for function and to assure there are no complications such as edema or skin irritation. The condom should be changed and the skin thoroughly cleansed daily. The use of any one type of external urine collecting device should be determined by the individual patient's needs.

Rubber incontinence urinals (Fig. 4-14) are available, but in using these to provide external drainage there is great danger of skin irritation due to maceration of the rather constantly moist prepuce and glans penis. Applications of tincture of benzoin help obviate this problem. Unless urinals are kept meticulously clean and are aired daily and deodorized there is the additional problem of odor. Nevertheless, this type of external drainage apparatus is often used by persons who are permanently incontinent and are unable to manage the problem completely by using a voiding schedule. The urinal is more secure if its sheath is held in place on the penis with liquid surgical adhesive. The procedure for using a rubber incontinence urinal is as follows: The penis should be clean and dry. Tincture of benzoin should be applied to the prepuce and glans and penile skin and allowed to dry. The sheath should then be placed over the penile shaft and compressed firmly with the hand. Placing a rubber strap with adjustable buttons about the penile shaft also helps to secure the sheath; the strap should not be tight enough to constrict the urethra. The urinal should be removed at least once a day and the penis washed thoroughly with mild soap and water. Benzalkonium chloride (1:750) should then be applied, and after it is dry, the penis should be powdered with stearate of zinc.

The patient may be able to apply his own external drainage apparatus. He must, however, be instructed in the proper method, and his technique should be supervised. It is also important to be sure that patients using external drainage empty their bladders completely. It may be embarrassing and upsetting to a man to have a young nurse apply external drainage apparatus or teach him to do this. If there is no male member of the nursing team, an older more mature nurse may be called upon. At other times the doctor may be willing to do this. A member of the patient's family such as wife, brother, or son may be taught to help him care for this personal need.

External drainage is not feasible for a woman. If incontinence in a woman cannot be controlled with a voiding schedule, the doctor should be consulted. He may order the use of an indwelling urethral catheter since women seem to be somewhat less susceptible to infection from its use. This is probably because the urethra of a woman is so much shorter than that of a man and has no direct communication with the reproductive system.

Improvised protection. To improvise protection for the incontinent male patient, a shower cap can be used. The *procedure for using a shower cap to collect urine drainage* is as follows: Cut a hole big enough to fit around the penis near the elasticized edge of the cap. Bind the opening of the hole with adhesive tape to prevent tearing of the cap and skin irritation. Fill the inside of the cap with absorbent material placed in doughnut fashion. Then slip the penis through the hole and pin the edges of the cap together. If more support is needed, the cap may be pinned to a belt. A deodorant can be added to the cap.

This improvization may be used if skin irritation has resulted from the use of other measures since it allows for more frequent cleansing of the area. The pads should be frequently changed to keep the skin as free from urine as possible. This method may also be used when every effort is being made to have the patient void normally. Other methods that give more protection may decrease his efforts to achieve continence; this method sometimes reduces his anxiety so that he is more successful in maintaining urethral sphincter control.

Penile clamp. A man may use a penile clamp (Cunningham) to maintain continence of urine (Fig. 4-15). This device mechanically compresses the urethral wall. A doctor's order must always be obtained for its use. Penile clamps are often uncomfortable, and they must be released and repositioned at least every 2 hours to prevent circulatory obstruction. Most patients who use clamps alternate them with an external drainage apparatus and use the clamp primarily for short periods such as when they are going out.

Indwelling catheter. As a last resort an indwelling urethral catheter may be used to control incontinence. However, instead of urethral catheterization a cystostomy is frequently performed on a man and a cystostomy tube inserted into the bladder. This type of intubation decreases the incidence of urethritis, epididymitis, and urethral fistulas and diverticula.

Bladder training. Injury to the spinal cord impairs the bladder reflex mechanisms. This type of difficulty is known as *neurogenic* or *cord bladder* and will develop into one of two syndromes, *spastic* or *flaccid*, depending on the level of the cord lesion. In neither instance does the patient have the normal urge to void and consequently he has no way of knowing when he will be incontinent. This is most upsetting to patients. A flaccid bladder occurs when the lesion is at the level of the sacral conus or below. The bladder becomes distended, overflows periodically, and does not empty except by the conscious effort of the patient. After initial treatment with an indwelling catheter, this is accomplished by scheduled voiding combined with abdominal straining and manual compression. Many patients with atonic bladders can become catheter free. Spinal lesions above the bladder reflex centers in the conus medullaris

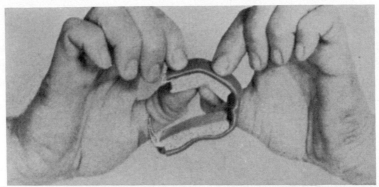

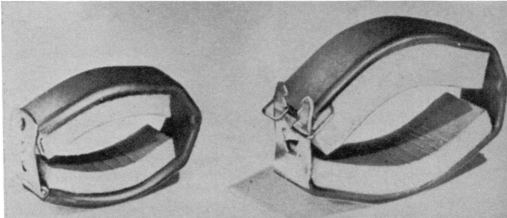

Fig. 4-15. Cunningham clamp used to compress urethra within penis for control of incontinence. Note that wings of clamp are malleable.

result in an automatic (spastic) bladder. Voluntary control of micturition is lost and automatic emptying occurs when the detrusor muscles are sufficiently stretched during bladder filling to trigger the reflex arc. Therefore bladder capacity determines frequency of micturition. To maintain continence under these circumstances, the patient must carefully regulate the amount of fluid he drinks during each interval between bladder evacuations and must plan to empty his bladder voluntarily a short time before the end of the interval at which it would empty automatically. The patient with an automatic bladder may need to trigger micturition reflexly by pinching or stroking trigger areas on the thigh or by anal stimulation.

If an automatic bladder cannot be developed, the use of an indwelling urethral catheter or a cystostomy tube may be necessary to ensure adequate urinary drainage and control of incontinence. If the patient is able to keep the bladder emptied by the use of manual expression, an external drainage apparatus may be used to cope with the incontinence.

The complex problem of the neurogenic bladder and the program of care by which it is managed is discussed in greater detail in Chapter 12.

Incontinence caused by damage to urethral sphincters

Cutting or tearing of the urethral sphincters causes urinary incontinence. The torn sphincter usually cannot be repaired so the problem is a permanent one.

If the external sphincter in the male has been severed, the patient will be totally incontinent and will require the use of an external drainage apparatus. At times an indwelling urethral catheter or a cystostomy tube may need to be used.

If only the internal sphincter is damaged in the male, and this is deliberately done in a transurethral resection of the bladder neck, the patient should not be incontinent. He may need to use perineal muscle exercises to strengthen and maintain the tone of the external sphincter, especially if it has been weakened by surgery.

Sometimes there is malfunction of the urethral sphincters resulting from relaxation of both the sphincters and the perineal muscles. If malfunction of the urethral sphincters is caused by infection, scar tissue, or other lesions, it is frequently alleviated by medical or surgical treatment of the predisposing condition. If it is the result of relaxation of the sphincters or perineum, the use of perineal exercises may improve the situation.

Perineal exercises consist of contracting the abdominal, gluteal, and perineal muscles while breathing normally. However, unless the patient has the sensation of the need to void and has some ability to control the urinary stream, these exercises are useless. The exercises can be explained by asking the patient to hold himself as he would if he needed to void very badly and there were no available facilities. Strengthening of the gluteal and levator muscles helps, and this can be done by having the patient squeeze a piece of paper or cloth in the fold between the buttocks. Stopping and starting the urinary stream during voiding will give additional exercise. The patient should strive eventually to learn to maintain a constant muscle tone.

Operations designed to tighten the muscles are sometimes performed. These are described in the discussion on stress incontinence in Chapter 13.

Incontinence from fistulas and ostomies

Traumatic openings into the urinary tract often present serious problems of incontinence. Many times these are best controlled by catheter drainage. At other times this is not desirable.

Perhaps one of the most common and difficult situations caused by urinary incontinence from a fistula occurs in women who have *vesicovaginal fistulas.* The treatment of this condition is surgical repair (Chapter 13), but frequently this cannot be undertaken for several months because of tissue induration. Therefore these women must usually endure long periods of complete incontinence through the vagina. Since catheter drainage is contraindicated, *perineal pads and plastic-lined pants must be used.* A special catheter attached to a contraceptive diaphragm can be used by some women to keep dry. These patients need much encouragement and should be urged to continue their usual activities insofar as possible. If they plan to be away from home for a period of time, it is wise to limit fluids for about 4 hours before leaving. The use of scented soaps and baths may help their morale.

Rectovesical fistulas present fewer problems of incontinence. The anal sphincter will usually retain urine and the patient will void through both the urethra and the anus. If a large amount of urine drains into the rectum, however, the patient should be instructed to evacuate it every 2 hours. If urine stays in the rectum for long intervals, electrolytes may be reabsorbed through the rectal mucosa and upset the electrolyte balance of the body.

Care of artificial openings (such as nephrostomies, cystostomies, and urethrostomies) when tubes are present is the same as for any indwelling catheter. The patient with temporary or permanent ostomies (such as cutaneous ureterostomies or the more common ileoconduit) will need special care and observation of the stoma and skin area indefinitely. Prior to surgery resulting in either a temporary or permanent ostomy, the nurse should assess the patient both physically and emotionally in an effort to anticipate postoperative problems that can be prevented. Assistance can be given the doctor in choosing the site of the ostomy, particularly if it is to be permanent. Most generally the site may be pinpointed in the center of a line drawn from the umbilicus to the anterior superior ileac spine or slightly below. However, because of individual differences as to age, weight, stature, body creases, previous scars, and activities, it is advisable, after selecting the site, to fit the patient with the appliance he will be wearing postoperatively. The patient should wear the appliance at least 1 day preoperatively to ascertain if cutting or discomfort occurs when he or she is in various positions of sitting, reclining, and walking. If any discomfort occurs, the site of the stoma should be adjusted. Consideration should also be given to the female who may want to wear bare midriff styles and both male and female who wear bikini-type garments. Every effort should be made to keep the site at least 2 inches below the waistline.

Upon return from surgery, the patient with an ileostomy for the purpose of urinary drainage will most likely have two ureteral catheters draining via the ileostomy for several days. Mucus secreted from the ileum

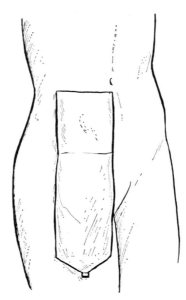

Fig. 4-16. Plastic bag may be applied to any urinary outlet on trunk of body for temporary collection of urine.

will be secreted via the ileostomy stoma also. While in the hospital, the patient is usually fitted with disposable-type bags (Fig. 4-16) that may be connected to a leg bag or straight drainage while the patient is reclining. The nurse must carefully watch for any signs indicating distention of the isolated segment of ileum since this may cause the suture line to break or it may cause back pressure on the kidneys. Swelling about the stoma may also prevent emptying of the conduit. Swelling about the ureteroileal anastomoses or pressure of distended organs against the conduit may prevent drainage from the ureters into the conduit.

Symptoms of ileus or peritonitis (fever, abdominal pain) should be carefully watched for and reported at once. After this type of surgery the ileal conduit may leak urine into the peritoneal cavity. If this happens, an emergency operation to repair the leak must be performed.

The stoma itself can be cleansed with saline solution or water. When changing an entire appliance, cleanse the stoma and then hold a piece of clean tissue or gauze over the opening to keep the surrounding tissue dry while attaching the appliance. Tincture of benzoin is generally used to protect the skin surrounding the stoma and under the appliance. Skin cement or self-adhesive disks are available for attachment. Properly applied and formed to the individual patient's body contour, the appliance will provide a leakproof seal. The patient may then bathe in a tub or shower with the appliance attached.

If skin irritation occurs, a substance such as *karaya gum powder* may be applied.

Various types of commercially made appliances and accessories are available to meet the individual patient's needs. As with the home care of the patient with catheter drainage, careful instruction, demonstration, and return demonstrations by the patient and/or family member should be initiated in the hospital. Contact with and a written referral to the public health nurse should be made in the same manner. Care of the drainage equipment is the same as that for catheters. For the patient with a permanent ostomy it is wise to have two permanent bag units so that a clean one is always available.

Helpful and detailed educational material for instructing the patient about ostomies and their care is available.* Local ileostomy and colostomy clubs have been formed in many communities, usually under the sponsorship of the American Cancer Society. Members meet to exchange ideas, discuss mutual problems, and give support to each other. Nurses are welcome to attend their meetings. Educational materials are available through these clubs and also the United Ostomy Association, Inc., who publish the *Ostomy Quarterly*. It is also suggested that inquiry be made as to the availability of an enterostomal therapist who may be employed in the community. The enterostomal therapist may or may not be a nurse; however, he or she has been trained in the care of patients with all types of ostomies and can offer practical advice in regard to individual patient problems.

Written guidelines are helpful for the patient learning to care for his own drainage.

Care of ileal conduit with an ileostomy bag

You are being sent home with an ileostomy bag because your doctor believes this is the most convenient way to allow for adequate drainage of urine. It is extremely important that you follow this plan of care in order to keep the opening and the skin in good condition.

Equipment needed for changing bag (some ileostomy sets are complete)
1. Disposable plastic bags
2. Double-sided adhesive disks
3. Q-tips or cotton-tipped applicators
4. Tincture of benzoin (do not use compound)
5. Can of adhesive remover (do not use acetone, ether, or benzene)
6. Absorbent cotton and mesh gauze
7. Small tube brush
8. Clean soft rags or cheesecloth
9. Paper bag for waste
10. Distilled vinegar
11. Deodorant powder or tablets

---

*Material may be obtained from United Surgical Co., Inc., Port Chester, N. Y. Also available are two pamphlets by Katherine Jeter entitled *Management of the Urinary Stoma* and *Count Your Blessings,* which may be obtained by writing the Department Of Urology, Columbia-Presbyterian Medical Center, New York, N. Y. 10032.

Other equipment needed (for night drainage)

1. Floor bag or bottle
2. Tubing (8 mm. in diameter), 4 feet

Procedure for changing permanent rubber bag (at least every 5 days)

1. Collect all equipment on a tray and go to the bathroom.
2. While running the bath water, sit near the tub and, with a small cloth saturated with adhesive remover, rub along the upper edge of the cuff until it begins to separate from the skin. **Note:** *Adhesive remover may be inflammable; do not smoke or be near an open flame (such as the pilot light on the stove) while using it.*
3. Grasp loosened edge of the cuff and gently pull away from the skin, continuing to apply adhesive remover until bag is completely separated from the skin.
4. Clean the skin with mild soapy water.
5. Wash bag thoroughly with warm soapy water. Soak it in vinegar solution (4 tablespoons of vinegar to 1 pint of water) for 15 minutes. Run tube brush through the opening at lower end of bag. Rinse with cold water containing deodorant. Dry bag thoroughly.
6. Get into bathtub with the water at waist level and bathe thoroughly; a shower may be used.
7. After stepping out of the bath and drying yourself completely, you are ready to reapply the bag. (If your skin around the ostomy is irritated, however, you should apply karaya powder or use a bag with a karaya gum ring.)
8. Place bag over the ileal opening with the opening in the center of the opening of the bag. A good fit prevents skin problems.
9. Holding bag in position, dip a Q-tip in tincture of benzoin and trace the outline of bag on the skin.
10. Removing bag, place a tightly rolled piece of gauze over or in the ileal opening. **Note:** *If at any time during the following steps the gauze becomes saturated, change quickly to a dry piece. Any urine running over the skin will cause your bag to leak.*
11. After making sure the inside cuff of the ileal bag is clean and dry, remove the backing from one side of an adhesive disk and apply to bag cuff. Press firmly to make sure disk is securely attached to bag. Now remove exposed disk backing and, without touching adhesive surface, lay bag aside.
12. Paint the area within the circle that you traced on the skin with tincture of benzoin.
13. When the tincture of benzoin becomes sticky, immediately place the lower cuff of the bag (with outlet in downward position) on the benzoin and press firmly. Remove gauze and bring upper part of bag into position. Apply pressure with fingers around outside of cuff to affix bag firmly to disk and skin. (When applying bag, make abdomen firm by taking a deep breath and holding until bag is secure.) **Note:** *If the bag begins to leak at any time, dry the loosened area under the cuff with a Q-tip and try to patch it by putting tincture of benzoin on with a Q-tip. If unsuccessful, remove cup and reapply. The edges of the bag may be sealed and reinforced with paper tape.*

Emptying the bag

1. Standing over the toilet, turn the screw on the bottom of bag.
2. Allow the bag to drain and retighten the screw.

Preparation for sleep

(*When you lie down, your drainage apparatus must be at a level lower than the tube or you will have pain because your kidneys cannot drain properly. You may also have leakage.*)

1. Unscrew the bottom of your bag and attach it to tubing draining into the floor bottle.
2. Allow 1 foot of tubing to go into the bottle and keep 2 feet between the bag and the bottle. Pin the tubing to the mattress to prevent pull on the bag.

Care of night equipment

Daily. Wash bottle and tubing thoroughly with soap and water. Soak for 15 minutes in vinegar or deodorant solution. Rinse with cold water.

Twice a week. Boil the drainage bottle and tubing for 10 minutes. This will control odors and ensure cleanliness.

The following suggestions may be provided for the patient who has an ileostomy.

Suggestions

1. To add extra support to the bag, sew a pocket in which the bag may be slipped in the appropriate place on the inside of the patient's undergarment.
2. It will be easier to change your bag if you have not had any fluids for 3 or 4 hours because there will be less urine flowing. However, you must still plan to drink between 2 and 3 quarts of fluid daily.
3. If your bag leaks:
   a. Review the method of changing it carefully. You may not be getting the skin cleansed and dried properly.
   b. Check to see that no part of the bag is kinked and that clothing is not constricting it. It may be preferable to wear suspenders rather than a belt and to wear a girdle with an opening over the bag.
   c. Check to see that you have your bedside drainage container at a level lower than the ileal opening.
   d. If leaking persists, return to the clinic or see your private doctor.
4. If skin irritation (redness and soreness) is not relieved by the prescribed substance, contact the clinic or your private doctor.
5. If stoma becomes swollen or irritated:
   a. Check to see if any untoward pressure is being applied to the stoma.
   b. Contact the clinic or your private doctor for advice.
6. Your ileal conduit should not keep you from participation in sports, including swimming, unless you are limited by your doctor for some other reason.
7. Most persons simply carry an extra disk, tincture of benzoin, and several applicators in their pockets or bags at all times. They seldom need to use these, but it is reassuring to have them.
8. If you are going on a trip, you will need to remember to pack a supply of equipment to change the bag and your night drainage equipment.
9. If you follow the directions for caring for the equipment, there should be no problem of odor; a deodorant can be used.
10. If you have back pain or any other unusual symptoms, return to the clinic, call your private doctor, or go to a hospital emergency room.
11. Protect your mattress with a full-length piece of plastic. Occasionally you may kink a tube by lying on it if you are restless. This might cause a slight leak. Some people prefer to use plastic-lined pants, which can be obtained in any large department store.
12. Special instructions (any special instructions should be added here).

Dilatation of ileal stoma. In dilating the ileal stoma, a finger cot should be slipped on the finger to be inserted into the ileostomy opening and the finger cot should then be well lubricated with a water-soluble jelly. The finger is gently inserted through the opening and into the conduit. Once-a-week dilatation is usually sufficient; however, the need for dilatation will be determined by the doctor.

Measuring for ileal bladder bag. A permanent ileal bladder bag should be ordered after surgery. The stoma should then be carefully measured and a pattern of the exact size of the opening needed should be given to the surgical supply house. There should be no pressure on the stoma and no skin surface exposed. Bags are custom made so patients usually like to have two or more available. The stoma may shrink slightly after a few weeks.

See Chapter 11 for more details concerning urinary ileostomy and appliances.

Management of urinary drainage from wounds

It is not necessary nor is it good practice to allow dressings to become saturated with urine. Not only is the patient made very uncomfortable, which interferes with his rest, but also the surrounding skin becomes irritated and decubitus ulcers may result. Infection of the wound itself may also occur.

There are many ways to prevent the patient's dressing from being constantly wet. The first thing to consider is whether the cavity draining urine is intubated or whether a tube is in place above the point of the draining wound. If either situation exists, the tube should be checked to ascertain whether it is draining. If drainage is not readily reestablished, the doctor should be consulted since the tube may be blocked or may have slipped out of place. A wound opening from an intubated cavity should drain very little urine.

If the urinary drainage from a wound is uncontrolled by catheterization, the nurse must study the type of wound, the placement of the incision, and the contour of the surrounding tissue to determine the most satisfactory method for keeping the particular patient dry. None of the following methods always works well with every patient.

Superficial suction drainage

A small, sterile, many-eyed catheter coiled inside one sterile 4 by 8 inch dressing may be placed over the wound with the eyes directly over the draining site. The catheter and gauze can be held in place with a strip of adhesive tape; the end of the catheter should be attached to Gomco suction drainage. As an alternative, a disposable-type plastic ostomy bag with an adhesive surface may be applied over the drainage site and changed once or more daily. Bags with karaya gum rings are also available.

These methods not only keep the patient dry but also permit the amount of drainage to be recorded. The patient may be out of bed but only within range of the suction.

Another improvised method. A 12-inch square of sterile plastic wrap may be used to collect urinary drainage from a wound. An opening large enough to fit around the draining wound is cut in the center of the plastic.

Dressings are then placed over the drainage site, and the plastic is folded over them in envelope style. Montgomery straps will be needed to hold a dressing such as this in place. When this method is used, dressings still require frequent changing. Although the patient may be dry externally, the urinary drainage lies in a pool over the incision. Unless the dressings are frequently changed, the wound will become infected from organisms growing in the stagnant urine. Patients kept dry by this method can easily be taught to change their own dressings as necessary.

Uncontrolled urinary incontinence

Despite all efforts, some patients will have uncontrolled urinary drainage. It is important that they are kept clean, odorless, and free from decubiti. Bedding and furniture can be protected by rubber, plastic, or oilcloth lined with absorbent material. Newspaper pads covered with soft absorbent material also provide protection. Pants with waterproof backing and lined with a removable absorbent material may keep the patient more comfortable. These can be purchased commercially or a resourceful person can improvise them. Cellu-cotton is a relatively inexpensive type of disposable absorbent material and is less expensive if purchased in large rather than small rolls. Washable materials such as baby diaper cloth may be used.

Regardless of what method is used, *scrupulous care of the skin* is essential. Urinary drainage is frequently infected and malodorous. The padding must be changed frequently, and the skin must be thoroughly washed and dried each time. If possible, the patient should be bathed in a tub of warm water at least once a day. Zinc oxide powders or karaya powder applied to skin areas subjected to urinary drainage are beneficial for the patient, but care must be taken not to allow the powder to cake on the skin. Commercial preparations such as Diaparene chloride, which control urine odor and to some extent lessen the irritating properties of urine, may be used on the skin and pads. Protective ointments are useless since urine, being either acid or alkaline, seeps through them onto the skin. Fluids should be taken freely because this keeps the urine less concentrated.

If the draining area must be kept surgically clean, the skin around it should be washed well with an antiseptic solution each time the dressings are changed. More distant skin should be cleansed as described in the preceding paragraph. It is important to remember that urine runs freely and dependently; skin on the back, thighs, perineum, in the inguinal area, and between the folds of the buttocks usually becomes wet.

Deodorants for freshening room air are often needed. An electric deodorizer is especially effective, but deodorant spray and wicks also work quite well. Frequent washing and airing of the water-repellent materials in use and disposal of waste materials in closed containers help to reduce odor.

If the female patient is out of bed and is incontinent from the urethra, a chair or wheelchair prepared as a commode is especially helpful in keeping her dry for periods of time. This makes her more comfortable and often makes it possible for her to mingle socially with others without anxiety about incontinence. The patient may do well to drink fluids freely during the early hours of the day and to take no fluids for 2 or 3 hours before retiring. This method also can be used for men but usually is unnecessary if external drainage apparatus is applied.

The *incontinent bed patient* can sometimes be kept relatively dry by improvised bed arrangements. The bed can often be built up so as to leave a depressed area beneath the portion of the body draining urine. (This method is discussed fully under the section on collection of 24-hour urine specimens in children in Chapter 6.)

A *Stryker frame* or *CircOlectric bed* can also sometimes be modified for use with the incontinent patient.

The nurse should remember that the use of methods that keep the patient dry does not preclude the need for the patient to be moved about in bed at intervals. Therefore it may only be possible to keep him completely dry for part of the day, but even this is helpful. Local areas will be moistened with urine regardless of the method used and these must be frequently cleansed.

Children with urinary drainage

Children may have any or all of the problems of incontinence and the problems are handled in much the same manner as with the adult. Variations will depend on age. The boy too young or too ill for "training" will, of course, require an external drainage apparatus adapted for his size. For example, a finger cot or the finger of a rubber glove may be used in place of a penile sheath. Most commercial equipment comes in sizes for children. Small girls will need to be managed by methods similar to those described for uncontrolled incontinence in women. The nurse must be responsible for routinely expressing the urine for any child requiring manual expression methods to ensure complete bladder emptying.

Home care of incontinent patient

Whenever a patient will have a continuing problem with incontinence of urine from the bladder or elsewhere after discharge from the hospital, he and his family should be instructed about management of the problem. The practicality of home care will be determined many times by whether methods acceptable to both the patient and his family can be established to manage the incontinence. Incontinence of urine can be so objectionable that the patient may refuse to go home or his family may refuse to care for him at home. The patient may be so depressed by the problem that it is unsafe for him to be left alone lest he attempt suicide.

The nurse's interest and skill in determining methods for coping with incontinence of urine that are relatively simple and yet provide security for the patient may be crucial in the adjustment of the patient and his family to the situation. The family may need help in learning to control their own reactions as well as in understanding the patient's feelings. The nurse's attitude as she cares for the patient and teaches him and his family can have a positive effect. Her skill in arranging materials for cleansing the patient and for disposal of excreta often sets a practical example of how to handle the situation.

Most of the methods described for the care of incontinent patients can be adapted for use in the home. In determining the method best suited for the particular patient, the nurse must consider the patient's home situation as well as his physical and emotional needs. Planning with the patient and his family is essential. After the plans are developed, whoever is to assume responsibility for the care should be urged to practice the method under the nurse's guidance. It is usually advisable to have a public health nurse make several visits in the home to give additional help. She should be completely informed of the plans and methods instituted by the hospital nurse.

If equipment will be needed for home care, the patient should be discharged with adequate supplies for at least 48 hours. He should know where to obtain additional supplies and, if necessary, arrangements should have been made to obtain these. The social service worker may help with these arrangements. Some patients may need supplies delivered; others need money to pay for supplies. Whenever possible, readily available and inexpensive materials should be used. Often the resourceful nurse can teach the patient satisfactory ways of improvising equipment.

CARE OF PATIENT WITH PAIN

Pain is a common complaint of urologic patients. It is important for the nurse to specifically determine the type of pain, its location, and with what activities it is associated. Pain may be described as sharp, stabbing, burning, aching, dragging, boring, or spasmlike. It may be constant or intermittent; it may be relieved by analgesics, rest, a particular position, or by some activity. Frequently the pain is associated with voiding. Close observation of the patient often gives clues to the severity of pain. Pinched faces, wrinkled brows, clenched teeth, and tightened fists may indicate severe pain. Profuse diaphoresis and a rapid pulse may also occur. A person curled up tensely in bed or tossing about usually has severe pain.

People vary in the manner in which pain is expressed. This depends on their emotional reaction to pain. Some persons tolerate severe pain and discomfort with little complaint; others tolerate pain very poorly. The infant and the elderly patient are least likely to react acutely to pain because they both have less acute sense organs. Therefore no indication of pain, no matter how slight, should be ignored in these patients. Young children often withstand pain poorly. Since tolerance of pain is influenced by emotional and social factors, the nurse should observe the patient's emotional response to painful situations. This will guide her in judging complaints of pain and in determining the nursing measures needed.

Complaints of pain should never be ignored. The specific observations made by the nurse will help the doctor to make a correct diagnosis and to prescribe appropriate treatment. Before giving treatment for pain the nurse should determine whether the pain is that for which the treatment was ordered. If not, new orders should be obtained as necessary.

The use of analgesic drugs is not always the treatment of choice for pain. Burning sensations in the bladder and urethra may be best relieved by dilution of urine through more ample hydration (forcing fluids) and by local application of heat with hot-water bottles, heating pads, or sitz baths. Urinary infection may be the etiology of the discomfort and antibiotics are then in order. The discomfort caused by overdistention of the urinary tract is relieved by drainage of the tract; this is a particularly urgent consideration postoperatively. Measures should be taken to empty the bladder within 8 hours postoperatively in an adult who has no indwelling catheter. A child should not be allowed to go more than 6 hours without voiding. Provided drainage is adequate, relief from spasms such as occur in the bladder may be better obtained by using antispasmodic drugs than by using analgesics. Pain in an incision and ureteral colic, however, usually require the use of narcotics. Morphine or meperidine hydrochloride (Demerol) is frequently prescribed for adults; codeine for children. Occasionally, pain in the incision is caused by the dressing becoming too tight. This may be the result of swelling about the wound, and if this occurs, the doctor should be notified. A "sticking" pain in a portion of the incision frequently occurs when the wound becomes infected. It may be relieved by the doctor opening the wound edges to provide for drainage of pus pockets. Sudden, sharp pain causing the patient to complain of a popping sensation is typical of rupture of the wound or of some internal organ. The dressing may become saturated with peritoneal fluid. If this type of pain occurs, the patient should be put flat in bed and a tight abdominal binder applied. A doctor should be summoned at once and no medication should be given for pain until he has seen the patient.

The nurse should remember that emotions such as fear tend to increase the degree of pain. It is often helpful to explain to patients why they have pain and what can be done to relieve it. If pain or discomfort is usual during or after a procedure, the patient who is prepared for this prior to the procedure often reacts less violently to it. Pain is less tolerable at night because there is less activity to distract the patient. The use of sedatives or tranquilizers in conjunction with analgesic medication may help the patient relax, sleep, and get effective relief of pain. Often the patient needs no more than a chance to talk and assistance in finding a comfortable position in bed. Always examine the site of pain to rule out foreign objects or unforeseen circumstances causing the discomfort.

Extreme lethargy may result from the use of opiates and tranquilizers. This should be reported to the doctor at once. No patient receiving large doses of sensorium-dulling drugs should be allowed to get in and out of bed without assistance lest he fall and hurt himself. He should also be attended while he is up.

Patients in pain are likely to be quite irritable. Noise and excessive talking may annoy them. If the patient desires, visitors should be restricted; his reactions often may need to be interpreted to his family. Treatments should be planned during periods when the analgesic is at the peak of its effectiveness. Rest periods between necessary activity should not be interrupted. Reading, listening to music, or other pleasurable activities may help to divert some patients and may lessen the sensation of pain; others prefer to be left completely alone. Patients who have prolonged periods of pain may desire visits from their clergyman. Patients knowing they are dying of cancer tolerate pain poorly.

CARE OF PATIENT REQUIRING SURGERY

The patient undergoing urologic surgery will require either general, spinal, or local anesthesia, depending on the extent of the operation. An exception may be a very young baby who requires a minor procedure such as circumcision. Since the nerve endings are not yet completely functional, the only aid necessary in this instance may be giving the baby his formula or a pacifier during the procedure.

The basic needs of the patient with urologic disease that requires surgery are the same as those of any other surgical patient. Considerations especially pertinent to the urologic patient will be discussed next, but the nurse needing greater detail should see a surgical nursing textbook.

Preoperative care

The preoperative care starts as soon as the patient and/or his family have been told by the doctor that surgery is necessary. The doctor will explain the operation contemplated, why it is necessary, the expected outcome, and perhaps some of the hazards. The nurse must know what the patient and his family have been told since she is often asked to clarify this. It may be anticipated that the patient or family will not remember all that he or she has been told.

Any patient may be upset by the need for surgery; the patient with urologic disease, however, is often quite upset. Since urologic surgery may necessitate substantial alteration of the genitourinary anatomy, the patient may have to adjust to the problem of "being different" (having a new route of urinary excretion). The male patient may be made sterile, impotent, or both by some operative procedures. If a radical operative procedure is contemplated, the doctor usually discusses the implications in detail with the patient and his family. Many doctors feel that the patient should participate in making the final decision to undergo such an operation.

While attempting to reach a decision, the patient often is very depressed. During this stage the nurse can give moral support by providing for privacy, allowing extra family visits if these seem to help the patient, caring for his physical needs, and answering or channeling to appropriate persons the questions raised by either the patient or his family. The patient also is often helped by talking with his clergyman, with understanding members of his family, and with patients who have made good adjustments following similar surgical procedures. The nurse should be alert for changes in mood or behavior that might indicate the need for psychiatric guidance.

During the preoperative period the patient is maintained in the best possible physical condition. He should be encouraged to eat a well-balanced diet and additional protein, and vitamin C may be given to enhance postoperative wound healing. Vitamin K is often ordered since bleeding is a common postoperative complication of a clotting deficiency. The patient is examined for any coexisting problem such as cardiac, vascular, or pulmonary diseases or diabetes mellitus. These disorders are controlled prior to surgery.

A *permit for operation* must be signed prior to the patient's surgery. Depending on the policies of the individual hospital, this may or may not be a nursing responsibility. In some instances a permit that covers all procedures and operations may be signed routinely upon admission of the patient, or it may be necessary to sign an informed consent for each procedure or operation performed. A parent or legal guardian must sign permits for minors. Occasionally a minor may be considered emancipated (married, mature, and earning his own living); he may then sign his own permit.

Urologic procedures occasionally involve sterilization of a male patient, either as a primary operation or in conjunction with other surgery. Whenever bilateral ligation of the vas deferens or bilateral orchiectomy is contemplated, the patient must sign a permit for sterilization as well as the operative permit. He is urged to discuss this with his wife and, depending on his religious beliefs, he may want to discuss it with a member of the clergy. The wife should sign a primary sterilization consent, properly witnessed.

Although the doctor usually discusses the anticipated operation with the patient, the nurse should sit down with him well in advance of surgery to discuss the expected preoperative and postoperative routines. He and his family should know if he can expect to have catheters or other tubes in place; he should know what type of sensations (pain, pressure, soreness) to expect and what can be done to relieve them. He should be instructed in how to cough and breathe deeply, how to help turn himself, and how to exercise his arms and legs. This period also gives the patient a chance to ask any questions, to express any apprehension, and to be reassured. If the nurse feels that the patient needs further medical explanation or reassurance, she should refer his questions to the doctor.

In the immediate preoperative period the skin about the operative area must be cleansed and shaved with few exceptions. Care must be taken to prevent accidentally nicking the skin in shaving. An autoclaved razor and a new blade should be used for each patient since there is evidence that viral hepatitis is transmitted through razor cuts. Disposable razors or dipilatories are preferable.

A detergent containing hexachlorophene is generally used to cleanse the skin. It has antibacterial properties that have a cumulative effect and make the skin relatively germ free. Neither casual rinsing with water nor drying will remove hexachlorophene from the skin; organic solvents such as alcohol or ether will remove it, however, and should not be used. Hexachlorophene preparations are irritating to the scrotum and, if used, should be rinsed off well. Thorough washing with a mild soap and water is preferable in preparing the scrotum; the doctor should be consulted about this. An excellent movie, *Disinfection of the Skin,* is available.*

The surgeon will usually leave instructions on how large a skin area he wishes prepared. In other instances the nurse prepares an area specified by hospital procedure for a particular operation. The area to be prepared will be more extensive than actually required for the incision. This will include areas where adhesive tape will be applied to secure dressings. The following guide may be used in preparing the skin for specific operations.

Abdominal operations. If the patient is female, shave the skin from below the breasts to and including the pubic area; if a male, shave from the nipple line to and including the pubic area. Cleanse the umbilicus with soap and water and remove any material collected there.

Perineal, urethral, penile, and scrotal operations. If the patient is a

---

*ANA-NLN Film Library, 267 West 25th St., New York, N. Y.

female, shave the skin from the umbilicus to and including the pubic area, the perineum, and adjacent thighs. If a male, include the penis and scrotum; hair is rarely present except at the base of the penis. All areas should be thoroughly cleaned. No shaving is necessary for cystoscopy, and many urologists do not desire shaving prior to transurethral surgery.

Kidney operations. Shave the skin on the affected side from the spine to beyond the midline anteriorly and from the nipple line to the pubic area.

Preanesthesia care. Patients often fear anesthesia; the reasons for this vary, but the patient should be encouraged to express his fears and should be given truthful reassurance. It is helpful for the patient to know that the anesthesiologist studies his situation and gives him the anesthetic best suited for him and his operation. The anesthesiologist may not always visit the patient, but he consults the patient's doctor and studies his chart. Continuing fear and apprehension should always be reported to the doctor and the anesthesiologist.

The nurse helps to ensure safe anesthesia by carefully preparing the patient. Since many anesthetics are given according to body weight, the nurse should be sure that an accurate weight is recorded on the chart. Adults and children over 7 years of age who are to receive a general anesthetic usually are given no food or fluids by mouth for at least 6 hours previously. Younger children and infants may be given food up to 4 hours before anesthesia and fluids up to 2 hours beforehand. If the patient has taken food or fluid after the prescribed time limit, the doctor and anesthetist must be notified because the patient may vomit during anesthesia and aspirate vomitus into the lungs. This can be fatal.

If the anesthetic is being given for a cystoscopic examination, the patient should have an empty bladder before being anesthetized so that an estimate of his residual bladder urine can be made by the cystoscopist. This is best achieved by asking the patient to void just before he is premedicated. If a catheter is in the bladder, it should be left connected to drainage apparatus unless otherwise ordered. Cleansing enemas may also be ordered since the patient is often constipated or has difficulty in defecation postoperatively.

Preoperative medications should be given on time. If delayed for any reason, the doctor should be consulted before their administration since he may prefer to give the drugs intravenously. The type of medications and dosage should be carefully checked and if the nurse questions the advisability of giving the prescribed medications, she should consult the doctor. (See discussion of therapeutic care under the various age groups in Chapter 5.)

Mouth care should be given before general anesthesia to reduce the danger of surgical parotitis. All dentures and removable bridges must be taken out prior to anesthesia to prevent their being aspirated or broken.

Any other prosthetic parts such as eyes or limbs should also be removed; hairpins should be removed to prevent accidental injury. Nail polish should be removed since the nail beds are used as indicators of adequate oxygenation.

The patient should have all his valuables put safely away before leaving his bedside. Religious medals, rosary beads, and wedding rings may be retained, but they must be securely tied or taped to the patient at a site that will not interfere with the incision.

Care during anesthesia. The nurse should know what anesthetic is going to be used and the precautions necessary for safety. Many volatile anesthetics are inflammable. Cardiac and respiratory failure are untoward effects of some anesthetics, and emergency equipment such as oxygen, cardiac and respiratory stimulants, and a cardiac resuscitation tray should be readily available. (Consult a standard medicosurgical textbook for details.)

When a *general anesthetic* is being given, there should always be provision for head-low position, suction, endotracheal intubation, and oxygen administration. Cardiac and respiratory stimulants should be available.

When a *spinal* or *local anesthetic* is used, the nurse is often responsible for assisting the doctor in its administration and for observing the patient for untoward reactions. An occasional patient may have an untoward systemic reaction to local or spinal anesthetic agents such as procaine. The patient should be watched for signs of excitability, twitching, pulse or blood pressure changes, pallor, or respiratory difficulty. At the first signs of any toxic symptoms, the doctor should be notified. A short-acting barbiturate such as thiopental sodium (Pentothal) should be available for the doctor to administer. Oxygen equipment should be set up and ready to be used if necessary. The nurse assisting the doctor should know how to maintain an airway and how to give artificial respiration. (Excellent movies on this are available from drug companies and from civil defense organizations.) Since the patient receiving this type of anesthetic is awake, the room should be quiet, and unnecessary conversation or inadvertent reference to frightening information should be avoided. The patient should not experience pain, but he will have pressure and pulling sensations. Spinal and local anesthesia are used frequently for elderly patients who, because of lung disease such as pulmonary emphysema, tolerate inhalation anesthesia poorly.

The patient having general or spinal anesthesia should be carefully moved with the body well supported. In placing him on the treatment table or returning him to bed, care must be taken to maintain proper body alignment and to avoid pressure or pull on any body part; improper movement may cause nerve damage.

For more specific information concerning various anesthetics the nurse should consult textbooks of surgical nursing, operating room nursing, and anesthesiology.

Operative care

The nurse with the patient during surgery is responsible for his safety. She should remain with the patient until he is anesthetized, at which time the anesthesiologist assumes primary responsibility for his safety. It is unsafe to leave the patient alone after he has been premedicated since he may be quite groggy. He is also likely to be apprehensive. During the induction of the anesthetic the nurse may be needed to help the anesthetist, especially if the patient resists the anesthetic.

The nurse is responsible for ensuring that the patient is properly lifted and placed in a position that will provide the doctor adequate exposure but will prevent unnecessary strain on the patient's muscles and joints. The positions needed for urologic operations often place the patient in an unusual position for long periods of time. Renal surgery necessitates hyperextension in a side-lying position (see Fig. 10-6); bladder, urethral, and prostatic surgery may require the dorsal recumbent (lithotomy) position (see Fig. 6-1); and for some prostatic, perineal, and transrectal or transsacral procedures the patient may be placed on his abdomen and "jackknifed" at the hips. Specific positions used for operations are described in the discussion of specific disorders requiring surgery. The judicious use of pads to support and separate body parts prevents pressure ulcers of the skin and many postoperative aches and pains caused by minor (or sometimes major) degrees of nerve and musculoskeletal injury. Pressure on soft tissues must also be avoided.

The nurse who is present during the procedure is responsible for making sure that all the equipment needed for the procedure is ready, in good working condition, and sterile. In this way she prevents unnecessary delays in the operation and reduces the amount of time the patient will be under anesthesia and subjected to trauma. This frequently influences the postoperative course. Maintenance of strict aseptic techniques to reduce the incidence of postoperative infection is absolutely mandatory. In urologic surgery the danger of infection is great. Bacteria can invade the bloodstream through cut surfaces of the kidneys, bladder, or prostate gland and cause septicemia. Local infections in any part of the urinary tract may eventually impair the renal function. Great care must be exercised in making a correct sponge count at the conclusion of an operation (Fig. 4-12). Many surgeons have an x-ray film made as an additional check. For complete descriptions of the operative procedures and the equipment used, the nurse should see books on operating room technique and atlases of surgical urology.

Postanesthesia care

The patient should always be accompanied to the unit in which post-anesthesia care will be given by the anesthesiologist or some member of the medical or professional nursing staff. The nurse in the postanesthesia unit should be carefully briefed on the condition of the patient. She should know the type of anesthetic used, whether or not the patient was or is intubated, any complications or hypotension occurring during anesthesia, and the procedure performed while the patient was anesthetized.

Until the patient is completely awake, he must be constantly attended. He should be protected from physical injury and care must be taken to prevent displacement of any tubes or dressings.

The patient should be placed in a position that will ensure a patent airway and prevent aspiration. He can usually be placed on his side or in a semiprone position. If he must remain on his back, the head should be turned well to one side or placed in slight hyperextension with the chin up and jaw forward. Excessive mucous secretions may occur especially when ether or vinyl ether has been used, and the posterior pharynx should be kept well suctioned. If the secretions are in the tracheobronchial area and cannot be removed by regular suctioning, the anesthesiologist or a doctor should be called to do intratracheal suctioning. Ether and cyclopropane often cause vomiting and care must be taken to prevent aspiration.

If thiopental sodium has been used, the patient should be observed carefully for laryngeal spasm. If restlessness, apprehension, stridor, retraction of the soft tissues about the neck, or cyanosis occur, the doctor should be notified immediately. A laryngoscope of the proper size, tongue blades, and an endotracheal tube should be at the bedside and an emergency tracheostomy set and oxygen should be available. The patient's head should be held with the chin up and the jaw forward until the doctor arrives. Mouth-to-mouth resuscitation may be necessary. If so, the nostrils should be closed by pinching or covered by the mouth if the patient is an infant. Care must be taken with infants and young children not to breathe too strongly since it is possible to rupture the alveoli.

The patient's blood pressure and pulse should be checked frequently following anesthesia and discontinued only after the vital signs have been stable for an hour or more. Cyclopropane may cause rate and rhythm irregularities in the heartbeat. The doctor should be notified about any changes in quality, rate, or rhythm of the pulse. Thiopental sodium, tribromoethanol (Avertin), and spinal anesthetics frequently cause the blood pressure to drop. Elevation of the feet and use of stockinettes help alleviate this.

Blood pressure measurements are difficult to take on infants and therefore are rarely ordered. The pulse rate and quality must be carefully noted, however, for any signs indicating shock. The pulse rate of an infant may normally be quite rapid (120 to 180), but it should not be weak and thready as well as rapid. This may indicate shock or hemorrhage.

Although it is common practice for patients to be placed in the Trendelenburg position (head low) when the blood pressure drops, patients who have had a spinal anesthetic should never be placed in this position without a specific order. Spinal anesthetics may travel up the spinal canal and paralyze the diaphragm.

Oxygen may be ordered for some patients after anesthesia; this is especially true for children and older persons. Children who have had endotracheal intubation are frequently put in a humidifying unit because they are prone to tracheitis. They should be watched carefully for any signs of respiratory obstruction since tracheal edema is not uncommon after intubation and an emergency tracheostomy may need to be performed.

After recovery from anesthesia, deep breathing and coughing should be encouraged for 24 hours or until respiratory exchange is normal. If mucus is not being raised and respirations sound moist, the doctor should be notified. The patient should turn or be turned every hour while he is in bed and should be encouraged to be up and about as soon as ordered.

Following spinal anesthesia the patient may be kept flat in bed for 6 to 12 hours; he can be turned from side to side. It is thought that keeping the head flat may reduce the possibility of a "spinal" headache. This is a severe throbbing headache that usually appears after 24 hours and lasts for variable lengths of time. The headache may be caused by leakage of spinal fluid from the puncture in the dura or by sterile chemical meningitis. It is worse when the patient is upright. It is best relieved by his remaining flat in bed and moving about as little as possible. Analgesics and sedatives may give some relief and should be given as ordered. Fluids may be forced and vasodilating drugs given to stimulate production of spinal fluid. The nurse should *not* suggest the possibility of this phenomenon to the patient; it does not always occur.

The nurse unfamiliar with the care of an anesthetized patient should consult a surgical nursing textbook or a book on care in the recovery room for a more detailed discussion than that given here. Special considerations related to the age of the patient should always be considered.

Postoperative care

The care needed by a patient following urologic surgery does not differ greatly from that needed by any surgical patient. Immediately postoperatively he will need postanesthesia care and, in addition, one of the first responsibilities of the nurse is to check the dressings and to see that all indwelling catheters and any other drainage tubes such as gastric tubes are patent and connected to the appropriate drainage apparatus.

Hemorrhage. Hemorrhage may follow any urologic operative procedure, but it is especially common after transurethral prostatectomy, suprapubic prostatectomy, and nephrolithotomy (especially if the kidney is completely split). It is uncommon after nephrectomy, but if it occurs, it is a serious emergency. Tachycardia, hypotension, and other signs of shock such as apprehension, pallor, and cold clammy skin, under any circumstances, should alert the nurse to the possibility of serious hemorrhage. The nurse should always note the preoperative blood pressure because if the patient was hypertensive, the blood pressure may be relatively high but still represent a marked drop relative to his usual pressure. In elderly patients, hemorrhage may occur with only a very slight drop in pressure until the blood volume is drastically reduced. This is because of the inelasticity of their vessels. Small changes in the pressure therefore are of significance. The source of the bleeding in patients with closed incisions may not be readily visible. In patients with drains in the wound or with catheters the blood is usually visible on the dressings or in drainage tubes and bottles. No sign of hemorrhage should be ignored.

After surgery involving the urinary system, urine is usually dark red to pink, but it should not be bright red or viscid. Following urologic surgery, wounds may drain copious amounts of light red urine. Bright red blood on dressings, however, indicates hemorrhage. Following surgery on the kidney the nurse should look along the posterior edge of the dressing for blood because it tends to drain toward the sacral area. If the patient has a suprapubic incision, blood may be noted along the side of the dressing and in the inguinal region.

If hemorrhage occurs, the doctor should be called at once. If the bleeding is external and from an incision, a pressure dressing should be placed over the site until the doctor arrives. The patient should be placed flat in bed and equipment obtained to put him in the Trendelenburg position; he should not be put in this position, however, without a doctor's order. If the patient is lying in a pool of blood, some absorbent material should be slipped under him after the doctor has seen how much blood there is. This will make him less apprehensive and more comfortable. Dressing materials and material for intravenous therapy should be at the bedside. If the patient has a catheter in place, materials for irrigation should be prepared; in addition, a suction syringe, several bottles of sterile physiologic saline solution, and several large sterile basins should be available.

Temperature control. The patient who has had transurethral surgery is likely to be more chilled than the usual patient because large amounts of cold irrigating fluids may have been used during the operation. The bed into which he is placed should be warm and he may need extra covers until his body temperature becomes readjusted. His temperature should be checked (by mouth) as soon as he has revived from the anesthesia, and if it is above or below normal, it should be rechecked every 2 hours until it has returned to normal limits. External heat should be removed or applied as necessary. It is not unusual for the patient to have a shaking chill postoperatively.

The loss of body heat following any tissue trauma is a special problem with infants, whose temperature may drop to as low as 92° F. Special care should be taken that the drapes used during the operation do not become wet since this will cause dissipation of body heat. Postoperatively an infant should be placed in a flannel gown, wrapped in a blanket, and placed in a crib that has been warmed. A heating lamp may be ordered to be placed over the crib. It should contain a bulb no stronger than 60 watts and should be placed 2 feet above the crib. Care must be taken not to overheat the baby since his temperature-regulating mechanism is quite labile. Rectal temperature is usually taken every hour until it stabilizes, and the amount of external heat is adjusted according to the temperature.

Pain. During the first 48 hours postoperatively most urologic patients, except those having cystoscopy or transurethral operations, will require narcotics for relief of pain in the incision. Elderly patients and infants need less than other age groups. An analgesic should be given before the pain is severe because its effectiveness is reduced otherwise. Narcotics should be given with caution to patients with depressed respirations or blood pressure without first consulting the doctor. Oxymorphone hydrochloride (Numorphan) is an excellent analgesic in the immediate postanesthetic period. It is much more potent than morphine or meperidine but lacks their soporific effect. It acts quickly (20 to 30 minutes) and lasts 3 to 6 hours. (See Chapter 5 for precautions to take with infants, children, and elderly patients.)

Ambulation. Following urologic operations, patients are usually gotten out of bed within 24 hours. Unless otherwise ordered, the patient should be encouraged to walk about with assistance. He should not sit in a chair for long periods of time because this position causes more stasis of blood in the venous system than does bed rest. Elastic knee-length stockings are ordered for most patients. They are usually worn for a week. While the patient is in bed he should be encouraged to exercise to prevent stasis of blood and thrombus formation in the veins of the legs. He should flex his knees, rotate his ankles, and press the back of his knees against the mattress ten times every 2 to 4 hours while he is awake. These exercises should be supervised to make sure they are effective. The patient should also be urged to move from side to side in bed and to use his upper extremities for such activities as eating, bathing, and combing his hair.

Maintenance of fluid and electrolyte balance. Although many patients can ingest normal amounts of food and fluids the day after surgery, others cannot, or the urologist may not want them to have an oral intake. A careful record of the patient's intake and output for at least 3 or 4 postoperative days is necessary, especially if calories and fluids are given intravenously and if nasogastric suction is instituted. In the latter situation, electrolytes such as sodium, chloride, and potassium are lost and must be replaced. Although there is a tendency for water and sodium to be retained by the body in the immediate postoperative period, fluid and some salt must be given. Patients suffering from cardiac or renal insufficiency pose special problems, and the reader is referred to the specific disease entity for greater detail as to management. The hourly (or 4- or 8-hour) urinary output should be recorded. A high output may cause an excessive loss of electrolytes, and if fluid intake does not keep up, the patient may become dehydrated. More often a low output is encountered due to faulty intravenous administration, renal shutdown, or excessive loss through lungs and skin caused by fever, perspiration, or a hot environment. Blood transfusions, while necessary to replace blood loss or correct anemia, are also prone to overload the circulation in some patients and elevate the serum potassium level in others (old blood has more free K^+ from red cell breakdown). The nurse should be familiar with the signs of fluid and electrolyte imbalance. *Dehydration* may be noted by loose, dry skin of poor turgor. The tongue looks shriveled and dry, and the eyes are soft. Urine output is low, and its specific gravity is high. *Overhydration* may result in dependent edema, pulmonary rales, dyspnea, restlessness, and cardiac failure. Acute pulmonary edema is an emergency requiring Fowler's position, oxygen, tourniquets on the extremities, and phlebotomy (withdrawal of blood). The physician may administer narcotics, diuretics, or cardiac-strengthening medicine. *Sodium depletion* is not uncommon after major surgery, especially when gastric suction or diarrhea removes salts, and sodium-poor intravenous fluid is given. The patient exhibits nausea, headaches, muscular weakness, hyporeflexia, vomiting, or abdominal cramps. Convulsions, coma, and shock may occur. *Sodium retention* occurs after surgery if fluid output is low. Restlessness, tachycardia, edema, and hyperreflexia are warning signs. *Potassium depletion* (hypokalemia) is suggested by weakness, apprehension, paralysis, nausea, vomiting, abdominal distention, convulsions, or coma. It may be preceded by excessive loss of gastrointestinal fluid. *Potassium excess* (hyperkalemia) causes nausea, diarrhea, abdominal cramps, muscular weakness, and irregular pulse and may result in cardiac standstill. It frequently follows excessive tissue destruction, multiple transfusions with old blood, and renal failure. The patient responds to ion exchange resins given orally or by enema, intravenous glucose, and cessation of K^+ intake. *Calcium loss* is seen in renal failure and may result in paresthesias, irritability, tetany, or convulsions. Reflexes become hyperactive. Calcium should be replaced orally or intravenously. *Excessive serum calcium* seen in hyperparathyroidism and widespread malignancy causes excessive thirst, lethargy, mental confusion, nausea, vomiting, and constipation. A high acid-to-base ratio is known as *acidosis*, and the patient may breathe deeply, giving off a "fruity" odor. Disorientation, coma, and death may occur. It is a common sequel to vomiting, diarrhea, and renal failure. Acute acidosis responds to intravenous sodium lactate. *Alkalosis* (too much base) produces slow, shallow respirations and may accompany electrolyte deficits; it responds to intravenous ammonium or sodium chloride. In electrolyte and fluid imbalances, the underlying cause must be diagnosed and corrected and the proper antidotes administered.

Gastrointestinal function. Hiccoughs and abdominal distention may occur. The nurse should see a surgical nursing textbook for detailed discussion of these problems. When extensive abdominal surgery or renal surgery is performed, a gastric tube may be inserted and connected to suction drainage to prevent vomiting and distention.

The first spontaneous bowel movement may not occur until 4 or 5 days after surgery. Mild cathartics or stool softeners may be given on the doctor's order before this, but enemas are rarely ordered prior to this unless symptoms of fecal impaction or intestinal distention occur. Infants and young children may, however, be given mild cathartics or a small enema as early as 24 hours postoperatively. The patient who has had prostatic or bladder surgery should be advised not to strain very hard in an attempt to evacuate his bowel; straining may cause bleeding from the operative site. If enemas are ordered after prostatic surgery, a soft rectal tube and very low pressure should be used. Only about 250 ml. of enema fluid are usually given.

The incision. Often following urologic surgery there is urinary drainage from the wounds. Because of this, the nurse working with these patients is more likely to have an order to change postoperative dressings more often than is the case when she cares for other surgical patients. However, copious leakage of urine from an operative wound should be reported to the doctor immediately because it may represent blockage of normal urine flow that can often be corrected by unblocking a catheter. Occasionally it does have disastrous results if not treated at once.

DRESSING THE WOUND. The equipment used for dressing a wound should always be sterile, and aseptic techniques should be observed. A separate sterile field should be used for dressing wounds opening into separate cavities. Each kidney and the bladder are considered separate cavities. If a wound must be dressed and a catheter opening into the same cavity irrigated, the same sterile field may be used, provided the field is kept dry. The catheter irrigation should be done before the wound is redressed. Montgomery straps are often used to hold the dressings in place. Many acceptable methods are available to manage wounds from which large amounts of urine drain. These are described in detail in the preceding discussion on management of urinary drainage from wounds. Wet dressings are a source of wound infection and cause the patient to be very uncomfortable.

WOUND COMPLICATIONS. Any redness of the wound or temperature elevation should be reported to the doctor since these may indicate wound infection. Purulent drainage from a wound or catheter also indicates infection. A large amount of straw-colored drainage from an abdominal wound or protrusion of bowel from it is serious. The former is symptomatic of wound dehiscence and the latter of evisceration. These conditions are discussed in detail in books on surgical nursing. They occur more often in children and the elderly than in adults and are more prevalent in patients with malnutrition, cancer, and wound infections.

Allergy to tape manifested by redness, blisters, or pruritus should be noted. Paper tape or nonallergic tape may be substituted. Application of tincture of benzoin protects the skin.

CARE OF THE PATIENT DURING DIALYSIS THERAPY

Dialysis, an accepted and effective procedure in the treatment of uremia, has opened up new hope for patients whose life-span was previously limited. Within the past 20 years the techniques have continually been improved and simplified. Nurses' roles in relation to such procedures have changed from one that was primarily of a technical nature to one that requires expertise in therapeutic techniques, diagnosis of nursing needs, and teaching the patient and his family. In addition, the nurse works as an associate and consultant to the physician and other members of the health team within the hospital setting and with appropriate community agencies. The nurse who is interested in this type of nursing usually receives special guidance and instruction in medical centers that have special dialysis and/or transplant units. Much is being written in the literature describing in detail the various aspects of caring for patients undergoing dialysis and renal transplant surgery. The nurse who is interested is encouraged to explore such resources frequently as changes are rapidly taking place.

Peritoneal dialysis

The purpose of peritoneal dialysis is usually to correct electrolyte and fluid imbalance or to remove toxic substances and metabolites ordinarily excreted by normally functioning kidneys. (See Chapter 7 for a detailed explanation.) The method is relatively simple and may be performed anywhere within the hospital without the use of elaborate equipment.

Commercially prepared administration sets are now available along with dialyzing solutions. As with any procedure, a clear explanation should be given to the patient and his family. Prior to peritoneal dialysis the dialyzing solution, if not at room temperature, should be slightly warmed. Warming the solution causes dilatation of peritoneal vessels and increases urea clearance. The bladder of the patient should be emptied just prior to the procedure to avoid possible puncture. The patient is weighed and vital signs are taken to establish base-line measurements. He is placed in a supine position, with the head of the bed elevated approximately 45 degrees. Some patients are allowed to sit in a chair. Bed covers are draped to expose the abdomen, which is cleansed with tincture of Zephiran, and sterile drapes applied. Appropriate dialysis solutions are attached to tubing and the tubing filled. The physician inserts an 18-gauge needle percutaneously into the peritoneal cavity. The filled tubing is attached to the needle and the dialysis solution allowed to flow as rapidly as possible (usually 15 to 20 minutes to instill 2100 ml.). The tubing is then clamped. This step is called "priming the patient" and facilitates insertion of the peritoneal catheter by providing a distended area of fluid, thus preventing possible perforation of the bowel. The patient should be closely observed, and signs of abdominal or respiratory distress should be called to the attention of the physician.

It is essential to record the exact starting time of instillation and amount of solution instilled on the peritoneal dialysis record (Fig. 4-17). After priming the patient, the physician will reprep the abdomen with tincture of Zephiran and insert the peritoneal catheter. Dialysis tubing is then attached to the catheter. The catheter should be securely fastened to avoid loss into the abdominal cavity. The physician will designate a period of time to wait before syphoning. Bottles used for dialyzing solutions are then placed on the floor, preferably in a metal tray or basin, the tubing unclamped, and the airway dislodged (see Fig. 7-1). An alternative method would entail the use of a Y connector to which tubing, a clamp, and a separate collection receptacle are attached. Movement of the patient side to side, pressure on the abdomen, and coughing, laughing, or deep breathing will sometimes facilitate syphoning. The catheter may also be irrigated with 30 ml. of normal saline solution. If the syphon cycle exceeds 2 hours, the physician should be notified, as repositioning of the catheter may be necessary. Dialyzing solution bottles if filled to the top will contain 1200 ml. Any excess solution in the basin should be carefully measured and the total amount recorded. Dialysis cycles are repeated as ordered by the physician; however, thirty-six cycles is the

Peritoneal Dialysis

Patient's Name: ....   Date: ....

Case No.: ....   Diagnosis (1).............................

Age: ....   (2)..............................

(3)..............................

Time	Dialysis No.	Volume		Fluid Balance	Previous	Present	Remarks
		In	Out				

MEDICATION

Fig. 4-17. Example of peritoneal dialysis fluid-medication data sheet.

usual number. When removing the catheter, the nurse may note resistance at first; if marked resistance continues, however, the physician should be notified. The tip of the catheter is usually cut off with sterile scissors and sent to the laboratory in a culture tube for culture and sensitivity tests. Neosporin ointment is applied to the site of insertion and a dry sterile dressing applied. Saturated dressings should be changed p.r.n. The patient should then be reweighed. The nurse must remain alert for postural hypotension.

During the procedure the patient should be encouraged to carry out normal activities; however, assistance may be necessary for meals, bathing, occupational therapy, etc. Close observation as to bleeding and changes in vital signs is important. If a great deal more fluid is removed than added, it is possible, although unlikely, that the blood pressure may decrease. Reduction of potassium may cause muscle cramps and increased weakness. Extravasation of fluid into the tissues may also occur. Small amounts are of little concern; however, large amounts should be called to the attention of the physician. Strict attention to aseptic technique and possibly shorter dialysis times will prevent many infections and the possibility of peritonitis. Perforation of the bowel may occur, particularly in patients with intra-abdominal adhesions or late in the cycle of dialysis because of the pressure of the catheter on an edematous bowel. In such instances the patient would have large amounts of watery diarrhea or cloudy and fecal-type return when syphoning. Wound evisceration is possible, as are pulmonary complications. Because of an upward displacement of the diaphragm and shallow respirations, pneumonia, atelectasis, or bronchitis may result. Control of the fluids in both amount and rate is essential to avoid overhydration or hypotension.

Hemodialysis

What previously was an extremely elaborate and expensive procedure is now simplified to the point where many patients and families dialyze themselves in their homes. The cost of hemodialysis is slowly decreasing because of research and new developments. Bringing the cost from over $1000 to within a $20 range now seems realistic and means a greater number of patients will reap the benefits.

Selection of peritoneal dialysis or hemodialysis for treatment of acute renal failure is based on many individual patient factors. What might be the choice for one patient may be contraindicated in another. The very obese patient who has had abdominal trauma or surgery, multiple adhesions, or an aortic aneurysm would be a poor candidate for peritoneal dialysis, and hemodialysis would be the preferred procedure. In contrast to peritoneal dialysis, hemodialysis is about four to five times more effective; however, age, body size, urine volume, additional disease processes, complications, general physical condition, irreversible acute renal failure, and suitability for renal transplantation, in addition to psychosocial factors, must be weighed. (See Chapter 7 for further implications in choosing dialysis.)

Basically, hemodialysis is accomplished by drawing blood from an artery, circulating it through a membrane dialyzer for purification, and returning it to a vein (see Fig. 7-2). When forearm vessels are not available, large vessels such as the brachial or femoral vessels may be used. The most recent technique developed is that of an arteriovenous fistula in which an anastomosis is made between the radial artery and the cephalic vein. With this method, the patient is free of tubes in his arm. When being dialyzed, two venipunctures are necessary. The patient using home dialysis may have a leg fistula, which he can be taught to puncture himself. The text will not cover the detailed procedures for the various types of dialyzing apparatuses since new improvements are being made so rapidly.

As a therapeutic technician and as a teacher, the nurse should be aware of complications that can occur during hemodialysis. Both hypotension and hypertension should be noted, the former being due to excessive ultrafiltration or possibly other medical problems such as bleeding and the latter probably due to the underlying disease. Drowsiness, headache, confusion, convulsions, or vomiting may be symptoms of too rapid a correction resulting in cerebral edema. Infection of shunts can lead to severe septicemia or septic embolization; thus well-supervised instruction in care of the shunt is essential. Pruritus is frequently a symptom that is difficult to treat. Cleansing with vinegar solutions, hot baths, and antipruritic agents is sometimes helpful. Burning of the feet is also a frequent complaint. General complaints of fatigue, insomnia, malaise, weight loss, etc. may be due to malnutrition, infection, and/or poor dialysis techniques. Deviations in a patient's usual behavior may be expected, particularly in the patient who is being maintained for a prolonged time, and may become a way of life. Concerns as to dependency on other family members, physical limitations, and economic factors may force the patient into phases of rejection, denial, and withdrawal. Each patient's reactions will differ and need to be met on an individual basis, the nurse participating as an active member of the health team. (See Chapter 7 for further detailed care of patients with renal failure.)

SPECIFIC DRUG THERAPY

The drugs most commonly employed in urology are those used in antibacterial therapy and those used in cancer therapy.

Antibacterial therapy

The prophylactic use of antibiotics and sulfonamides exposes the patient to the hazards of drug toxicity, superinfection, and the development of drug-resistant urinary flora. The injudicious use of these drugs may prevent treatment of subsequent acute infections by the usual measures. Consequently, many doctors are now using antibacterial therapy only when the patient manifests symptoms such as fever, tissue inflammation, or purulent drainage that suggests the development or presence of infection. The use of prophylactic therapy is a decision for the attending urologist.

For effective antibacterial therapy, control of the pH of the urine is often necessary. Some antibiotics are much more effective in an acid environment (nitrofurantoin, penicillin, mandelic acid), whereas others are more effective in an alkaline environment (sulfonamides, streptomycin, kanamycin). Still others are more effective at a normal pH (colistin, polymyxin, tetracycline). The nurse should test the urinary pH frequently and instruct the patient carefully if it will be necessary for him to continue his therapy at home. Potassium acid phosphate, ascorbic acid, and ammonium chloride act as acidifying agents. Alkalinization may be accomplished with sodium bicarbonate.

Any obstruction to urinary flow must also be eradicated prior to antibacterial therapy. Although antibacterial therapy may control the acute complications, the infection can seldom be entirely eliminated from the urinary tract until catheter drainage is no longer necessary. A urine culture with drug sensitivity tests is usually ordered for any patient being treated for a urinary tract infection. This test will indicate the type of organism causing the infection and the drugs to which the organism is most susceptible. The results of the test can be reported within 36 hours. Meanwhile, antibacterial therapy based on the doctor's clinical observation and judgment is usually started. After the laboratory report becomes available, a different drug may be used.

Antibacterial agents should never be given until it has been ascertained that the patient has no history of sensitivity to similar drugs and that there are no other contraindications for giving the drug. Excesses of many drugs (for example, streptomycin and kanamycin) are eliminated from the body through the kidneys and therefore cannot be given safely to patients with impaired renal function. When a patient has acidosis, the kidneys are not functioning to capacity, so any excess drug will not be excreted. Therefore those drugs eliminated by the kidneys are contraindicated or must be given in reduced doses for acidotic patients. Excesses of some drugs must be broken down by the liver before they can be excreted; these drugs cannot be given safely to patients with liver disease. The nurse as well as the doctor should know the drugs with similar chemical structures (drugs of the same family), symptoms of sensitivity to the various antibacterial drugs, and contraindications to their use. If the nurse has any information that causes her to question the use of a prescribed drug, she should give this information to the doctor. Table 3 gives the average doses of some of the antibacterial drugs and symptoms of adverse reactions.

The follow-up of patients who have required antibacterial therapy may be continued for several months after treatment has been discontinued. The nurse should urge the patient to return to the doctor regularly until he is discharged since asymptomatic recurrences of the bac-

Table 3. Antibacterial therapy (average 24-hour dosage; should be titrated according to weight)

Drug	Average dose		Adverse reactions
	Adult	Child	
Methenamine mandelate (Mandelamine)	1-1.5 Gm. q. 6 hr. (oral)	6-10 mg./lb. q. 6 hr. (oral)	Nausea, vomiting
Sulfonamides			
Sulfisoxazole (Gantrisin)	1 Gm. q.i.d. (oral)	10 mg./lb. q.i.d. (oral)	Nausea, vomiting, headache, skin rash, sore throat, fever, pallor, jaundice, purpura
Sulfamethoxazole (Gantanol)	1 Gm. b.i.d. (oral)	12 mg./lb. b.i.d. (oral)	
Sulfamethizole (Thiosulfil)	1 Gm. q.i.d. (oral)	10 mg./lb. q.i.d. (oral)	
Penicillin V	500 mg. q.i.d. (oral)	250 mg. q.i.d. (oral)	Dermatitis, anaphylactic shock, nausea, vomiting, fever
Ampicillin (Polycillin, Omnipen, Penbritin)	500 mg. q.i.d. (oral)	250 mg. q.i.d. (oral)	Same as for penicillin
Streptomycin	250-500 mg. q. 6 hr. (I.M.)	2-5 mg./lb. q. 6 hr. (I.M.)	Fever, rash, dizziness, deafness, vertigo
Tetracyclines			
Chlortetracycline (Aureomycin)	250-500 mg. q. 6 hr. (oral)	5 mg./lb. q. 6 hr. (oral)	Nausea, vomiting, anorexia, glossitis, diarrhea, rash, azotemia
Oxytetracycline (Terramycin)	250-500 mg. q. 6 hr. (oral)	5 mg./lb. q. 6 hr. (oral)	(same for all tetracyclines)
Demethylchlortetracycline (Declomycin)	300 mg. q. 12 hr. (oral)	2.5 mg./lb. q. 12 hr. (oral)	
Doxycycline (Vibramycin)	100 mg. q. 24 hr. (oral)	0.5 mg./lb. q. 24 hr. (oral)	
Erythromycin	250-500 mg. q. 6 hr. (oral)	3-4 mg./lb. q. 6 hr. (oral)	Nausea, vomiting, diarrhea, rash, fever
Chloramphenicol (Chloromycetin)	250-500 mg. q. 6 hr. (oral)	5-10 mg./lb. q. 6 hr. (oral)	Rash, fever, may cause aplastic anemia

Drug			
Polymyxin B (Aerosporin)	30 mg. q. 6 hr. (I.M.)	0.25 mg./lb. q. 6 hr. (I.M.)	Albuminuria, fever, dizziness, weakness, azotemia
Colistimethate (Coly-Mycin)	0.25-1.5 mg./lb. q. 6 hr. (I.M.)	0.25 mg./lb. q. 6 hr. (I.M.)	Itching, tingling of extremities, circumoral or lingual paresthesia, azotemia
Kanamycin (Kantrex)	1.5 mg./lb. q. 6 hr. (I.M.)	1.5 mg./lb. q. 6 hr. (I.M.)	Azotemia, deafness
Nalidixic acid (NegGram)	500-1000 mg. q. 6 hr. (oral)	8 mg./lb. q. 6 hr. (oral)	Rash, fever
Cephalothin (Keflin)	250-1000 mg. q. 6 hr. (I.M. or I.V.)	5 mg./lb. q. 6 hr. (I.M.)	Neutropenia, rash
Cephaloridine (Loridine)	500-1000 mg. q. 6 hr. (I.M.)	5 mg./lb. q. 6 hr. (I.M.)	Rash, fever, azotemia
Cephaloglycin (Kafocin)	250-500 mg. q.i.d. (oral)	5 mg./lb. q. 6 hr. (oral)	Nausea, vomiting, diarrhea
Cephalexin (Keflex)	250-500 mg. q.i.d. (oral)	5 mg./lb. q. 6 hr. (oral)	Nausea, vomiting, diarrhea, rash, pruritus
Clindamycin (Cleocin)	300 mg. q. 6 hr. (oral)	4 mg./lb. q. 6 hr. (oral)	Nausea, vomiting, diarrhea, abdominal pain
Gentamicin (Garamycin)	0.6 mg./lb. q. 8 hr. (I.M. or I.V.)	1.3 mg./lb. q. 8 hr. (I.M. or I.V.)	Deafness, azotemia, vertigo
Disodium carbenicillin (Geopen)	½-1 Gm. q. 6 hr. (I.M. or I.V.)	5-10 mg./lb. q. 6 hr. (I.M. or I.V.)	Nausea, rash, pruritus, fever, anaphylaxis
Nitrofurantoin (Furadantin) Macrocrystals (Macrodantin)	100 mg. q. 6 hr. (oral)	1 mg./lb. q. 6 hr. (oral)	Nausea, vomiting, skin rash, headache, hemolytic anemia, peripheral neuritis

terial growth with the risk of chronic pyelonephritis and renal damage are possible. Serious consequences of inadequate treatment may eventually lead to hypertension, renal failure, and death.

Mandelic acid and methenamine mandelate. Methenamine mandelate (Mandelamine) is the preparation commonly used. This drug acts only on bacteria in urine by releasing formaldehyde in an acid medium, and it has no effect on bacteria within the body tissues. It is particularly effective against *Escherichia coli* and *Streptococcus faecalis.* Patients taking this drug must test their urine four times a day with nitrazine paper. If the pH is more than 5, ascorbic acid, 100 to 500 mg. four times daily, or potassium acid phosphate is given to increase the acidity of the urine. Fluids must be reduced to around 1500 ml. a day since the drug is effective only in concentrated urine. This drug has an unpleasant flavor that cannot be disguised. It often causes nausea and vomiting and should be given after meals to reduce its irritating properties. If given in liquid form, the use of a drinking straw held well back on the tongue reduces the unpleasant taste. For adults the usual dose of methenamine mandelate is 1 to 1.5 Gm. four times daily. It is contraindicated for patients with acidosis or renal damage.

Phenazopyridine hydrochloride. The drug phenazopyridine hydrochloride (Pyridium) is used primarily for its analgesic effect in the urinary tract. It has no bacteriostatic action. It may be used safely for long periods of time. The patient should be informed that it will give a reddish color to the urine. The usual dose for adults is two tablets three times a day. It is contraindicated in severe renal damage and hepatitis.

Sulfonamide drugs. Sulfisoxazole is the drug in this group most commonly used. However, many other forms of the drug may be ordered. The sulfonamide drugs have a wide bacterial spectrum, but bacterial strains resistant to these drugs can develop. Sulfonamides may cause nausea and vomiting; this is more common in children than in adults. For adults the usual dose of most sulfonamides is 2 to 4 Gm. daily for 7 to 10 days. If the drug is to be continued beyond this time, periodic determinations of the white blood cell count are usually made since leukopenia may occur. Sulfonamides are marketed as palatable syrups for children. Sometimes sodium bicarbonate is given with these drugs to reduce the incidence of acetylated sulfonamide crystallization in the urine with blockage of the renal tubules. This is not required with the newer preparations. Sulfamethoxazole needs to be given only twice a day.

Penicillin. Penicillin V has been found to be effective for long-term prophylaxis against streptococcal infections such as might occur in pyelonephritis. Oral divided doses totaling 1 to 2 Gm. daily may be given. Penicillin is also used for the treatment of gonorrhea or to supplement other antibiotic drugs such as erythromycin or streptomycin. Severe dermatitis and even anaphylactic shock are side effects. The average daily dosage for an adult with gonorrhea is 600,000 to 1,200,000 units of a long-lasting preparation given in a single dose. It is often given intravenously and intramuscularly, but forms for oral use are available.

Ampicillin. Ampicillin has been found to be effective against many strains of *Escherichia, Salmonella,* and *Shigella* and *Proteus mirabilis.* It has been used for both upper and lower urinary tract infections, the usual dosage being 250 to 1000 mg. orally every 6 hours. Toxicity is the same as for penicillin.

Streptomycin. This drug is effective against tubercle bacilli and coliform bacilli. Except in the treatment of tuberculosis, it is usually continued for only a few days. Fever, rash, dizziness, deafness, and vertigo are possible side effects. The average daily adult dosage is 1 to 2 Gm. in divided doses. Its use is contraindicated by obstructive uropathy or azotemia. In long-term therapy the dosage schedule is markedly reduced.

Tetracycline drugs. Chlortetracycline (Aureomycin), oxytetracycline (Terramycin), tetracycline (Achromycin), demethylchlortetracycline (Declomycin), and doxycycline (Vibramycin) are the commonly used drugs in this group. These drugs have a wide antibacterial spectrum but may cause nausea and vomiting. Glossitis (sore tongue) and proctitis (inflammation of the bowel) may also occur. Administering the drug after meals or with milk and crackers decreases gastrointestinal symptoms. If diarrhea occurs, the doctor should be consulted before the next dose of the drug is administered since he may wish to discontinue its use. The average adult dose of these drugs is 250 mg. four times a day with the exception of doxycycline, the dosage of which is 100 mg. once daily.

Erythromycin. This antibiotic is especially effective in treating staphylococcal infections and seems to have few side effects. The usual adult dose is 250 mg. four times a day. It is available in a cinnamon-flavored syrup for children.

Chloramphenicol. Although organisms in the urinary tract are very susceptible to it, chloramphenicol (Chloromycetin) is not used as often as indicated because rarely it may cause aplastic anemia. It is used, however, when no other preparation is effective and the patient is acutely ill. The usual daily adult dosage is 1 to 4 Gm. given orally in four divided doses. It may be administered intramuscularly and intravenously. Its use is continued 5 to 7 days.

Polymyxin B and colistimethate. These drugs are used with caution because they may cause nephrotoxic and neurotoxic side effects. Polymyxin B is occasionally used for a resistant *Pseudomonas aeruginosa* (pyocyaneous) infection. The usual adult dose is 30 mg. four times a day: the maximum dosage is 200 mg. per day. The drug should not be used longer than 2 weeks, and if the order for it is not discontinued after this time, the nurse should consult the doctor. It is contraindicated for patients with depressed renal function. Colistimethate (Coly-Mycin) is particularly effective against *Pseudomonas* and bactericidal against *Escherichia, Aerobacter,* and *Klebsiella.* Symptoms such as itching and tingling of the extremities and circumoral or lingual paresthesis may be expected and should be carefully recorded and reported to the doctor. The adult dose is 1.5 to 0.25 mg. per pound of body weight. Colistimethate sulfate pediatric suspension is also available.

Kanamycin. Kanamycin (Kantrex) is primarily used against *Proteus* and *Pseudomonas.* Although it may produce irreversible kidney damage, it is considered safe for short-term treatment. Increased fluid intake is necessary when administering this drug. Hearing loss may also occur; therefore frequent observations should be made by the nurse. For an acute infection, 1.5 mg. per pound of body weight is given four times a day (less when kidney function is impaired).

Nalidixic acid. Nalidixic acid (NegGram) is unrelated to any other type of chemotherapeutic agent. It is most effective against gram-negative organisms. It is given in doses of 500 to 1000 mg. four times a day to the adult; for the child, 6 mg. per pound of body weight four times daily is given. It too is useful for chronic pyelonephritis. Toxic effects are limited. Since it is metabolized by the liver, periodic liver function tests may be carried out.

Cephalothin. Cephalothin (Keflin) is bactericidal against gram-negative and gram-positive organisms. *Pseudomonas* organisms are notably resistant. Caution should be exercised if the patient is known to be sensitive to penicillin. It may be administered intramuscularly or intravenously, the intravenous route being preferred for severe infections such as septicemia and bacteremia. Stability can be preserved for up to 48 hours if the drug is kept refrigerated after reconstitution; otherwise it should be given within 6 hours. It is highly effective against a wide spectrum of gram-positive and gram-negative organisms. It is safe in patients with reduced renal function.

Cephaloridine. Cephaloridine (Loridine) is one of the cephalosporin family of broad-spectrum antibiotics especially effective against urinary tract organisms such as *Proteus mirabilis, Escherichia coli,* and *Klebsiella.* It must be given intramuscularly or intravenously. (See Table 3 for average dosage schedule.) Adverse reactions include hives, rash, fever, and renal impairment. If used at all, great caution should be exercised in giving this drug to patients with reduced renal function.

Cephaloglycin. Cephaloglycin (Kafocin) is indicated for acute and chronic infections of the urinary tract such as cystitis, pyelitis, and pyelonephritis when caused by strains of *Escherichia coli, Klebsiella-Aerobacter,* and *Proteus* species. Culture and sensitivity tests should be initiated prior to and during therapy. Patients should be watched closely for allergic symptoms, particularly if they are known to be sensitive to penicillin.

Cephalexin. Cephalexin in the monohydrate form (Keflex) is the oral equivalent of Keflin and has been used effectively in both acute and chronic urinary infections such as cystitis and pyelonephritis. Although it is to be used with caution, success has been achieved in treating infections in patients with impaired renal function. Less adverse reactions such as gastrointestinal and allergic reactions occur. Doses of 250 to 500 mg. every 6 hours are usual for adults.

Clindamycin. Clindamycin (Cleocin) is a relatively new semisynthetic antibiotic. As with all new drugs, precaution should be taken in regard to hypersensitivity. As yet it is not indicated in newborn babies or infants under 30 days of age. It is effective against gram-positive organisms and may be used in anuric patients. Dialysis does not effectively remove it from the blood; therefore in patients with severe renal insufficiency, serum levels should be determined periodically and dosages adjusted.

Gentamicin. Gentamicin (Garamycin), another relatively new bactericidal antibiotic, is effective in infections caused by susceptible strains of gram-negative bacteria. Its use should be limited to treatment of serious infections. Its greatest benefit is in treating infections caused by *Pseudomonas*. In patients with impaired renal function and serious infection, serum concentrations rise; consequently, the risk of nephrotoxicity, deafness, and vertigo is increased.

Disodium carbenicillin. Disodium carbenicillin (Geopen) is a semisynthetic penicillin that is particularly effective against gram-negative organisms such as *Pseudomonas*. It may be administered intramuscularly or intravenously. Toxic effects are not readily demonstrated in patients with normal renal function. Severely uremic patients may develop hemorrhagic manifestations, however. As with other penicillins, there is the possibility of anaphylactic reactions and/or fever.

Nitrofurantoin. Nitrofurantoin (Furadantin) may be given by mouth or intravenously. It has a wide spectrum of activity against gram-positive and gram-negative organisms and therefore is a good urinary antiseptic. It is both bacteriostatic and bactericidal and is indicated for pyelonephritis and cystitis. The principal side effects are nausea and vomiting, but skin rash and headache may occur. If given intravenously it should be administered in two divided doses and the infusion should never be allowed to run faster than 35 to 40 drops a minute. Prochlorperazine dimaleate (Compazine) may be given intramuscularly to counteract the gastrointestinal effects. The average adult dose is 100 mg. every 6 hours. It is contraindicated for patients with severe renal impairment or acidosis. Hemolytic anemia may occur in Negroes or in persons of Mediterranean or Near Eastern origin who receive this drug. Peripheral neuritis is occasionally found in patients on long-term, high-dosage therapy. Macrodantin, a newer preparation, is touted to be less disturbing to the gastrointestinal system although as effective.

Drugs used in cancer chemotherapy

There is a continuing search for drugs that will selectively control and inhibit the growth of neoplasms without destroying normal tissue. It appears that carcinogenic agents produce disturbances in cells. These disturbances may be derangements of the cellular function or faulty synthesis of nucleic acid (basic genetic material of the cell) and other essential cellular components. Therefore the goal in chemotherapy for cancer is inhibition or interference with the function or synthesis of nucleic acids present in the tumor cells.

Since most of the drugs being used in cancer chemotherapy are experimental, the nurse should carefully note and report signs and symptoms relative to any system in the body, not only the cancerous system. Cardiovascular, pulmonary, renal, and gastrointestinal symptoms and weight changes should be anticipated. It is frequently impossible to know what side effects may be expected. However, the nurse should get as much information as possible from the doctor and the pharmacist about the drugs being used.

Some of the *drugs* used for treatment of cancer are *given into the arterial supply to the tumor*. A cutdown is usually done on the artery and a polyethylene catheter is left in place until the therapy is completed. If the tumor is deeply seated, an operative procedure may be required to place the catheter. It is extremely important that the catheter not be dislodged or blocked before the therapy is discontinued. A continuous perfusion (fluid given under pressure) or infusion (fluid given by gravitational flow) must be run; the fluid is given only fast enough to keep the catheter patent except during periods when the drug is being given. To provide perfusion, a Bowman pump that can be adjusted to pump the fluid at the prescribed rate is ordinarily used. It is attached below the fluid flask. The nurse is responsible for keeping the catheter anchored and the fluid running at the prescribed rate between administrations of the drug.

The patient may become rapidly toxic while receiving the drug. He should therefore be attended, preferably by the doctor, during the period the drug is being given. If a nurse is assigned to this, she should watch the patient carefully for toxic symptoms of the drug being used. If toxic symptoms appear, the fluid containing the therapeutic drug should be removed, but kept sterile, and a flask of the prescribed maintenance fluid, usually 5% glucose in water, should be attached. The doctor should be called immediately to give specific orders.

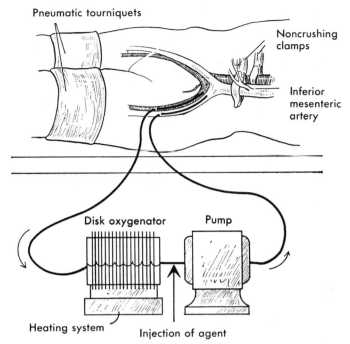

Pneumatic tourniquets

Noncrushing clamps

Inferior mesenteric artery

Disk oxygenator   Pump

Heating system   Injection of agent

Fig. 4-18. System used for perfusion of chemotherapeutic agents into pelvic area. Note pneumatic tourniquets on legs and noncrushing hemostats on vena cava and aorta to prevent drugs from circulating outside region of treatment. Blood from vein is oxygenated, drug is added, and blood is then pumped back into pelvic circulation.

Occasionally *extracorporeal perfusion* is used to instill drugs into pelvic tumors. This treatment requires an operation. A laparotomy is done to reach the blood vessels in the abdomen. The pelvis is then isolated by clamping the aorta and inferior vena cava just above the iliac bifurcations. Cannulas are inserted into femoral artery and vein and then attached to an oxygenator and sigmamotor pump so that relatively normal oxygenation of the lower extremities continues during the procedures. Pneumatic tourniquets are placed on both legs (Fig. 4-18). The drug is then perfused into the pelvic area, and after its action has dissipated, the vessels are unclamped, the cannulas removed, and the abdomen closed.

This method causes less systemic side effects from the drug than do regular perfusion methods. Longer acting drugs that are unsafe to give by regular perfusion can also be used. Postoperatively the patient should be observed for symptoms of phlebitis, thrombus formation, and septicemia as well as delayed reactions to the drugs used.

Antimetabolites. These drugs are chemically similar to some normal metabolic substance in the body and the tissues tend to use both the metabolite and the antimetabolite indiscriminately. Therefore the drug can inhibit an enzyme system or metabolic process for which the metabolic substance is necessary. In this way the formation of nucleic acids can be impeded at various stages of development.

Purine, pyrimidine, and uracil are basic genetic substances. They are essential components of nucleic acids. The purine antagonists (6-mercaptopurine and thioguanine) interfere with the use of purine in nucleic acid synthesis. The pyrimidine antagonists (6-azauracil, 5-fluorouracil [5-FU], 5-fluorouridine [5-FUR], 5-fluorodeoxyuridine [5-FUDR]) interfere with the use of uracil in synthesizing nucleic acids. These drugs may be used in the treatment of metastatic cancer of the bladder. They may be given orally or intravenously. The usual dose is 15 mg. per kilogram of body weight for 5 days; a half dose is then given every other day until the thirteenth day. Depression of the white blood cell count, anorexia, stomatitis, and diarrhea are toxic symptoms. The folic acid antagonists (aminopteroylglutamate sodium [aminopterin] and methotrexate) block the synthesis of both purine and pyrimidine. They may be used in the treatment of testicular tumors, especially of chorionic carcinomas, which appear to require folic acid for their growth. These drugs are usually given in 25 mg. doses for 5 days. After a rest period of 7 to 10 days to allow normal tissue to recover, the treatment may be repeated. The amino acid antagonists (azaserine [O-diazoacetyl-L-serine] and DON [6-diazo-5-oxo-L-norleucine) are antibiotics that inhibit the formation of nucleic acid.

Polyfunctional alkylating agents. These drugs react with a variety of organic and inorganic materials by the process of alkylation. They attack all cells indiscriminately, but neoplastic cells are more severely damaged. The drugs in this group are nitrogen mustard, chlorambucil, triethylenemelamine (TEM), dimethanesulfonoxybutane (Myleran), and triethylenethiophosphoramide (Thio-Tepa). The drugs are generally given in infusions, but some are available orally. Thio-Tepa, when instilled repeatedly in the bladder, is known to eradicate superficial neoplasms. In solution these drugs cause local skin reactions, and rubber gloves should be worn by those preparing and administering them. Care should be taken to prevent any of the drug from getting on the patient's skin. If this happens, the skin must be washed at once with copious amounts of water. Since these drugs cause nausea and vomiting a few hours after injection, administration should be carefully planned so that the height of the reaction does not coincide with mealtime. The white blood cell count is decreased for a time after treatment. During this period, precautions should be taken to avoid infections. Gown-and-mask technique may sometimes be ordered to protect the patient from organisms carried by others.

Steroid hormones. Steroid hormones are given as chemotherapeutic agents because of their specific effects on specific tissues. Cancer arising from tissues modified by steroid hormones may retain some of the tissue's original hormonal responsiveness; therefore giving of the steroid hormone may increase the growth rate or cause regression. Such drugs are classified as androgens, estrogens, progesterone, adrenocortical compounds, and adrenocorticotropic hormone (ACTH). Some are given orally and others intravenously or intramuscularly. The estrogens (diethylstilbestrol and ethynylestradiol) are effective in the treatment of carcinoma of the prostate. Provera (a progesterone) is used for metastatic carcinoma of the kidney, as is testosterone.

Antibiotics. Among the antibiotics prescribed in cancer therapy are actinomycin D or IV, mitomycin C, and streptonigrin. Actinomycin D is given intravenously for children with Wilms' tumor or for patients with lymphoma or choriocarcinoma. In combination with methotrexate and chlorambucil, it is useful for testicular tumors. The usual adult dose is 0.5 mg. daily for 5 days; for children, 15 mg. per kilogram of body weight. This treatment is repeated every 3 to 5 weeks until a therapeutic response is obtained or toxicity occurs. Toxic symptoms are exhibited by the decrease in number of white blood cells and platelets, ulceration of the tongue and mouth, nausea, vomiting, loss of hair, and excoriation of the skin. Prochlorperazine dimaleate (Compazine) may be given to control nausea and vomiting. Hair begins to grow again within 2 weeks after treatment has been discontinued, and the patient should be told this. Meantime a woman or female child may wish to wear a turban or a wig. The drug should be stopped if ulcerations of the mouth occur since gastrointestinal bleeding soon follows. The nurse should therefore check the patient's mouth daily and should report any ulceration to the doctor. The drug is also stopped if the blood count departs from normal. Special care should be taken to prevent infection. Skin abrasions should be prevented if possible; if they occur, they should be cleaned and dressed. Contact with anyone who has an upper respiratory or other communicable infection should be avoided.

Other drug therapy

When the bladder is hypertonic and irritable, the patient will complain of frequency, burning, and bladder spasms. For relief, tincture of hyoscyamus and its natural alkaloids may be employed. Methantheline (Banthine), propantheline (Pro-Banthine), and valethamate (Murel) may also provide relief. When the bladder is lacking in muscle tone, neostigmine (Prostigmin) and bethanechol chloride (Urecholine chloride) are used to improve the atonic condition, to encourage micturition, and/or to eliminate the need for a catheter. Neostigmine is available in 15 to 30 mg. tablets; there are also preparations for subcutaneous, intramuscular, and intravenous administration. Care should be taken with asthmatic patients and those with hypothyroidism. Urecholine is available in 5, 10, and 25 mg. tablets. It is given in oral doses to the point of tolerance. Caution must be used in the parenteral route of administration (2 to 5 mg. subcutaneously only) since pulmonary paralysis can occur.

Diuretics, the purpose of which is to increase the net loss of water, may be indicated for various conditions, including urologic disorders. They may be divided into two categories, those that increase the glomerular filtration rate and those that increase the renal solute excretion. They may again be subdivided according to their specific action to achieve diuresis. Mercurial (Mercuhydrine, Thiomerin, Neohydrin) and xanthine diuretics promote diuresis in adults with the nephrotic syndrome but are less effective with the child. Urea and mannitol are used for patients with renal vascular hypertension. Mannitol is also used in oliguric renal failure, to prevent uric acid nephropathy, to prevent acute renal failure during attacks of paroxysmal myoglobinuria, to irrigate the operative field in transurethral resection, and to prevent hemolysis, hemoglobinuria, and acute renal failure. No more than 100 Gm. is given daily when the urinary outflow is less than 100 ml. per hour. Urinary loss of sodium and potassium and congestive heart failure are possible side effects. Furosemide (Lasix) and ethacrynic acid (Edecrin) are two relatively new, powerful diuretics. Because of their potency, they are used only when there can be close observation clinically and control by laboratory results. Both drugs have been used in the management of acute and chronic renal insufficiency. Ethacrynic acid has more adverse gastrointestinal effects than furosemide. Deafness may be a major side effect with either drug, the incidence being less with furosemide.

IRRADIATION THERAPY

X-ray therapy and radioisotopes are the most common forms of irradiation used in urologic therapy. Radiotherapy is effective in curing cancer in some instances; in others it limits the growth of cancer cells for a time.

X-ray therapy

The patient who is to have x-ray therapy should know what to expect before, during, and after treatment. The untoward effects of x-ray therapy are usually not mentioned to a patient, but he may have heard that "burns" and nausea occur. If he asks, the nurse should explain simply why these *sometimes* occur or refer his questions to the doctor.

The patient should know that he will be placed on a table in a room by himself. The equipment will be similar, although larger and more complex, to that he has seen during routine roentgenographic examinations. He should know that the radiotherapist will be stationed outside the room, will observe him throughout the treatment, and will communicate with him if he desires. The patient should understand that the treatment will not be painful and that he must remain in the exact position in which he is placed. If the patient asks how many treatments he will receive, a definite answer should not be given. Treatments may have to be discontinued because of side effects or more treatments than originally planned may be given.

Prior to the first treatment, the patient's skin should be thoroughly cleaned. After this, nothing should be used on the area being irradiated unless specifically ordered. Medicated ointments and powders may contain heavy metals that would increase the radiation dosage. The area to be irradiated is marked by the radiologist and these markings must not be washed off until the treatment is complete since they are important guides to the therapist. Sponge baths must replace showers or tub baths.

Skin reactions invariably occur during irradiation therapy but are much reduced with cobalt therapy. Reddening may be seen on about the tenth day, and the skin may turn a dark reddish purple after about 3 weeks. The skin is usually dry and it cracks easily; application of a vegetable fat may be ordered. Itching and burning may occur, and the skin may actually slough and ooze. If this occurs, treatment may be discontinued until healing takes place. The doctor will order the ointments he wishes used on the sloughing area. Dressings should be loosely applied and anchored to healthy skin; it is advisable to use paper tape rather than adhesive; aseptic technique should be used.

Gastrointestinal reactions to radiation therapy are more common when the x-ray ports (the areas where the x-rays enter the body) lie over some part of this system. Nausea, vomiting, anorexia, malaise, and diarrhea may occur. Liver extract, vitamin B, and intravenous solutions of glucose in physiologic solution of sodium chloride may be given for nausea, anorexia, and dehydration. Antiemetic drugs such as dimenhydrinate (Dramamine) may give symptomatic relief. Camphorated tincture of opium (paregoric) is used to control diarrhea; bismuth subcarbonate or other drugs containing heavy metals are contraindicated. Resting before and after meals helps some patients control nausea and vomiting. It is often helpful to withhold food for 2 hours before and after the treatment. Breakfast is usually the meal best tolerated, and the patient should be encouraged to eat as much at this meal as possible.

Irradiation over the bladder gives severe symptoms of cystitis. Forcing fluids may relieve this. Heat over the area is contraindicated because irradiated skin tolerates excesses of heat or cold poorly. The treatment may have to be discontinued because of hematuria. The urinary output of a patient having radiation therapy to any part of the urologic system should be measured since tissue edema caused by response to the irradiation may lead to urinary obstruction.

The patient having irradiation treatment may not be hospitalized. If not, he and/or his family should be taught to recognize the untoward symptoms that may occur and advised to report these to the doctor. Appropriate preventive nursing measures such as the timing of meals, forcing fluids, and skin care should also be taught.

Radioisotope therapy

Radioisotopes are being used increasingly not only for diagnostic purposes but for therapeutic purposes as well. The action of radioactive isotopes is much the same as that of x-ray therapy: destroying tissue by ionizing radiation in the tumor area. A radioactive isotope releases excess energy in the form of nuclear radiation because its nucleus is unstable and is attempting to reach a more stable state. A physician will be responsible for the administration of radioactive isotopes in one of two ways; as a drug, which will be incorporated into the biologic system, or as encapsulated sources, which will be removed after a specific time elapse. The potential hazard lies in the fact that they emit one or two types of radiation that can be detected only by special equipment. General rules to follow are to keep as much *distance* from the center of radioactivity as possible and spend as little *time* in the vicinity of the radioactive source as is consistent with adequate patient care. Wearing rubber gloves when handling excreta or vomitus is also recommended. The nurse should check with the individual institution's policies and procedures regarding safety precautions in caring for patients receiving radioisotope therapy. The nurse should explain to the patient and his family and visitors any precautions being taken and the reason for them. The patient and his family should also be told that the danger to others will be negligible before he leaves the hospital. The patient should know he may summon the nurse whenever necessary.

Among the drugs used are chromic radiophosphate (P^{32}) given in approximate doses of 5 to 40 mc. It has been found to be effective occasionally for carcinoma of the prostate. Untoward effects include leukopenia, anemia, and thrombocytopenia. Also effective in the prostate is radiogold colloid (Au^{198}) in approximate doses of 75 to 200 mc. Radium-226 in the form of needles or capsules can be used for removable implants, and it has the advantage of a long half-life that eliminates the need for adjusting the dose. It is one of the most dangerous because it emits a high degree of gamma energy if the capsule is broken. Cobalt-60 is another of the radioisotopes used as a removable implant. It has the same disadvantages as radium. In addition, dosage adjustments must be made periodically. Radiotantalum needles (Ta^{182}) have been used effectively on bladder tumors, the dose being variable.

For permanent implants in a cancer that cannot be surgically removed, Radon-222 and gold (Au^{198}) seeds are used. Radon seeds are tiny sealed tubes (usually gold) that contain the emanations of radium. The half-life of radon seeds is about 4 days, and most of the emanations have disappeared at the end of a month. As with all such radioactive isotopes, radon seeds should be handled with a long-handled forceps and should be kept well above the waist to prevent irradiation of the ovaries or testicles of the handler. Techniques for handling and sterilizing radon seeds should be determined in consultation with the doctor in charge of radioisotopes.

Severe cystitis usually results from the implantation of radon seeds in the bladder. Sedatives, antispasmodic drugs, fluids, and local heat give symptomatic relief. Sloughing of tissue and subsequent hemorrhage may occur and should be reported to the doctor at once. The patient should be cautioned that he may pass a seed on voiding. Although the emanations may be relatively harmless, the seed should not be flushed into the sewage system. It should be retrieved with a long-handled implement such as a spoon and placed in a metal container and returned to the hospital or the doctor's office.

CARE OF PATIENT OUTSIDE THE GENERAL HOSPITAL

Urologic disease is often a chronic illness. Sometimes, however, it may be an acute, completely curable condition that can become chronic unless the person receives proper treatment over an extended period of time. Many patients will be treated for extended periods of time as outpatients. Many of the patients receiving medical care outside the hospital still require rather complex nursing procedures such as care of a catheter or other measures for the control of urinary drainage.

Home care

Since the patient with a urologic disorder may require much care at home, the nurse has a responsibility to teach the patient and/or his family about his disease and the hygienic and therapeutic measures pertinent to his proper care. A person who understands what he should do and why this is necessary is more likely to follow instructions.

Many patients are given medications and special diets. All too often the patient does not take the prescribed dosage of medications. He may not understand or may not accept the need to take them at specific intervals. He may cut down the dose or stop taking the medication entirely for several days. This may destroy the therapeutic effects of the drug. The patient should always be strongly urged to consult the doctor before making any changes, and he should know how to reach the doctor. Often the patient is not aware of ways to prevent side effects (for example, taking a certain medicine before or after meals). He should know about side effects that should be reported to the doctor. It is helpful to allow the hospitalized patient to take his own medications for several days prior to discharge. This provides opportunity for the nurse to supervise him and to foresee and prevent problems that might otherwise arise.

A patient may fail to take medications because he cannot afford to buy them. The nurse should know the approximate cost of drugs and should try to determine with the patient whether the cost will be prohibitive. If so, the assistance of the social service department is indicated. Sometimes mentioning the patient's concern over the cost to the doctor is advisable. He may be able to prescribe another drug that is equally effective but less costly.

Patients are more likely to follow diet instructions if the diet is planned to fit the usual food patterns of the family. The one who cooks the meals as well as the patient should always be included in the planning. If patients do not eat at home, they should be helped to plan for selection of food in restaurants. Sometimes hospitals provide menus from which the patient can practice food selection. The nurse and dietitian should assist the patient in selecting the proper foods.

Provision should be made for the patient who must perform procedures involving urologic nursing techniques to practice the procedures prior to leaving the hospital, clinic, or doctor's office. Whenever possible, written instructions should be available. The patient should be guided as to where necessary equipment can best be obtained and how to obtain emergency care.

It is advisable to have a nursing follow-up clinic staffed by a nurse competent in urologic nursing to which the patient can return for consultation and assistance when problems arise. If this is not available, the patient should be allowed and encouraged to visit or call the nurse on the inpatient urologic unit. He may be given the phone number and extension before he leaves the hospital. This would prevent many patients from becoming depressed and hopeless about their condition since frequently the management of nursing techniques is more troublesome to the patient than symptoms of the disease itself.

Referral of the patient to a public health nurse is often indicated. The visiting nurse may give further instructions and supervision of nursing techniques or she may need only to make a visit to supervise the patient in carrying out medical orders such as medication or diet prescriptions.

Nursing homes

Not all patients can be cared for at home and yet they may not need hospitalization. The family of these patients will need help in selecting a suitable nursing home or related facility. The doctor and social service department are often helpful in this but the nurse, too, should be able to give some guidance in suggesting to the family what to look for in selecting a nursing home.

The family who must take the responsibility for selecting a nursing home should be helped to realize that nursing home facilities vary widely. The type of care needed by the patient must first be determined by the doctor. A list of licensed nursing homes in the area should then be obtained from the local health or welfare department or the state department of health. Licensure, unfortunately, does not guarantee good care. It is therefore advisable to visit the nursing home during a busy period of the day. It is also a good plan to make inquiries about the reputation. It is wise to look into the medical and nursing supervision, the food service, the homelike qualities, the fire protection, and the cost of service. An excellent guide to help a family is the brochure *Thinking About a Nursing Home.** In making a final placement, some compromises may have to be made; the family must not expect perfection. Nursing-home care is *not* home care.

A nursing referral that outlines the nursing needs and the methods being used to meet these needs may make the transition from hospital or home to nursing home easier for the patient. The hospital nurse or public health nurse should make these referrals.

QUESTIONS

1. What should be included in a good nurse's notes?
2. By what routes are fluids lost from the body?
3. What is included in a good fluid data chart?
4. How does one compute the drainage lost in dressings?
5. What is the difference between a Rochester needle and a cutdown?
6. What hazards are involved in the use of the catheter?
7. What is the usual cause of epididymitis?
8. What are the usual indications for the use of a catheter?
9. What is the difference between a pyelostomy and a nephrostomy?
10. What is the difference between a cystostomy and a perineal urethrostomy?
11. Describe the care of the urethral meatus in a patient with an indwelling catheter.
12. What size catheter should be used routinely in the male? In the female?
13. How are filiform and followers used?
14. What is the difference between Pezzar and Malecot catheters?
15. List three types of self-retention catheters.
16. Describe two methods of aseptic catheterization.
17. Why should a catheter be anchored?
18. Why is it dangerous to have alcohol or other strong urinary antiseptics at the bedside?
19. Differentiate between an ambulatory, daytime catheter drainage setup and a nighttime catheter drainage setup.
20. Describe several types of bedside catheter drainage systems.
21. Describe a sterile closed drainage system.
22. Describe a method of catheter irrigation.

---

*Available from American Nursing Home Association, 1346 Connecticut Ave., N.W., Washington, D. C.

23. What do we mean by scheduled voiding?
24. Describe an external catheter drainage system for the male. How can this be improvised?
25. What is a Cunningham clamp?
26. What is meant by bladder training—with and without a catheter?
27. Describe perineal exercises.
28. How can one manage incontinence from fistulas or ostomies?
29. What is the difference between a regular ileostomy and a urinary ileostomy?
30. List several methods of managing urinary drainage from wounds.
31. How can one manage uncontrolled urinary incontinence?
32. What factors increase a patient's pain?
33. How much should the nurse tell the patient preoperatively about the anticipated surgery and its outcome?
34. Describe good mouth care postoperatively.
35. List several important postoperative nursing functions.
36. Why should sterile gloves always be used in handling any type of dressing on a patient's wound?
37. What is the difference between peritoneal dialysis and hemodialysis?
38. Describe a peritoneal dialysis system.
39. Describe a hemodialysis system.
40. List six different antibiotics, their routes of administration, and adverse reactions that might be anticipated.
41. What is the mechanism of methenamine mandelate action?
42. Name three antibiotics in the cephalosporin family.
43. Name two drugs highly effective against *Pseudomonas* organisms.
44. Describe a chemotherapy perfusion system.
45. List four chemotherapeutic agents used to combat cancer.
46. What is the most common danger in the use of chemotherapy?
47. Name four types of chemotherapeutic agents.
48. Name three different diuretic agents.
49. Name two types of irradiation therapy.

REFERENCES
Urinary output and catheter care

Andriole, V. T., Stamey, T. A., Kunin, C. M., and Martin, C. M.: Preventing catheter-induced urinary tract infections, Hosp. Prac. 3:61, 1969.

Campbell, M., and Harrison, J. H.: Urology, ed. 3, Philadelphia, 1970, W. B. Saunders Co.

Clifton, J.: Collecting 24-hour urine specimens from infants, Amer. J. Nurs. 69:1660, 1969.

Finkelberg, Z., and Kunin, C. M.: Clinical evaluation of closed urinary drainage systems, J.A.M.A. 207:1657, 1969.

Guarding against retrograde infection in urinary drainage (editorial), Nation's Hosp. 1:17, 1968.

Krisman, A. M., and Henderson, R. B.: Suprapubic bladder drainage following anterior vaginal wall repair, Canad. Med. Ass. J. 101:164, 1969.

Krusen, F. H., Kottke, F., and Elwood, P. M.: Handbook of physical medicine and rehabilitation, Philadelphia, 1965, W. B. Saunders Co., chap. 31.

Linden, R., and Keane, A. T.: The catheter team, Amer. J. Nurs. 64:128, 1964.

MacKinnon, H. W.: Urinary drainage: the problem of asepsis, Amer. J. Nurs. 65:112, 1965.

Martin, A. M.: Nursing care in cervical cord injury, Amer. J. Nurs. 63:60, 1963.

Prather, G. C., and Sears, B. R.: Pyelonephritis. In defense of the urethral catheter, J.A.M.A. 170:1030, 1959.

Santora, D.: Preventing hospital-acquired urinary infection, Amer. J. Nurs. 66:790, 1966.

Shafer, K. N., Sawyer, J. R., McCluskey, A. M., Beck, E. L., and Phipps, W. H.: Medical-surgical nursing, ed. 5, St. Louis, 1971, The C. V. Mosby Co.

Smith, L. H., and Martin, W. J.: Infections of the urinary tract, Med. Clin. N. Amer. **50:**1127, 1966.

Thompson, L. R.: Evaluating disinfectants, Amer. J. Nurs. **62:**82, 1962.

Zinner, N. R., Kenney, G. M., and Weinstein, S.: Effect of bladder irrigation during indwelling urethral catheterization, J. Urol. **104:**538, 1970.

Urinary incontinence

Hill, M., Shurtleff, D. B., Chapman, W. H., and Ansell, J. S.: Bowel and bladder control, Amer. J. Nurs. **69:**545, 1969.

Middleton, P. M.: A dignified future for the incontinent, Canad. Psychiat. Ass. J. **13:**269, 1968.

Robertson, C.: Manual expression of urine, Amer. J. Nurs. **59:**840, 1959.

Trainham, G., and Montgomery, J. C.: Developmental factors in learning bowel and bladder control, Amer. J. Nurs. **46:**841, 1946.

Fluid and electrolyte balance

Anthony, C. P.: Fluid imbalances—formidable foes to survival, Amer. J. Nurs. **63:**75, 1963.

Berry, M. A., and Kerlin, C. B.: The drops of life: fluids and electrolytes, RN **33:**35, 1970.

Burgess, R. E.: Fluids and electrolytes, Amer. J. Nurs. **65:**90, 1965.

Deane, N.: Kidney and electrolytes. Foundations of clinical diagnosis and physiologic therapy, Englewood Cliffs, N. J., 1966, Prentice-Hall, Inc.

Fielo, S. B.: Teaching fluid and electrolyte balance, Nurs. Outlook **13:**43, 1965.

Matheny, N. M., and Snively, W.: Nurses handbook of fluid balance, Philadelphia, 1967, J. B. Lippincott Co.

Potassium imbalance (programmed instruction), Amer. J. Nurs. **67:**343, 1967.

Shafer, K. N., Sawyer, J. R., McCluskey, A. M., Beck, E. L., and Phipps, W. H.: Medical-surgical nursing, ed. 5, St. Louis, 1971, The C. V. Mosby Co.

Taylor, W. H.: Fluid therapy and disorders of electrolyte balance, Dorking, England, 1965, Adlurd & Son, Ltd.

Watt, B. K., and Merrill, A. L.: Composition of foods, raw, processed, and prepared, Agriculture Handbook No. 8, Washington, D. C., 1963, Agriculture Research Service, United States Department of Agriculture.

Urinary ostomies

Andersen, L.: Care and management of ostomies, Bedside Nurse **3:**24, 1970.

Hungleman, J., and Kolba, M. T.: Bridging the gap between hospital and home, RN **32:**56, 1969.

Shaw, B. L.: Current concepts of stoma care, RN **32:**52, 1969.

Care of patient with pain

Davis, J. E.: Drugs for urologic disorders, Amer. J. Nurs. **65:**107, 1965.

Jourard, S. M.: The bedside manner, Amer. J. Nurs. **60:**63, 1960.

Kaufman, M. A., and Brown, D. E.: Pain wears many faces, Amer. J. Nurs. **61:**48, 1961.

Knowles, L. N.: How can we reassure patients? Amer. J. Nurs. **59:**834, 1959.

Pain. I. Basic concepts and assessment (programmed instruction), Amer. J. Nurs. **66:**1085, 1966.

Pain. II. Rationale for intervention (programmed instruction), Amer. J. Nurs. **66:**1345, 1966.

Shafer, K. N., Sawyer, J. R., McCluskey, A. M., Beck, E. L., and Phipps, W. H.: Medical-surgical nursing, ed. 5, St. Louis, 1971, The C. V. Mosby Co.

Webb, C.: Tactics to reduce a child's fear of pain, Amer. J. Nurs. **66:**2698, 1966.

Care of patient requiring anesthesia and surgery

Adriani, J.: Anesthesia for infants and children, Amer. J. Nurs. 64:107, 1964.
Benz, G. S.: Pediatric nursing, ed. 5, St. Louis, 1964, The C. V. Mosby Co.
Cambell, M. B.: Anesthetist should visit the patient before surgery, Southern Hosp. 3:28, 1970.
Carnevali, D.: Preoperative anxiety, Amer. J. Nurs. 66:1536, 1966.
Clemons, B.: The OR nurse in the patient care circuit, Amer. J. Nurs. 68:2141, 1968.
Depee, J.: A critical time for preoperative patients; effective therapeutic communication in nursing, Monograph 8, New York, 1964, American Nurses' Association.
Dumas, R. G.: Psychological preparation for surgery, Amer. J. Nurs. 63:52, 1963.
Edgeworth, D.: Nursing and asepsis in the modern hospital, Nurs. Outlook 13:54, 1965.
Healy, K. M.: Does preoperative instruction make a difference? Amer. J. Nurs. 68:62, 1968.
Johnson, J. E.: The influence of purposeful nurse-patient interaction on the patient's postoperative course. Exploring progress in medical-surgical nursing practice, New York, 1966, American Nurses' Association.
Leithhauser, D. J., Gregory, L., and Miller, S. M.: Immediate ambulation after extensive surgery, Amer. J. Nurs. 66:2207, 1966.
Mousel, L. H.: Correlation of the old and new in anesthesia, J. Amer. Ass. Nurs. Anesth. 34:30, 1966.
Owens, E. J.: From one operating room nurse to another, Amer. J. Nurs. 63:106, 1963.
Payn, J. P.: Modern concepts of anesthesia, Nurs. Mirror 121:242, 1965.
Sawyer, J.: Nurse's preoperative visit can help allay urological patient's fears, Hosp. Top. 43:108, 1965.
Schroeder, L. M.: Immobility effects on urinary function, Amer. J. Nurs. 67:790, 1967.
Scully, H. F., and Stevens, M. J.: Anesthetic management for geriatric patients, Amer. J. Nurs. 65:110, 1965.

Dialysis

Cummings, J. W.: Hemodialysis—feelings, facts, fantasies, Amer. J. Nurs. 70:70, 1970.
Dunea, G.: Peritoneal dialysis and hemodialysis, Med. Clin. N. Amer. 55:155, 1971.
Foy, A. L.: Dreams of patients and staff, Amer. J. Nurs. 70:80, 1970.
Halper, I. S.: Psychiatric observations in a chronic hemodialysis program, Med. Clin. N. Amer. 55:177, 1971.
Hinckley, B.: The changing role of the dialysis nurse—her place in the structure of nursing service, Nurs. Clin. N. Amer. 4:395, 1969.
Kossoris, P.: Family therapy—an adjunct to hemodialysis and transplantation, Amer. J. Nurs. 70:1730, 1970.
Lennon, E. M.: The surgical dialysis patient, Nurs. Clin. N. Amer. 4:443, 1969.
Potter, D. J., Johnson, K. E., and Markovitz, M.: Maintenance home dialysis and the organ replacement era, Arizona Med. 26:29, 1969.
Schlotter, L.: Learning to be a home dialysis patient; trials and tribulations, Nurs. Clin. N. Amer. 4:419, 1969.
Schlotter, L.: What do you teach the dialysis patient, Amer. J. Nurs. 70:82, 1970.
Schockley, D. B., and Stiehl, R. R.: Hemodialysis in a community hospital, Nurs. Clin. N. Amer. 4:409, 1969.
Shafer, R.: Chronic uremia: Is death inevitable? Hosp. Manage. 109:34, 1970.
Stewart, B. M.: Hemodialysis in the home—the value of house calls by training personnel, Nurs. Clin. N. Amer. 4:431, 1969.
Two days of every week (editorial), Amer. J. Nurs. 70:77, 1970.
Wang, F.: Conservative management of chronic renal failure, Med. Clin. N. Amer. 55:137, 1971.

Antibiotics and chemotherapy

Aaron, H.: Drugs: some adverse interactions, Amer. J. Nurs. 65:1545, 1966.
A.M.A. drug evaluations, Chicago, 1971, American Medical Association.

Bergersen, B. S., and Krug, E. E.: Pharmacology in nursing, ed. 11, St. Louis, 1969, The C. V. Mosby Co.

Brand, L., and Komarita, N. I.: Adapting to long-term hemodialysis, Amer. J. Nurs. **66:** 1778, 1966.

Conn, H. F.: Efficacy of new drugs, Med. Clin. N. Amer. **48:** entire issue, 1964 (symposium issue).

Cox, C. E. O'Connor, F. J., and Lacy, S. S.: Clinical effectiveness of intramuscular sodium nitrofurantoin against urinary tract infections, J. Urol. **105:**113, 1971.

Davis, J. E.: Drugs for urologic disorders, Amer. J. Nurs. **65:**107, 1965.

Donaldson, S. S., and Fletcher, W. S.: The treatment of cancer by isolation perfusion, Amer. J. Nurs. **64:**81, 1964.

Downing, S. R.: Care during the exchange, Amer. J. Nurs. **66:**1572, 1966.

Fitzpatrick, G. M., and Shotkin, J. M.: Pelvic perfusion, Amer. J. Nurs. **61:**79, 1961.

Fox, J. E.: Reflections on cancer nursing, Amer. J. Nurs. **66:**1317, 1966.

Goldberg, L. I.: New potent diuretics, Hosp. Top. **46:**77, 1968.

Hall: J. W., III: Drug therapy in infectious diseases, Amer. J. Nurs. **61:**56, 1961.

Kautz, H., Storey, R., and Zimmerman, A.: Radioactive drugs, Amer. J. Nurs. **64:**124, 1964.

Levin, N. W.: Furosemide and ethacrynic acid in renal insufficiency, Med. Clin. N. Amer. **55:**107, 1971.

Levine, L. A.: Intra-arterial chemotherapy for the cancer patient, Amer. J. Nurs. **64:**108, 1964.

Murphree, H. B.: The use of potent analgesics, Amer. J. Nurs. **63:**104, 1963.

Physicians' desk reference to pharmaceutical specialties and biologicals, ed. 25, Oradell, N. J., 1971, Medical Economics, Inc.

Rodman, M. J.: Drugs for urinary tract infection, RN **28:**61, 1965.

Schneider, W., and Boyce, B. A.: Complications of diuretic therapy, Amer. J. Nurs. **68:** 1903, 1968.

Spicher, C.: Nursing care of children hospitalized with infections, Nurs. Clin. N. Amer. **5:**123, 1970.

Irradiation therapy

Boeker, E. H.: Radiation safety, Amer. J. Nurs. **65:**111, 1965.

Kautz, H. D., Storey, R. H., and Zimmerman, A. J.: Radioactive drugs, Amer. J. Nurs. **64:**124, 1964.

Renal transplantation

Felix, K.: Total patient care—the team approach to transplantation, Nurs. Clin. N. Amer. **4:**451, 1969.

George, C. R., Tiller, D. J., and Burrows, S. M.: Life with a transplanted kidney, Med. J. Aust. **1:**461, 1970.

Jonasson, O.: Renal transplantation: certain immunological considerations, Med. Clin. N. Amer. **55:**193, 1971.

Manax, W. C.: Human renal transplantation: progress in organ preservation in vitro, Med. Clin. N. Amer. **55:**205, 1971.

Short, M. J., and Alexander, R. J.: Psychiatric considerations for center and home hemodialysis, Southern Med. J. **62:**1476, 1969.

Tapor, M. A.: Nursing the renal transplantation patient, Nurs. Clin. N. Amer. **4:**461, 1969.

Care of patient outside the general hospital

Fellows, B.: Hemodialysis at home, Amer. J. Nurs. **66:**1775, 1966.

Jourard, S. M.: How well do you know your patients? Amer. J. Nurs. **59:**1568, 1959.

Morris, E. M.: Choosing a nursing home, Amer. J. Nurs. **61:**58, 1961.

Rossman, I. J., and Schwartz, D. R.: The family handbook of home nursing and medical care, Garden City, N. Y., 1961, Dolphin Books, Doubleday & Co., Inc.

Shafer, K. N., Sawyer, J. R., McCluskey, A. M., Beck, E. L., and Phipps, W. J.: Medical-surgical nursing, ed. 5, St. Louis, 1971, The C. V. Mosby Co.
Walstrom, D. E.: Initiating referrals—a hospital based system, Amer. J. Nurs. 67:332, 1967.
Winter, C. C.: Practical urology, St. Louis, 1969, The C. V. Mosby Co.

5

Age—a factor in the nursing care of the patient

Genitourinary disease may occur at any age. The nurse working on a urologic service therefore should be prepared to give nursing care to patients of any age, from newborn infants to octogenarians. The age of the patient influences his needs and must always be considered in determining and giving nursing care.

CARE OF INFANT (BIRTH TO 2 YEARS OF AGE)

Occasionally a baby is born with or develops within a year or two a urologic condition that necessitates hospitalization for a period of time. The nurse caring for a sick baby must not only provide for his clinical nursing needs but also try to see that his total development progresses as well as possible under the circumstances.

Psychologic needs

It is normal and necessary for a baby to be fondled and loved. This is essential for his psychologic development. The plan for care therefore should include time for cuddling the infant of any age, and as the baby develops, some time should be taken each day to play with him. To develop normally, however, the infant needs love expressed in much more than a physical way. The baby needs "mothering." This is a period of life when the mother and baby are normally together and it is therefore preferable that whenever possible the mother be available to provide the infant's "mothering" needs. It is probably not essential for the welfare of a young infant that the mother be present 24 hours a day. However, as he approaches the age of 2 years, it becomes more necessary (see discussion of preschoolers). Arrangements such as those discussed in relation to preschoolers may need to be made to accommodate the mother on the nursing unit. If the mother can-

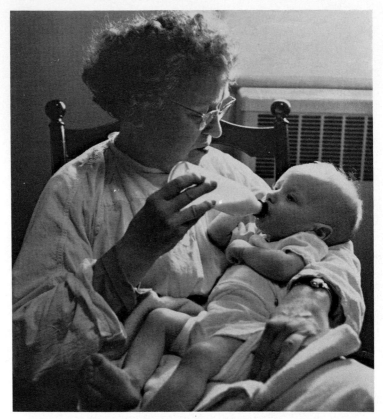

Fig. 5-1. Substitute mother gives infant bottle while sitting in rocking chair. (Courtesy Today's Health, American Medical Association, Chicago, Ill.; photograph by Dorothy Reed.)

not be with her baby, another family member such as a grandmother, a teen-age sister, or even the father may wish to assist with the care (Fig. 5-1). Sometimes a volunteer or paid worker may be assigned as "mother" for the infant whose family is not present. The nurse, of course, should herself provide some of the "cuddling" for infant patients as she gives them care, but her attention must by necessity be divided among many patients and therefore she is usually unable to be the mother-substitute.

It is possible to provide for the psychologic needs of infants in the busy hospital routine. Keeping a rocking chair available at the baby's bedside is helpful. Then, while the infant is being bathed and dressed or even while he is being given certain treatments, he can be held comfortably, talked to, and stroked. Some babies may have restrictions of movement and cannot be held. The resourceful nurse, however, will still find ways of providing loving care. Even a baby who cannot be held can be stroked and talked to; his crib can be wheeled back and forth in a rocking motion. The baby who has attached apparatuses such as catheters usually

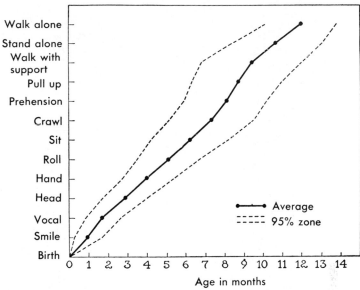

Fig. 5-2. Developmental graph for infant during first year of life. (From Aldrich, C. A., and Norval, M. A.: J. Pediat. **29:**306, 1946.)

can be moved safely provided those caring for him are properly instructed in the necessary precautions.

Physical development

Provisions should be made for the baby to have as much normal movement as possible. A firm mattress helps the sick baby who has poor muscle tone move about more easily. Any part of the infant's body that must be restrained should, if not contraindicated by his condition, be released at least every 2 to 4 hours day and night. At this time the baby should be allowed to move about freely for 5 or 10 minutes. No restraint should be removed without first consulting the doctor. If possible, the baby should be turned on his abdomen for about an hour twice a day. He may also be propped to either side for periods of time.

Although the sick baby may normally be somewhat retarded in development, it is inexcusable for this to be further delayed by failure to provide equipment and routines to facilitate normal development (Fig. 5-2). As the infant develops, he should begin to look about. At this time bright rattles or mobiles may be strung over the crib to provide exercise in eye movements. When the baby begins to clutch with his hands, a rattle or some similar toy should be provided. Normal development of the hands and of thumb apposition may otherwise be unnecessarily delayed. The baby may be hospitalized at the age when he begins to crawl and pull himself up. Unless it is contraindicated, provision should be made for a playpen

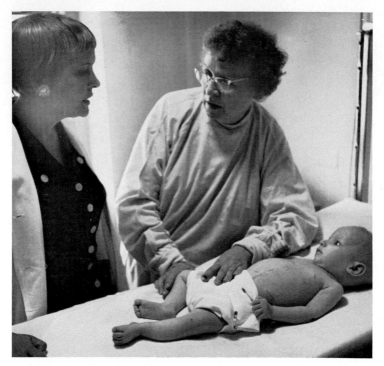

Fig. 5-3. Substitute mother changing infant's diaper when social service worker visits. Note well-healed wounds and that baby is being protected against accidentally rolling out of crib while side is down. (Courtesy Today's Health, American Medical Association, Chicago, Ill.; photograph by Dorothy Reed.)

or some other safe area where he may move about more freely than in a crib.

The nurse should be alert for any indications of abnormality in development and should report these to the pediatrician. If she has not had recent experience in caring for infants, the nurse may need to review child development in one of the many available textbooks on this subject.

Hygienic measures

Each day the infant's entire body should be thoroughly inspected. This is usually done during the bath. The eyes, ears, and nostrils should be inspected for discharges and cleaned as necessary. The skin and scalp should be observed for any lesions. Rashes on the back of the head, the buttocks, and perineum are rather common. These can be minimized by keeping the baby clean and dry (Fig. 5-3). If the baby has any urinary tract infection, special care needs to be taken since the urine is likely to be more acid or alkaline than normal.

When an infant is sick, the color, amount, and frequency of both his urine and his stools should be noted and recorded daily. The consistency of the stool should also be noted. Any changes in either urine or stool should be reported immediately to the doctor.

If the baby is hospitalized for a long period, plans should be made for him to be in the outside air and sun at intervals. Care should be taken not to chill the baby or to overexpose him to the sun, especially if he is on antibiotics.

Feeding

The infant must be given his regular feedings as well as fluids between feedings. Often an infant with a urologic condition will need extra fluid intake; the doctor should specify the amount and type of fluid. Plans must be made to space this extra fluid between feedings. Medications are usually dissolved in feedings; some may be given by medicine dropper. Even well infants usually receive vitamins A and D. A baby should be held for his bottles and medications since this prevents aspiration. It also may improve his appetite because most infants are used to being fed this way at home.

The nurse should consult both the urologist and the pediatrician about increasing the baby's dietary intake. There usually is no reason why the diet of a hospitalized infant should not progress with his age in the same way it would normally. Well babies, beginning soon after birth, usually receive prescribed formulas equivalent to 2½ ounces and 50 calories per pound of body weight a day. This is supplemented by orange juice and vitamins A and D. Solids in the form of the yolks of hard-boiled eggs and strained baby foods are usually started by the third or fourth month. Some doctors start babies on solids as early as 6 or 8 weeks of age. When the infant begins to get teeth and learns to chew, he is usually advanced to minced or chopped foods (junior foods). Most children go on an "adult diet" sometime between the eighteenth and twenty-fourth month. When a baby no longer takes a formula, his diet should include the "basic four elements."

Solid foods should be given before the bottle, and new foods should be started one at a time. If an infant rejects a food, a substitution should be made and the food tried again later. To train the child to chew, he may be given crackers or dry toast. Chopped food should never be given before he has mastered chewing.

Failure of the infant to eat properly may be a sign of any one of many serious disorders and should always be discussed with the doctor. Apathy to feedings and loss of appetite may signify uremia or incipient infection. Failure to gain weight in spite of taking feedings is always a serious sign. Unusual fussiness between feedings is often indicative of ill health. A satisfied and healthy baby usually sleeps soon after his feeding and awakens prior to the next one.

Changes in the character and timing of stools may indicate serious gas-

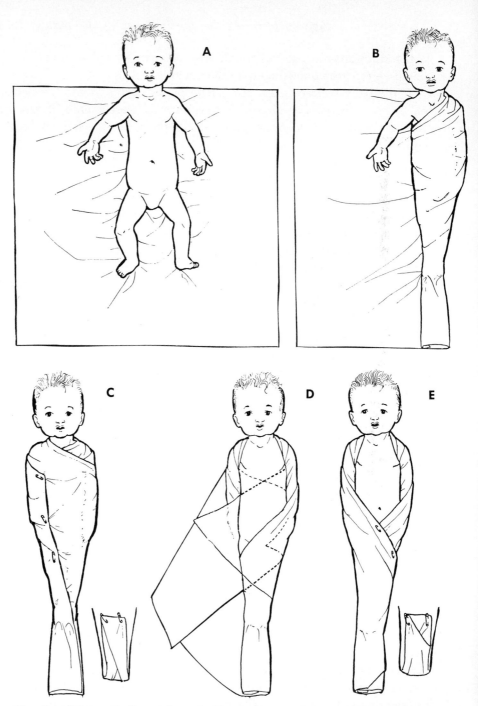

Fig. 5-4. "Mummying" an infant. **A,** Place infant on sheet or blanket to be used. **B,** Wrap one side of sheet snugly around and under baby so that one arm is at his side and legs are together. **C,** Bring other side of sheet across body, securing other arm at side. Pin securely at side and bottom. This method is often used when infusions are given into vessels in the scalp or neck. **D** and **E,** "Mummying" that may be used for abdominal dressings and other treatments. Note that arms are securely held at sides and legs are held out straight and are together.

trointestinal disease. Persistent vomiting, as contrasted with the normal occasional regurgitation that occurs in many well infants, nearly always is a serious sign and may be the first evidence of infections anywhere in the body or of intestinal obstruction. The infant cannot withstand inadequate intake of food and fluids nor the excessive loss of fluid for more than a few hours without developing signs of fluid and electrolyte imbalance. This is because only about 25% of the body fluid in infants is extracellular, as compared with about 33% in older children and adults.

Before the baby is discharged from the hospital, the nurse should be sure that the mother knows the formula he is receiving and how to prepare it. If no one is qualified to give this instruction, nurses from the nursery for newborn infants may be called upon or sometimes the nutritionist or dietitian will teach formula preparation. The visiting nurse can be asked to go into the home to give the mother additional help as necessary.

Safety measures

A baby, no matter how young, should never be left alone with the crib side down. If he is on a treatment or x-ray table, he should be held. For some treatments it may be necessary to "mummy" or place a blanket restraint on the baby to prevent him from moving his arms and legs. (See Fig. 5-4 for a description of this procedure.)

Since babies are usually quite active with their arms and legs, at times it may be necessary to use restraining measures to prevent a baby from pulling on catheters or dressings. Often elbow splints are sufficient; these prevent bending of the elbow but allow movement of the arm as a whole (Fig. 5-5). Since the baby is as agile with his feet as with his hands, a splint may need to be placed behind the knee. At other times it may be necessary to apply wrist or ankle restraints. These should be well padded and should allow for maintenance of correct body alignment and slight movement of the part (see Fig. 6-5). Special care must be taken to ensure that any splints are well padded and do not press into soft tissues lest ulceration of the tissue occur. No restraint should impede circulation to the part. Any type of protection restricting movement should be removed every 2 to 4 hours, and the baby should be encouraged to actively move the part while the nurse sees that dressings or tubes are not disturbed.

For a tiny baby a long gown, which fastens snugly in the back and can be tied below the feet, may suffice to keep dressings and catheters out of reach. A gown with mittens also may give adequate restraint.

When the baby begins to move about more actively, a harness restraint (Fig. 5-10) should be used to secure him in the crib. This slips over the shoulders and chest, fastens in the back, and is tied to the lower bar at the head of the crib with a square knot (this is secure but easily untied). Preferably the harness should be made like a vest, and its ties should be

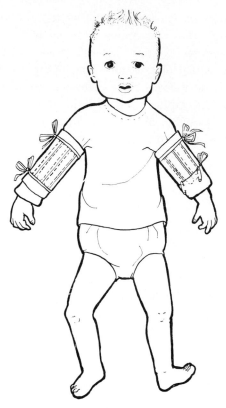

Fig. 5-5. Elbow splints prevent infants from pulling on catheters and dressings but permit free movement of shoulders and hands.

short enough to prevent the infant from becoming entangled in them and choking.

Care must be taken that no soft pillows, filmy plastic, blankets, or other material that might smother the baby is in contact with or anywhere near his face. Pins or any other objects such as glass connectors that he might accidentally swallow must never be left within reach.

Spiritual needs of the family

The religious or denominational affiliation of the infant's family should be ascertained, and the nurse should be meticulous in assuring that appropriate observances are carried out. She should always ask whether the baby has been baptized, and if not, whether the family wishes him to be. The family also should be consulted about their desire to have a priest, minister, or rabbi informed should the baby become critically ill. The nurse discussing the infant's progress with the family should assure them that their desires in these matters have been met.

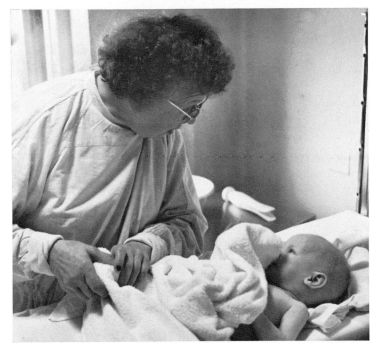

Fig. 5-6. Volunteer acts as substitute mother for hospitalized infant. Note she wears a gown and seems to be talking to baby as she bathes him. (Courtesy Today's Health, American Medical Association, Chicago, Ill.; photograph by Dorothy Reed.)

Therapeutic measures

In caring for an infant a cardinal rule to remember is "Babies are not little adults." Although an infant may have the same urologic condition as an adult, the disease commonly produces clinical manifestations different from those seen in an adult. Infants, when ill, often display a general systemic response such as fever, vomiting, and diarrhea; local manifestations are less prominent than in adults. Because of their extremely active metabolism, small size, and limited reserves (especially of fat and extracellular fluid), babies respond rapidly and critically to unexpected changes in the course of their illness. They may be apparently well one moment and an hour later, if symptoms are not observed, reported, and treated, they may be moribund. The younger the infant, the greater is the danger from generalized systemic involvement.

Young babies, especially ill ones, are very prone to *infections* and often die as a result of them. The nurse and others caring for a sick infant should wear an isolation gown (Fig. 5-6). Some clinics advise a mask and some use sterile masks and gowns. This is to protect the baby against organisms carried by those coming in contact with him. Careful hand-washing techniques are essential, and no one with an upper respiratory infection or any staphylococcal infection should care for the baby. The unit should be kept clean and dust free.

All treatments involving openings on the skin or entry into any body cavity should be carried out with utmost gentleness to prevent traumatizing tissues. Strict surgical aseptic techniques should always be followed.

Respiratory embarrassment is less well tolerated by a baby than by an adult. He is therefore more likely to develop hypostatic pneumonia and atelectasis. Following anesthesia the baby's position must be changed frequently (every hour), and it is desirable to invoke him to cry lustily since this aerates his lungs. The baby who has received an anesthetic often needs oxygen to make each inspiration more effective and to reduce the work of the heart in attempting to get adequate oxygen to all parts of the body. This is usually given by a small oxygen tent, head tent (Burgess box), or nasal catheter. Steam tents may be needed to loosen mucous secretions. (A pediatric textbook should be consulted for detailed discussions of these procedures.) Special care should be taken with an anesthetized infant to ensure that he does not swallow his tongue.

Any infant who is "croupy," has a dusky color, shows sternal retraction on respiration, or has irregular respirations (Cheyne-Stokes) needs immediate medical attention. The nurse caring for a sick baby should always know how to give mouth-to-mouth resuscitation. Excellent movies on this subject are available from civil defense organizations and drug companies.

A baby has greater nutritional needs than an adult and can survive for only a short time without nourishment and fluids. His glycogen reserves are minimal, and acidosis develops quickly. The skin surface is proportionately greater in an infant than in an adult and dehydration as well as chilling occurs readily. Diarrhea, persistent vomiting, and fever quickly dehydrate a baby. Flushed, dry skin, poor skin turgor, dry lips and tongue, sunken eyeballs, and general lethargy are indications of *dehydration* and should be reported to the doctor at once. If dehydration occurs, the baby will go rapidly into shock from loss of blood volume and death will soon follow. Because of the ease with which an infant becomes dehydrated and develops electrolyte imbalance, fluids and feedings are withheld only the minimal time necessary prior to anesthesia to ensure that the stomach is empty. Feedings are resumed as soon as possible and parenteral fluids are given until this time.

If a baby is too weak to take a bottle, he may be gavaged. (See a pediatric textbook for this procedure.) If he is unable to tolerate feedings by mouth, nutrition is maintained by giving parenteral fluids. Parenteral fluids are often given to infants by hypodermoclysis, injecting the fluid beneath the abdominal or scapular skin. A vein in the scalp, the femoral vein, or the jugular vein may be used as a site for intravenous infusions (venoclysis) given under pressure. A cutdown or Rochester catheter inserted into a vein in the leg or arm, similar to that done on adults, may be performed if a continuous drip infusion is to be given. Usually a 24-gauge needle with a short bevel is used for venoclysis in infants. If a baby needs additional electrolytes and tolerates fluids by mouth, oral formulas of electrolytic fluids are available. Otherwise, fluids must be given intravenously as with adults. (A pediatric textbook should be consulted for further details concerning the procedures used for administering fluids to children.)

Infants are rarely given cathartics or enemas to empty the bowel in preparation for radiography or surgery. Extensive purging often causes a loss of body fluids and electrolytes, especially potassium, in infants. Orders for cathartics and enemas should be carefully clarified with the doctor, and if either is given, the infant should be closely observed for signs of dehydration.

The infant is also more susceptible to *overhydration* than is an adult since his reserves of intracellular and extracellular fluid are proportionately less than those of the adult. If any signs of respiratory difficulty occur during an infusion, the rate of fluid flow should be sharply reduced and the doctor summoned immediately. The infant may be given fluids by continuous drip, but because of the danger of overhydration, he often receives them in small amounts by a drip-o-meter several times a day. If a continuous infusion is being given, the baby should be constantly attended lest signs of overhydration occur unobserved.

A restless, irritable infant may be manifesting *pain,* which he has no other way of expressing. The infant with severe intermittent pain usually cries sharply and his facial muscles contract. He is resistive to movement. Since pain is difficult to evaluate and localize in babies, any of these indicative symptoms should be reported in detail to the doctor. Narcotics are hazardous in infants and therefore are rarely prescribed. If a narcotic is given, the baby should be carefully observed since infants tolerate narcotics poorly. Codeine is usually the narcotic used for infants. Barbiturate preparations are considered the medication of choice.

The infant's family

The nurse should always remember that the baby usually belongs to a family who will be interested in the course of his illness and his general development. This is not information confidential to the nurse; she is responsible for sharing it with the family. Arrangements should be made for the family to speak with the doctor about the infant's medical progress and about plans for his continued treatment. The nurse can tell the family about any new symptoms displayed by the infant, signs of physical or psychologic improvement, and advances in normal development. She can also explain to the family procedures that the infant is undergoing.

When a family member is assisting in the nursing care of the infant, the nurse is still responsible for the care. She should specifically define that care for which the family member will be responsible and plan to teach her about the care and assist her with it as necessary. It is always best to assist the family member at least the first time she gives the care. When the nurse feels that her assistance is no longer needed, she should still plan to observe the care periodically and she should let the family member know she is always available to give assistance or to answer questions. The nurse usually gives the infant his medications and treatments, but if he will need continued treatment at home, the family member who will give this care should have the opportunity to learn and practice the procedures involved under the guidance of the nurse. Often a baby whose mother has been allowed to assist with his care in the hospital will be able to be discharged from the hospital sooner than otherwise because the family is less fearful and is prepared to provide continuing nursing care in the home.

Home care

It is usually advisable to arrange for a visiting nurse to make a home visit to any baby that has been hospitalized. Early referral should be made so that the nurse may visit the home before the baby's return to help the family make the necessary preparations. It may be helpful for the visiting nurse, before doing this, to visit the baby in the hospital. In writing the referral the nutrition, development, medications, details of dressings, and other treatments should be included so that the nurse in the home can give continuing follow-up and care.

CARE OF YOUNG CHILD

Young children include two age groups: those 2 to 5 years of age (preschoolers) and those in elementary school. The preschoolers, because of their age, do not express themselves with complete facility and often have not learned to cooperate with spoken instructions. They require a very different approach than the elementary schoolchild, to whom appeals can often be made with surprising effectiveness. The extent of development of the capacity to cooperate, of course, will vary; the needs and approach to each child will also differ in relation to his stage of development.

Psychologic needs

Separation from the mother is especially difficult and upsetting for the child between 2 and 4 years of age. Consequently, unless it is absolutely necessary, doctors do not like to hospitalize children in this age group but care for them whenever possible in the home, in an outpatient department, or in the doctor's office. The nurse in the doctor's office or outpatient clinic working with patients in this age group can be especially

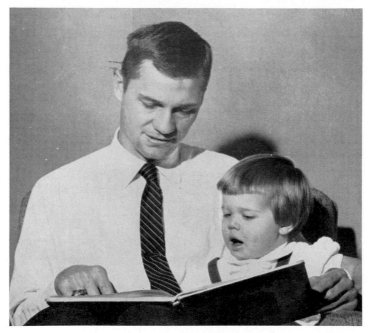

Fig. 5-7. Father spends time with his young daughter. (Bloom from Monkmeyer Press Photo Service.)

useful in helping parents understand the need for and details of procedures required by these patients. She should make referrals to public health nurses when further assistance is needed by the parents in providing the necessary care. If hospitalization is necessary, the child of any age should be prepared for the experience by his parents. The nurse in the doctor's office or clinic should be sure the parents know how to do this. It is helpful to the child if the parents tell him truthfully about the hospital and why he must go there. The child should be told about the high beds, bedpans, urinals, bed baths, eating in bed, the attire of nurses and doctors, and the play facilities in a matter-of-fact and reassuring way. He should not be frightened about the experience, but neither should he be led to expect the experience to be completely pleasant. If possible, the preparation for hospitalization should be done gradually. Well-written storybooks concerning hospitalization are available in bookstores and these may be helpful in introducing the topic.

The child of any age should know when his parents will be with him in the hospital so that he will not feel "deserted." Regular visits should never be missed (Fig. 5-7), and if frequent visits cannot be made, children seem to enjoy receiving some daily memento such as a brightly colored greeting card or a note from the family. Nurses should allow the child to keep the card with him and should be willing to read and reread it for youngsters of preschool age. When parents cannot visit, telephone conversations between the child and his parents give him some comfort.

Children, especially preschoolers, tend to form attachments with inanimate objects such as well-loved toys or blankets. The child should be allowed to bring a representation of home and comfort such as this to the hospital, and no one should worry if it is old or ragged. The object is the child's link with home and he should be free to take it with him wherever he goes, even to treatment rooms and to the operating room. This object, whatever it may be, is frequently an important comfort and security measure even for a sick child of school age.

It is important, too, for parents to allow children of any age, prior to their departure for the hospital, to help prepare for their return home. Often the child can pack a bag with clothes that he will wear on discharge from the hospital, or he may wish to help prepare the area of the house where he will stay while recuperating. This tells the child he is expected home again.

It is usually advisable, when facilities can be made available, for the mother to be allowed to "room-in" with her preschooler during the entire hospital stay. The elementary schoolchild will usually need her constant attendance only when he is to undergo anesthesia or an operation. Many hospitals have lounging chairs or cots placed at the child's bedside; some of these slide under youth beds and can thus be readily available. The mother's comfort should be considered and the thoughtful nurse will be sure that she knows the location of rest rooms, dressing and eating facilities, and a telephone booth. The mother should be informed about hospital regulations by which she is expected to abide so that upsetting incidences may be minimized. For example, it may be customary for the mother to leave the room during certain treatments or she may be forbidden in other children's rooms or in "workrooms" of the unit. Often, if the mother stays at the hospital with her child, plans must be made for the care of the rest of the family; the social service department of the hospital or of a public health agency may be helpful in this. It is certainly not always possible for a mother to stay with her child, and if she cannot stay, she should not be made to feel that she is a poor mother.

If the mother is unable to stay with the preschooler while he is hospitalized, his care should be assigned to as few nurses as possible so he can have a relatively permanent attachment to a few persons. This seems to add to his security. The "mothering" attendant, discussed in the section on care of the infant, is often useful. Frequent and regular visits from the parents are helpful, even though the child often ignores them during the visit and cries bitterly after they leave. The nurse should prepare the parents to expect this as the usual behavior; otherwise they are often most upset and feel tremendous guilt. They should realize that this is completely a "feeling" reaction on the part of the child and quite normal; no amount of reasoning with the child will change his reaction. He is angry at his parents because he thinks he has been deserted, but they should not add distrust to this by failing to visit at appointed times or by deceiving him in any way.

The preschool child has a tendency to show regression to earlier behavior patterns while in the hospital, on his return home, or at both times. This regression may take many forms. Some children return to earlier behavior of bed-wetting or soiling their clothes; others may have bad dreams and cry during sleep. Some refuse to eat; others revert to baby talk and whining or they may stop talking altogether. The child may be too good or he may be unusually naughty. Temper tantrums and clinging to the mother are common. If the child has to be separated from his mother, the regression may be more noticeable.

The parents often need guidance in handling the child of any age when he is discharged from the hospital. Both in the hospital and at home afterward every child needs to be assured by "mothering"; he is also reassured, however, by having to measure up to specific expectations in regard to behavior. The child of any age should be given some latitude of behavior, both in the hospital and at home, but some limits should be set and these should be made known to the child. On his return home the parents should resume their former expectations for his behavior.

The parents will want to know about their child's activities, behavior, and progress in the hospital. This is their prerogative, and although no child should be discussed with his parents when he is present, the nurse is responsible for keeping the parents informed and for making necessary explanations. This contact provides an excellent opportunity for instructing the mother in procedures she needs to know when the child is ready for discharge. Arrangements should be made for parents to discuss the medical aspects of their child's care with the doctor.

General care

Children respond best to as much normalcy as possible in hospital situations. There is rarely any reason why children who are not seriously ill or who do not have a fever cannot be dressed during the day. Most hospitals provide uniform suits and dresses as well as underclothing and night clothing. Children should be encouraged to continue activities they have learned to do for themselves at home such as dressing themselves, washing, and going to the toilet. It is helpful to learn from the child's mother what he does for himself and to make as few radical changes from the usual home routine as possible. Since children often are able to be up in the hospital unit, bathrooms should be adapted for their use either with low fixtures (Fig. 5-8) or by the use of sturdy step stools. Children usually

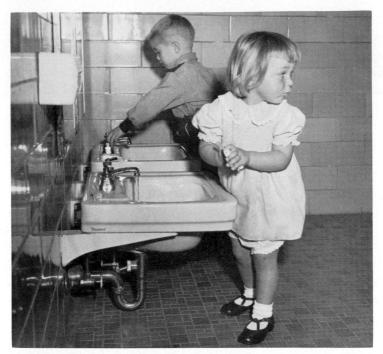

Fig. 5-8. Hospitalized children dressed and using bathroom adapted for their size. (Monkmeyer Press Photo Service.)

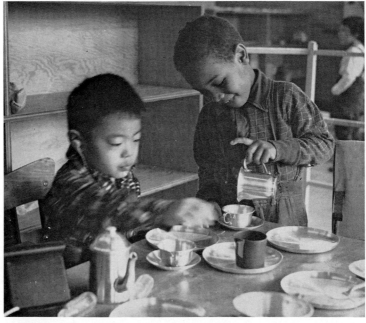

Fig. 5-9. Materials for make-believe play activities amuse many preschoolers. These two little boys are playing house. (Jan E. Ott from Monkmeyer Press Photo Service.)

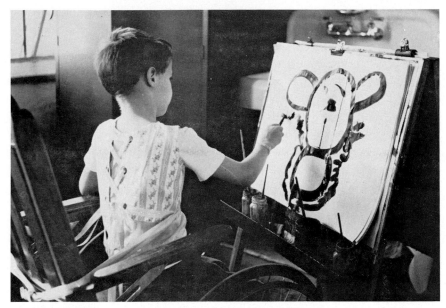

Fig. 5-10. Painting helps hospitalized child amuse himself. Note vest-type harness with back fastening used to hold him in chair. Note identification band on child's wrist. (Three Lions, Inc.)

eat better at a table with others. If the child must be confined to bed, the nurse should be sure he understands about the use of the bedpan, bed bathing, and eating from trays.

Eating during hospitalization may be a problem, but most children do better if not constantly coaxed. Many children in the younger age group are small eaters and finicky eaters. Making mealtime a party occasion is often helpful. Food likes and dislikes should be ascertained from the mother, and snacks between meals may supplement inadequate meals. The young child may be on a diet of chopped foods (junior foods); the child over 5 years of age usually is on an adult diet but servings need to be small. The older school-age child may have a voracious appetite. This is especially true if he is growing rapidly and is very active. Such a child needs foods high in protein and simple carbohydrates, but starches and fats should be avoided since overweight may become a problem.

Play should be provided and it should be suited to various age groups (Figs. 5-9 and 5-10). Preschool children often enjoy storytelling, crayoning, finger painting, and materials for make-believe play activities. The school-age child may be interested in reading, listening to records, observing and caring for birds or fish, making things such as model planes or jewelry, painting, or taking part in competitive activities.

If a child of school age is to be hospitalized or is sick at home for a long period of time (usually over 2 weeks), most boards of education provide visiting teachers and parents need to be reminded of this. Continuing with his schoolwork not only provides diversion for the child but also assures him of "keeping up" in school.

Any child who is confined to bed needs extra attention. Almost all children like to have stories read to them. Quiet play activities are also possible in bed. A variety of amusement is important because even the well child's span of attention is short; the sick child may tire of an activity even more readily. The child in the school-age group may prefer activities with others of his age, and this is usually possible but should be supervised to prevent undue activity for the bedridden child. A very sick child of any age may want little more than comfort, but this is just as important to him as is amusement.

Every child in the hospital and at home should receive some special attentions; the form will vary with the child. Many young children, even those of school age, need to be held and hugged occasionally; others respond better to interest in their activity or just quiet talking. Small tasks such as helping the mother or nurse pick up toys, clearing the table, or running an errand may also be assigned. Most children seem to enjoy this type of activity.

Discipline is necessary for the child in the hospital as well as in the home or school. The child should know the accepted limits for behavior and should be expected to observe them. Such a child is more likely to be a happy child.

Spiritual care

At the time of admission of a child the family should be consulted as to whether they desire a priest, minister, or rabbi called should the child require surgery or become critically ill. Visits from the clergy are enjoyed by many children, and often church groups are most helpful in providing volunteers to act as "mothers" or to organize play activities for hospitalized children (Fig. 5-11).

Therapeutic care

For painful procedures and for surgery, preschoolers and sometimes older children, too, may have to be *anesthetized*. A local or general anesthetic may be used, depending on the situation. The child should be told in simple terms what to expect before and after anesthesia. Storybooks about general anesthesia are available. Other children should not be permitted to observe a child receiving an anesthetic or any treatment, nor should they observe a child reacting from general anesthesia.

Children, especially those under the age of 5, like infants tolerate any systemic upset such as may occur with anesthesia and tissue trauma poorly. Their ability to withstand fluid and electrolyte loss is poor. (See this dis-

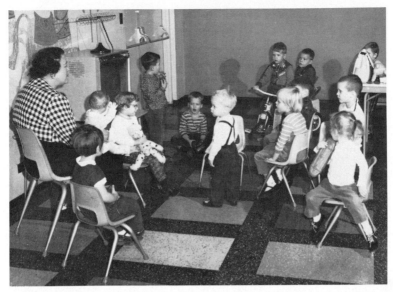

Fig. 5-11. This unit for preschoolers has volunteer who helps amuse children. Here, she is telling them a story. Note toys and television are available. (Courtesy Today's Health, American Medical Association, Chicago, Ill.)

cussion in section on infants.) Therefore the preparation of young children for anesthesia, surgery, or diagnostic procedures rarely includes extensive bowel preparation. An enema is often ordered, but if more extensive bowel preparation is undertaken, the child should be observed closely for signs of fluid or electrolyte imbalance (see section on infants). For the child under 7 years of age, doctors rarely order food or fluids withheld for extended periods of time. If the stomach must be empty for an early morning procedure, sometimes hard candy and fruit juice are given to the child at bedtime and again around midnight. Water is usually allowed until 1 or 2 hours before the procedure. Some doctors order sweetened fruit juice given in the early morning (6 A.M.) to children for whom a procedure is scheduled for late morning; those scheduled for afternoon procedures are often given breakfast. The child over 7 years of age frequently is prepared in a manner similar to an adult. If the child is dehydrated or has an abnormal electrolyte balance, measures are usually taken to correct the situation before the anesthetic is given or any extensive procedures undertaken. (See discussion on administration of fluids and electrolytes to infant.)

In preparation for anesthesia, children of any age are rarely given narcotics since they tolerate them poorly; small doses of phenobarbital sodium and scopolamine are usually given. Codeine, however, is sometimes used. Sometimes tribromoethanol (Avertin), prepared by the anesthetist but given by the nurse as a retention enema, may be administered before the child leaves his bedside to prevent his being unduly upset. A nurse whom the child knows or preferably one of his parents should always remain with him until he is anesthetized and should be with him as he awakens from the anesthesia. The child should be allowed to take a comforting toy along with him if he so desires.

During recovery from anesthesia, it is important to have the child breathe deeply to clear the lungs of anesthetic and to ensure full aeration. This can sometimes be best accomplished with preschoolers or even older children by playing a blowing game with them. Pieces of paper or lightweight objects may be blown across an overbed table (Fig. 5-12). Harmonicas or even blowing on combs covered with paper may give breathing exercise. Bottles arranged with tubes that allow water to be forced from one to the other by blowing (blow-bottles) provide another technique that may be useful. (See discussion of postanesthesia and postoperative care in Chapter 4 for additional information essential for providing adequate care.)

Many diagnostic, therapeutic, and nursing *procedures* are carried out *without anesthesia*. With preschool children, painless but strange procedures can often be accomplished most easily by the use of play techniques. The use of a rocking-horse seat for taking roentgenograms (Fig. 5-13) is an example. Devices of this sort are of value in many situations. For example, they may even be used for other things, such as holding a potty for collecting specimens. The resourceful nurse is able to devise many techniques of this type.

The procedure about to be performed and their part in it should be described to a child of any age. When they can assist in their own tests, older children are often more cooperative. Sometimes .they may watch the clock for the time to collect specimens or they may go with the nurse to prepare the materials for the test.

If the procedure will be uncomfortable, a parent or a nurse who is well liked by the child should be present to comfort and firmly hold him as necessary. If is often advisable to tell the child when he is about to be hurt. Restraining techniques such as "mummying" (Fig. 5-14) should be used as necessary for the safety of the preschool child. Restraints are rarely needed by school-age children who have been properly instructed. The child should be told truthfully what type of sensation he may expect. A matter-of-fact and straightforward approach usually gives the best results. Appropriate praise, comfort, and love should be given to the child of any age at the completion of a painful procedure.

Giving oral *medication* to children often requires an individualized technique. Forcing medications upon children should be avoided. If difficulty is encountered in getting the child to take a medication, the nurse should wait a few minutes and then try a new approach. It is helpful to ask the mother about methods she has found successful with her child.

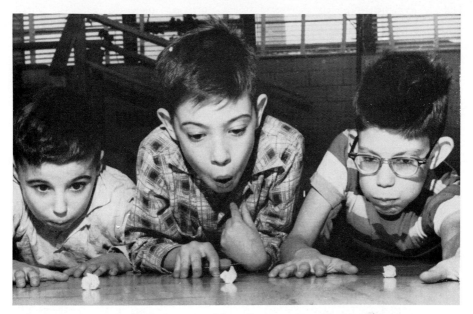

Fig. 5-12. These school-age boys need breathing exercise. They are competing to see who can blow his wad of paper farthest. (Courtesy Today's Health, American Medical Association, Chicago, Ill.; UPI Photo.)

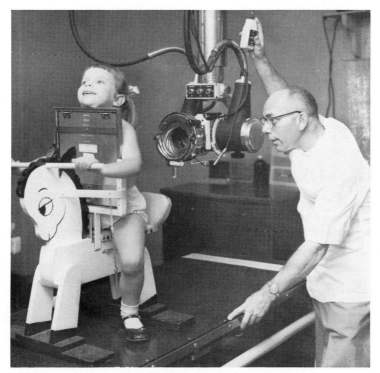

Fig. 5-13. A hobbyhorse to ride makes the chest roentgenogram a less upsetting experience for 4-year-old child. (Courtesy Today's Health, American Medical Association, Chicago, Ill.; UPI Photo.)

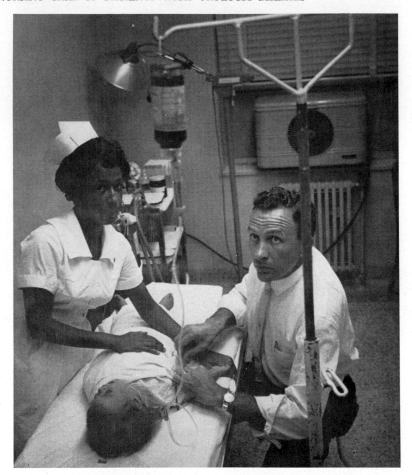

Fig. 5-14. Nurse comforts and holds little girl while doctor starts transfusion. Note this treatment is done in treatment room away from other children. (P.I.P. Photos by Bruce Roberts.)

Some children will swallow pills disguised with food; others will take them dissolved in small amounts of fruit juices, but care should be taken not to develop a food dislike by its use with medications. Children's medications often come in both liquid and pill form, and the child may accept one form better than the other. Usually children accept routines such as the taking of medicine better when they are among other children who are also receiving medications and treatments. Therefore it may be helpful to offer medications to children in a group situation. Special care must be taken, if this method is used, not to give drugs to the wrong child; the wearing of identification bands is advisable.

CARE OF TEEN-AGER

Teen-agers are usually assigned to an adult service in the hospital. Adequate handling of this age group offers a real challenge to the nurse

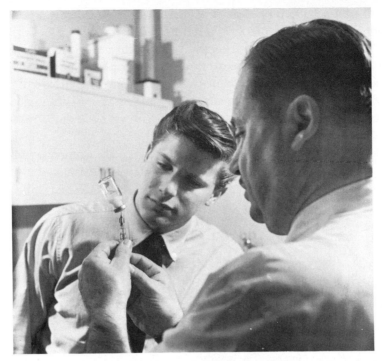

Fig. 5-15. Teen-agers are usually interested in learning. Male nurse is preparing drug for injection. Later, nurse will answer boy's questions. (Lew Merrim from Monkmeyer Press Photo Service.)

working in any situation. The teen-ager is neither a child nor an adult, and he may alternately respond and wish to be treated as either a child or an adult. This requires the nurse to "feel her way" and alter her approach accordingly.

Psychologic and spiritual needs

It is most important that the teen-ager's relative maturity be acknowledged by the nurse. She should talk to him as an adult. The teen-ager is likely to be flattered by this and is likely to cooperate well. Nevertheless, the nurse should be aware that the teen-ager has fears. She should anticipate these and by her manner let him know that she does not think less of him for showing them.

The teen-ager is usually interested in his disease and worried about his condition, even though he may appear very blasé and even disinterested. Unless the nurse makes a deliberate effort, this attitude may cause her to be negligent about exploring the true reaction of the patient to his condition and even about explaining procedures to him. Actually, the teen-ager is often eager for health teaching and is likely to accept it well. Teen-agers often enjoy discussions with a scientific flavor (Fig. 5-15).

Adolescents, both boys and girls, are likely to be quite modest. They should be ensured privacy, and any personal teaching or supervision such as that involving physical examination or the collection of urine specimens is more acceptable to them from a nurse of the same sex. If a male nurse is not available, the doctor will often give special attention to supervision of the boy. If a female nurse must attend to situations of this kind, an adolescent boy is much more at ease with a mature nurse than he is with a nursing student or a recent graduate who is near his own age. The nurse can help the teen-ager greatly by explaining factually what may be done by the doctor in the initial examination, the questions that will be asked, and diagnostic tests such as cystoscopy and radiography that he may undergo. He also usually wants to know who will be present during examinations.

Teen-agers worry most about being different from others in their age group. Surprisingly, many also worry about death, although they rarely mention this. The comfort and consultation of a priest, minister, or rabbi is therefore frequently desirable. The teen-ager should be allowed to express his fears freely and should be helped to explore them. The approach is similar to that described in the discussion of care of the adult.

Physical and developmental needs

Many boys and girls in their early teens are physically awkward and ill-coordinated since their growth during this period progresses in uneven stages. Care must be taken to place meal trays in a secure place and not to expect the young teen-ager to handle any tasks that would put him in the embarrassing position of "falling over" his hands and feet. Great tact is needed by the nurse to avoid being obvious about this.

The teen-ager, especially the young one who is growing rapidly, consumes large amounts of food. Girls between 13 and 15 and boys between 16 and 19 years of age need a greater caloric intake than at any other time during their life cycle. It is recommended that girls between 13 and 15 years of age receive 2600 calories daily; boys 13 to 15 years of age, 3100 calories; and boys 16 to 19 years of age, 3600 calories. Teen-agers often needed double or even triple servings of food at meals and nourishing snacks between meals. The nurse should see that the teen-ager gets enough food, and she should encourage good food habits to ensure an adequate nutritional intake as well as a filling one. Adolescent boys and girls need more iron and more protein in their diets than do adults.

Young teen-agers of both sexes are likely to be subject to disorders involving the skin. Acne vulgaris is a common condition at this age and is definitely related to the hormonal changes of puberty. There is no specific treatment for this condition, but washing the face well with a mild soap and water three to five times a day is recommended by many dermatologists. Vigorous scrubbing should be avoided and the pustules should not be squeezed. If possible, touching the face with the hands should be avoided. Blackheads can be safely removed by applying hot compresses for about 15 minutes and then using an instrument with a hole in a rounded metal tip that is especially made for this purpose. Drugstores stock this instrument. The doctor should be consulted about any infected lesion. Most doctors advise a diet low in starches, condiments, and fats. Rest seems to foster improvement. Illness may aggravate the condition and the teen-ager may need much reassurance that it will be self-limiting.

Teen-age girls often spend much time languishing and primping. They are flattered by attention by men but also enjoy "woman-to-woman" talk. The nurse should remember that illness may cause the menses to be skipped or to be premature. The girl should be told this, and she should be given instructions and necessary supplies for caring for her menses if they occur during her hospitalization. The teen-ager is often quite reluctant to broach this subject herself but may be, nevertheless, quite concerned by it.

Teen-age boys often try to get a "rise" from the young nurses by acting like a "man-about-town." At other times they may seem quite rude, failing to respond to people talking to them or responding curtly. If these reactions are handled in a matter-of-fact manner or ignored, they will usually pass. Boys, too, need to talk out their problems and feelings. The teen-age boy will often do this more easily with a mature nurse. Adolescent boys are often "panicky" about the effect of urologic disease on their sexual and reproductive activity. The nurse becoming aware of this should refer the problem to the doctor, who can give the best reassurance.

Teen-agers of both sexes usually enjoy reading, chatting, doing things with their hands, and participating in useful activities about the unit (Fig. 5-16). If they have hobbies such as stamp or coin collecting, the hospital stay often provides an opportunity for them to organize their collections (Fig. 5-17). The parents' cooperation in arranging for the necessary supplies should be enlisted. If the duration of the illness is longer than 2 weeks, plans should be made with the school to continue schoolwork unless this is contraindicated. There are various facilities available through the school. A teacher may visit the patient regularly for tutorial work, or some schools have an arrangement with telephone companies to set up an intercommunication system between the patient's bedside, whether at home or in the hospital, and the classroom. Television, especially educational programs, may also be helpful in profitably filling otherwise long and weary days for this normally active patient.

The teen-ager is usually considered an adult as far as physical aspects of preparation for diagnostic tests and therapy are concerned. There-

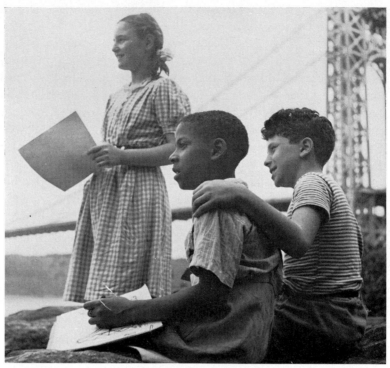

Fig. 5-16. Outside porch is available for use by hospitalized teen-agers. They find artwork a pleasant pastime. (Pinney from Monkmeyer Press Photo Service.)

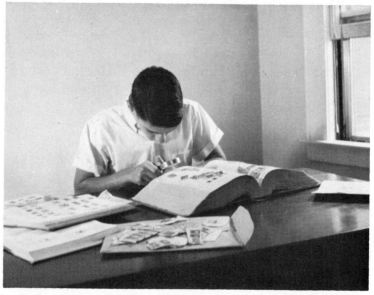

Fig. 5-17. Hobbies help teen-ager spend interesting hours while confined by illness. (Sybil Shelton from Monkmeyer Press Photo Service.)

fore all the general aspects of care discussed in Chapter 4 are applicable to the teen-ager.

In preparing for convalescent care, it is often helpful to discuss the plans with the teen-ager and his parents together. The teen-ager should participate in the planning because he is the one most affected by it; continuing progress will be dependent on his cooperation. He should be helped to make a realistic evaluation of his health situation and to set his short-term and long-term goals accordingly.

CARE OF ADULT

Too often the mature patient is considered to be one who, without outside assistance, can always handle all his problems except his medical one. Actually the adult often is confronted with the most acute socio-economic and psychologic problems of any patient, primarily because he is likely to have a spouse, children, or aging parents who depend upon him for support. Perhaps it is the complexity of the problems that makes nurses reticent about discussing them with patients. Nevertheless, the patient cannot settle down to the business of getting well if his mind is filled with anxieties.

Socioeconomic needs

The adult's major concern and worry may not be about himself. The patient may be the breadwinner for a family. How is the family being supported during his illness? How is he going to pay the doctor and hospital bills? The patient may be a mother with a family of small children at home. How are the children being cared for? The patient may have no family. Who will look in on him and help him "tie up the loose ends"? Who will care for him during convalescence? These are only a few of the pressing problems frequently facing the adult patient.

Help in planning to meet socioeconomic needs is available to patients through social work services in the hospital and of public health agencies. The nurse must become aware of the needs and make appropriate referrals. Since it is helpful if this type of assistance can be given to a patient prior to admission to a hospital, nurses in the doctor's office and in the clinic should be alert for patients who need this type of help.

Psychologic needs

The mature patient is often faced with the problem of being expected "to act like an adult." He may not feel free to show his emotions, believing that crying is for children. He may not feel free to express his fears or even to respond to pain by groaning or moaning. In consequence, he may unconsciously show his tensions in even less desirable forms—he may be extremely depressed; he may be demanding; or he may be overactive.

Fear is common in patients with urologic disorders. Although most laymen have only a vague understanding of the anatomy and physiology of the urinary system, they do know that the kidneys are essential to life. When told that they must have a nephrectomy, they may wonder whether they can live normally with only one kidney. Diseases that make voiding difficult not only cause discomfort but cause worry. Men are often fearful that disease or surgery involving the genitourinary system may decrease sexual capability. There is also a great fear of cancer among patients with urologic disease.

The patient who must look forward to a life that must be adjusted to intermittent dialysis will necessarily react in various ways. Inclusion of family members through all phases of such adjustment will be vital to both the patient's and his family's management and acceptance of his disease condition. Fear, anxiety, rejection, expression of anger, concerns of being a burden financially and physically, plus concerns about sexual activities must be expected and the patient and family allowed to express such feelings to the nurse and other team members. It should also be noted that those who work closely with this type of patient and family usually do so over an extended period of time. The nurse can become closely involved and may also experience feelings of anxiety and anger when a patient is uncooperative and refuses to follow instructions or the patient's condition progressively deteriorates.

The nurse should help patients by allowing them to talk out some of their feelings. This can often be done by simply taking the time to listen and by feeding back an occasional question such as "Why?" "What can be done?" or "What makes you feel this way?" She may propose, if it seems necessary, that the patient discuss these matters with his doctor, clergyman, or a social worker. Often providing for use of a telephone or for an unscheduled visit with a family member, friend, or business associate may alleviate a problem.

The nurse should always be sure that the patient knows how to obtain the medical care he needs. If he is an outpatient, he should know how and when to contact the doctor. The patient who needs special equipment for his care at home should be given guidance as to where to obtain this and he should be taught and supervised in the procedure he must carry out. If further nursing assistance is needed in the home, he should be given help in arranging for it. If the patient is to be admitted to a hospital, he should be advised as to when and where to go and what to bring with him. The nurse on the hospital unit to which he is assigned should tell him about hospital routines and the unit facilities.

Procedures that the patient is to undergo should be explained to him either by the doctor or a nurse. The patient should know when he

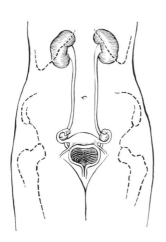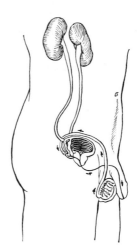

Fig. 5-18. Simple diagrams such as these may be used in teaching patients about female and male urinary and reproductive systems. (From Shafer, K. N., Sawyer, J. R., McCluskey, A. M., Beck, E. L., and Phipps, W. J.: Medical-surgical nursing, ed. 5, St. Louis, 1971, The C. V. Mosby Co.)

may expect to have pain, and measures should be suggested to minimize it. This also tacitly tells the patient that it is all right to express pain. The nurse should provide privacy for patients and should not show embarrassment if they cry; tears alleviate many tensions.

Patients are often too embarrassed to ask questions about which they are greatly worried. They may be inhibited by cultural background and emotional patterns in their discussion of the urinary and genital systems. Careful explanation of the procedures to be done helps to answer many of their unspoken questions and to allay many fears. For these explanations to be effective, some instruction in the anatomy and physiology of the genitourinary system may be helpful; simple diagrams can be used to advantage (Fig. 5-18). This instruction not only helps to overcome fear of the unknown but it also helps to make the genitourinary system a less unmentionable subject because the patient learns the terminology to use in asking questions.

Adults with illnesses of long duration also need *diversion.* It may be possible and desirable for them to carry on some of their usual business from their bedside. Provision should be made for some social contacts. Many adults relish the opportunity to just relax and read or watch television or listen to radio. Others are happier keeping actively busy; they may like some occupational therapy or they may prefer to do useful activities about the hospital unit or for their own homes.

Each patient is individual and his diversional activities should be determined by his own interests and his physical limitations. The nurse must be cautious not to force her own interests or those activities she thinks desirable upon a patient. For instance, not every patient is out-going; some may detest group activity and may be perfectly content and mentally healthy with more solitary activity. Others may dislike oc-cupational therapy activities and prefer to play cards or watch television. The main concern should be for each patient to find an activity to provide some diversion from his illness and to prevent him from becoming totally inactive and withdrawn.

The acutely ill patient rarely feels like participating in any diversion and often prefers to rest. Reading his mail or the headlines of the news-paper may suffice. Occasional short visits by the nurse or close relatives and the giving of necessary comfort measures such as turning a pillow, changing a damp gown, or giving oral hygiene are all the diversion he may wish.

Physical care

Occasionally a lactating mother is admitted to a urologic inpatient ser-vice. Measures then need to be taken to provide for breast pumping at regular intervals or for the milk to be dried up, usually by giving stil-bestrol. Doctor's orders for treatment should be obtained within a few hours after admission because unless treatment is started soon the breasts may become painfully engorged. The nurse may find it helpful to consult nurses on the obstetric service for information and help with these pa-tients.

The adult patient quite commonly has been taking medication or following a special diet for a condition other than his urologic one. The nurse should be aware of this and must be sure that this therapy is con-tinued or discontinued, as indicated, so the unrelated condition will not complicate the urologic disorder. She must be sure that the patient is not taking any medications of which the doctor is unaware and that a medication given by the nurse is not also being self-administered from the patient's personal drug supply.

CARE OF GERIATRIC PATIENT

Many patients admitted to the urologic inservice are in the geriatric age group. This is especially true of men since benign prostatic hyper-trophy usually accompanies aging.

Aging is a normal process. Tissues lose their elasticity and become less resilient; all physiologic processes gradually slow down. The speed with which this occurs varies, depending on hereditary factors and the stresses of life. The limitations imposed by the aging process, however, are often directly related to the general outlook of the patient. What are his interests in life? Is he a part of the mainstream of life?

In caring for patients in this age group, the nurse must carefully evaluate each patient in terms of his physical limitations and his social and psychologic assets and liabilities. How can he be helped to maintain his independence despite limitations, or perhaps how can he be encouraged to regain an interest in life? The nurse who herself sees aging as a normal inevitable process, one requiring adjustments in living patterns but not a withdrawal from life, is best prepared to work with the aging patient. Her philosophy needs to embrace the concept of ever-changing life, not of approaching death.

The basic needs of geriatric patients are no different from those of other adults. They need to be secure, to belong, and to have feelings of self-worth and self-respect. A major problem for many persons in this age group is satisfaction of their emotional needs. Physical disabilities impose limitations; the ever-changing social structure and the inevitable death of relatives and friends of their own age group also demand adjustments. Constant frustration in satisfying needs tends to cause some patients to give up. The major aim in caring for the elderly patient is therefore to help him make the adjustments necessary to make life worth living.

Psychologic and spiritual needs

The maintenance of individuality and a sense of worth is very important to elderly persons. The nurse can initially help with this by calling the patient by his name and thus implying respect for him as an individual. Such terms as "grandma" or "grandpa" should not be used unless the patient indicates a desire for this.

The nurse should get to know the patient as a person. This is often easily done by simply taking a sincere interest in his topics of conversation; older patients frequently talk at length about their families and the past. This may give clues as to interests to encourage and problems confronting the patient. It also affords an excellent opportunity for the nurse to vicariously broaden her own perspective of life and thus be more attuned to interests of elderly people.

Elderly patients are often lonely, and they may appreciate visits with the clergy or others from their church. Some prefer to see clergymen from their local church rather than those assigned to the hospital. The nurse should not hesitate to convey this wish to the patient's family or directly to his home church.

Individual attention should be given the patient whenever possible. The use of volunteers for visiting is sometimes desirable. When visiting with elderly patients, one should remember that they are interested in the activities of young people and of the world about them. These interests often must be satisfied for them through the eyes and ears of others. They rather commonly relate the events and activities to their own past; this is understandable because the past comprised their active years when satisfactions

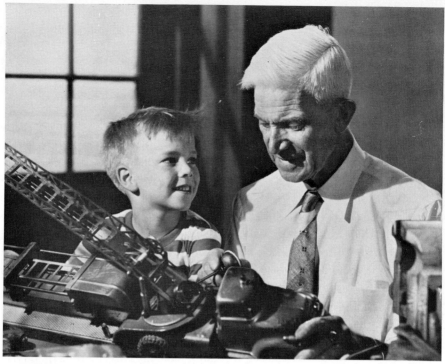

Fig. 5-19. This grandfather enjoys fixing grandson's toy. (© 1958, Parke, Davis & Co.)

were probably greatest and this should not be interpreted as disinterest in the present.

Provision should be made for the patient who requires long hospitalization to maintain his family contacts. Families, unfortunately, often tend to forget their older members when they go to the hospital. A grandfather or grandmother often wishes to see a grandchild and, if possible, this should be arranged (Fig. 5-19). Sometimes plans can be made for the patient to make a short visit outside the hospital. This is especially important if a wife or husband is physically unable to visit the patient. Arranging for telephone conversations with family members is also desirable.

Elderly patients are usually aware of death as an imminent possibility and often make surprisingly frequent and casual mention of death. The nurse should not avoid this issue. Nothing more may be needed than to quietly listen to the patient. A response such as "It's not unusual to feel this way when you are sick" does not prevent the patient from further exploration of his feelings nor does it give him false reassurance. After all, death is an inevitable part of life and becomes more inevitable with passing years. If the nurse senses that the patient is genuinely concerned about death, she may make a tactful inquiry as to whether he would like to see a clergyman, a family member, or the doctor or perhaps to arrange to trans-

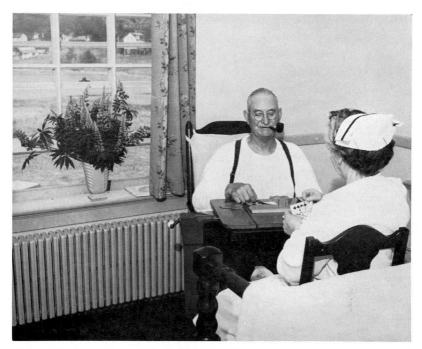

Fig. 5-20. Elderly patient enjoys game of cribbage with nurse. Note pants and suspenders being worn over hospital gown. (Brooks from Monkmeyer Press Photo Service.)

act some unfinished business. The nurse must never be unresponsive to such requests since they frequently are most important for the patient's peace of mind.

Most elderly persons want to feel useful. Depending on their abilities and interests, there are actually many tasks in which they can participate. Women may enjoy mending or knitting. If they are at home, they may be able to help with dishes or meal preparation. Men may be interested in repairing toys or making useful gadgets for the house. Many elderly persons enjoy painting. The older person may be quite slow in all his activities and great care must be taken not to show impatience since this often discourages further participation.

Chess, checkers, and cards are frequently enjoyed by elderly persons (Fig. 5-20). Many like to read; some are unable to see well enough to do so but are interested in listening to others read. Talking books, available through public libraries, may be appreciated. Television and radio may also provide desirable diversion.

Every means should be taken to keep the elderly patient as independent as possible, although physical limitations often necessitate some dependency. Totally dependent patients, however, often lose any desire to live; this tends to lessen the effectiveness of medical treatment in returning them once again to a more active life. Equipment that the patient may need should be placed conveniently within reach to prevent him from repeatedly having to ask for assistance. Self-help devices such as overbed trapezes or siderails that help him pull himself about in bed may be useful. Handrails along hallways and in bathrooms may allow him to walk about alone. Sturdy chairs with arms and wooden seats make it easier for many elderly persons to get in and out of chairs independently. Low beds also allow them to be more independent. If the patient normally uses a cane, glasses, or dentures, these should be readily available where he can find them.

Many geriatric patients can give most or all necessary physical care to themselves. Some may need encouragement to do so; others resent not being allowed to do for themselves. The nurse, however, must be patient and give them adequate time. The elderly patient often is exceptionally slow in the morning and it is therefore desirable to space activities accordingly. He may also tire easily.

Procedures should be explained to the elderly patient in the same way as one would explain them to any adult. Deafness is surprisingly common in persons of this age group, and care must be taken that the patient hears the explanations. It is always advisable to face the patient and to speak distinctly so that, if necessary, he may lip-read. If he wears a hearing aid, the nurse should be sure it is turned on. Many patients have better hearing in one ear than in the other, and if so, this should be noted on his nursing care plan. Written instructions are helpful for some older patients. One should also remember that the memory span tends to decrease with age and instructions may need to be repeated at intervals. It is unkind to show impatience with mistakes caused by failure to do this.

The elderly patient should be included in any discussion of plans for his future. After all, it is his future, not his family's or that of his doctor or others, that is being considered. His situation may require acquiescence to the wills of others, but he should at least be allowed to discuss plans with them.

Socioeconomic needs

The older person often lives on a limited income. All too frequently he has no medical or hospitalization insurance. An illness is therefore likely to cause financial worries. If a son or daughter is supporting him, he may feel that he is a burden and may worry about this. Accepting public financial assistance, although it alleviates immediate financial worries, may be a blow to the pride of many elderly persons and may markedly decrease their feeling of independence. It is sometimes helpful to remind them that the funds come from taxes and charitable contributions for which they, as citizens, have paid throughout the years.

The elderly patient may have a wife or husband whose security is in

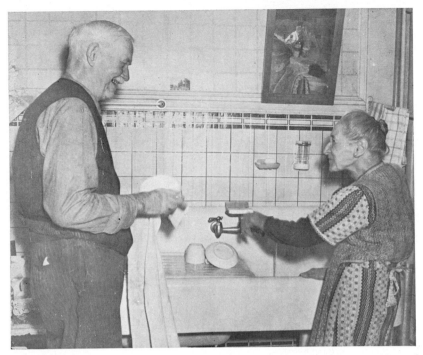

Fig. 5-21. Elderly husband and wife are often able to be helped to remain independent. Note heavy clothing and extra sweaters. (From Newton, K., and Anderson, H. C.: Geriatric nursing, ed. 4, St. Louis, 1966, The C. V. Mosby Co.; photograph by Anne M. Goodrich.)

some way threatened by the illness. He may have no family and perhaps no friends to turn to for consolation or help. An illness may mean he is no longer able to care for himself or to live in the same facilities; new living accommodations may be needed.

Facilities to meet many of the elderly person's needs are often available, but the nurse must assess the needs and make referrals through appropriate channels (Fig. 5-21). Needs may exist whether the patient is hospitalized, is being cared for at home, or is receiving care in a clinic or doctor's office. Referrals to social service agencies and to home nursing agencies are those most frequently indicated.

Physical needs

The aging process is one of physical deterioration. Because of this, the physical needs of the geriatric patient differ in some respects from those of younger patients.

General hygiene. The skin of elderly persons is thin and sensitive to pressure and trauma. The loss of subcutaneous fat and hardening of the surface blood vessels causes the skin to be wrinkled, sagging, and sallow. Seborrheic keratoses, lesions resembling darkened greasy warts, are com-

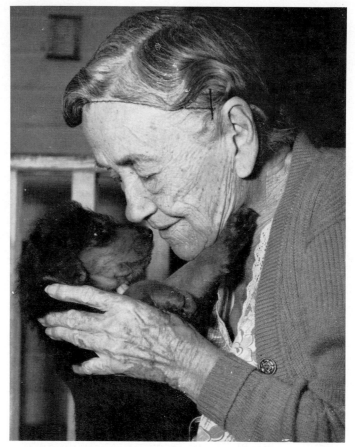

Fig. 5-22. Elderly patients retain former interests. Note discolored spots on skin and tiny raised area on eyelid. This is typical of skin changes frequently seen in geriatric patients. (VanDerMeid from Monkmeyer Press Photo Service.)

mon (Fig. 5-22). These are nonmalignant lesions but should be inspected frequently for any irritation or changes.

Because of dryness, poor circulation, and low resistance to infection, the skin of elderly persons readily becomes infected. Special care should be taken to prevent fungus infections such as epidermophytosis (athlete's foot). Elderly persons often need assistance in wiping their feet after bathing and cutting and cleaning their toenails. Nails are often hard and scaly; soaking the feet in warm water or applying oil to the nails for a day or two prior to cutting softens them and makes cutting easier and safer. A podiatrist should be called to care for very difficult nails.

Since the sebaceous glands in the skin atrophy with aging, the skin is likely to be very dry; daily bathing may be contraindicated. Usually a bath twice a week is sufficient. The use of mild superfatted soaps is advisable and after the bath, or more frequently if necessary, an emollient cream should be applied to the skin; the bony prominences should be lightly massaged. Washing of the hair should also be less frequent; shampooing only every 2 to 4 weeks with a mild soap solution or a shampoo with a nonalcoholic base is advised.

The incontinent patient should be kept clean by frequent sponging of local areas. Probably a daily tub bath is advisable in this instance. Tub bathing is desirable for most elderly patients to stimulate the circulation, but the tub must have sturdy handgrasps on both sides and a nonslippery surface to prevent falls. The patient often needs assistance in getting in and out of the tub.

If the patient is confined to bed, an alternating positive and negative pressure mattress may be extremely helpful in maintaining the skin in good condition. He should be encouraged to change position frequently, and bony prominences and weight-bearing areas should be massaged at least every 2 hours. Sometimes chamois skin or sheepskin pads placed under bony prominences prevent pressure sores.

Mobilization. If their physical condition does not contraindicate it, elderly patients should be encouraged to be active. Ambulation improves their general circulation and it improves their lung aeration. Older persons are susceptible to hypostatic pneumonia, and if they are confined to bed or chair, they should be encouraged to breathe deeply and to change position at least every 2 hours. They should sit and lie in positions that provide optimum chest expansion, and unless contraindicated, leg and arm exercises and full movements of joints should be encouraged. (See a textbook on fundamentals of nursing for a complete description of these exercises.)

Dress. When they are up and about, elderly patients should wear their shoes or supportive slippers. This decreases the possibility of accidental falls. Since they are likely to feel cold, these patients will usually want to wear socks or stockings. Many older patients will want to wear their socks in bed; some even wish to wear long underwear, flannel nightgowns, or sweaters. These seeming idiosyncrasies should be permitted when possible and plans should be made for laundry of this personal clothing. A family member may do this or it may be a nursing responsibility.

The patient usually has dentures and glasses; he may also have a hearing aid. Care needs to be taken to provide a safe place for the patient to leave these when he is not using them. He should also be given materials to clean his dentures and glasses and should be encouraged to wear them. Provision should be made for mouth care whether the patient wears dentures, has his own teeth, or has no teeth.

Diet. Eating may be a problem with geriatric patients. Many of their diets are habitually insufficient; others eat nutritionally inadequate diets. The older person needs fewer calories than a young adult since he is less active, but he does need a diet high in proteins and vitamins. Meat may need to be ground and vegetables may need to be pureed for patients with faulty dentitions. Using chopped (junior) foods may make preparation of meals simpler for the patient. If adequate food intake is a problem, food preferences should always be explored and an attempt made to provide foods palatable to the patient.

Elimination. Elderly patients may not completely empty their bladders or they may have some incontinence of urine. Bladder infection and cystitis are rather common problems. When a patient voids frequently in small amounts, his bladder should be palpated to be sure it is not distended and periodically overflowing. Toilet facilities should be readily available. Since nocturia is common, urinals and bedpans should be provided for night use or the patient should be in a low bed and night-lights should be left on to help prevent his falling enroute to the bathroom.

Constipation is another common problem and the patient may need a mild laxative routinely. Mild laxatives such as psyllium seed, colace, or milk of magnesia are usually given. Some patients may need small enemas or suppositories such as bisacodyl two or three times a week. A careful check should be made as to adequate bowel movements and fecal impactions should be avoided. A regular time for defecation and the drinking of prune juice is often beneficial.

Sleep. Older persons may often need to get up at night, thus interrupting a continuous night's sleep. Generally the desire to urinate is the reason. If the patient is allowed out of bed, this should not be discouraged. Safety precautions such as low beds, night-lights, and supervision should be employed, however. If the patient is not allowed up, siderails on the bed or even a Posey belt may be necessary to help the patient remember his surroundings if he is groggy on awakening. However, these devices may also exasperate and further confuse elderly patients.

For the elderly patient who is unable to sleep, nursing measures such as provision for planned activity during waking hours (walking, dressing self, etc.), warm milk, a soothing back rub, quiet surroundings, or a chance to talk are preferable to the use of sedatives. Afternoon naps can help break the elderly patient's rest pattern of arising at dawn and going to bed at dusk. Some patients may refuse the nap in the afternoon. In such instances very small doses of chloral hydrate may be prescribed. The enforced nap helps the patient stay awake longer in the evening so that some activity of interest to him can be planned.

Therapeutic measures

Elderly persons usually tolerate drugs poorly and may have bizarre reactions to them. Because of poor circulation, they are more likely than young patients to get a delayed cumulative effect from drugs. The nurse should carefully check for untoward reactions and report these to the doctor. Narcotics and sedatives are tolerated especially poorly. If the patient is emaciated or of really advanced years, the use of full adult doses of drugs should be questioned.

Older persons also tolerate loss of fluid and the withholding of food poorly. Their various body systems (circulatory, urinary, etc.) are likely to be functioning at maximum capacity with little marginal reserve; fluid and electrolyte imbalance readily ensues, with the patient going rapidly into shock. Caution must also be taken in giving fluids intravenously to elderly patients. Because of decreased elasticity of blood vessels and decreased cardiac output, the older patient who is given fluid rapidly may develop pulmonary edema.

Elderly patients who are undergoing diagnostic tests requiring withholding of meals or the use of enemas or cathartics should be attended unless they are in their beds because they often become quite weak and dizzy. No elderly patient should ever be left unattended on a treatment table and he should be helped on and off the table. Since he often is quite dizzy, it is advisable for him to arise slowly and sit on the edge of the table for a few moments before standing. Most elderly patients are less dizzy on resuming a standing position if the head has been elevated slightly while they are recumbent. The dizziness is caused by the slow compensation of their sclerotic blood vessels. Older patients with cardiovascular disease may also be orthopneic; that is, they may have to have their heads elevated to breathe adequately.

Because of the rapidity with which they develop decubitus ulcers, elderly patients who must lie on x-ray, treatment, or operating room tables for lengthy periods of time need thin pads placed under the "small" of their backs and a pad of material such as sponge rubber placed under bony prominences. Skin over bony prominences should be rubbed occasionally to improve the circulation to the area. On return to the unit the patient's skin should always be checked for pressure areas, and if any signs of pressure are evident, these areas should be massaged every hour until the tissue appears normal in color. If possible, the patient should be kept off these areas until signs of pressure disappear. If the patient is placed in a lithotomy position, care must be taken to place both legs in the stirrups at the same time to prevent undue pull on unresilient muscles; the backs of the legs should be padded carefully. Care must also be taken to prevent hyperextension and hyperflexion of the joints since many elderly patients have arthritic joints as well as osteoporotic bones that break easily.

The elderly patient, both before and after surgery, needs to be encouraged to eat a diet high in protein to aid wound healing; vitamin supplements are also often ordered because the elderly person is likely to absorb them from food less efficiently than younger patients. Since the older person has less resilient vasomotor control than the younger person and, at best, poorly compensates for even minimal drops in blood volume, he should always be well hydrated before anesthesia or surgery. A dehydrated older patient rapidly goes into shock although his blood pressure measurements may not show a precipitate drop as soon as it is apparent in younger patients.

The aging patient is less resistant to any infection than is a younger patient and he frequently develops a systemic reaction to it. Scrupulous care needs to be taken to prevent wound infection in these patients and to prevent the introduction of pathologic organisms into the urinary tract during catheterization and other procedures in which the urinary tract is intubated.

Geriatric patients usually have one or more chronic diseases in addition to their urologic problem. The nurse should be alert for the signs of chronic ailments such as cardiac decompensation, cerebral vascular accidents, diabetes mellitus, pulmonary emphysema, and arthritis. (See a medical nursing textbook.) Treatment of the coexistent chronic disease must be continued during the treatment of the urologic condition, and the nurse should be alert for accidental omission or discontinuance of necessary orders. Plans for nursing care of the elderly patient with urologic disease must often be modified according to his total limitations and therapeutic needs, that is, the urologic limitations and treatment and those limitations imposed by other coexistent diseases. Exacerbations of chronic diseases not apparent at the time of admission to the hospital often complicate urologic treatment in the geriatric patient, and the nurse should watch for and report symptoms suggestive of previously undiagnosed medical disorders.

The nurse in urology should be prepared to give care to patients with the chronic disorders listed in the proceding paragraph because they commonly coexist with urologic disorders in older patients. For the special nursing needs of patients with these and other medical disorders, a medical nursing textbook should be consulted.

QUESTIONS
1. How can the emotional needs of an infant be provided?
2. List the sequence of physical development in a baby through the first year and a half.
3. Why is it important to note the nature of the first urinary stream in a newborn infant?
4. Describe "mummying" an infant.
5. How do infants differ from adults in their response to illness and therapy?
6. Describe the needs of a preschool child.
7. Describe the emotional needs of a teen-ager.
8. What are some of the fears of an adult preoperatively?
9. Describe some of the problems in the care of elderly patients.

REFERENCES

Alexander, M. M.: Homemade fun for infants, Amer. J. Nurs. **70**:2557, 1970.

Ambler, M. C.: Disciplining hospitalized toddlers, Amer. J. Nurs. **67**:572, 1967.

Austin, C. L.: The basic six needs of the aging, Nurs. Outlook **7**:138, 1959.

Benoliel, J. Q.: Talking to patients about death, Nurs. Forum **9**:254, 1970.

Benz, G. S.: Pediatric nursing, ed. 5, St. Louis, 1964, The C. V. Mosby Co.

Berman, D. C.: Pediatric nurses as mothers see them, Amer. J. Nurs. **66**:2429, 1966.

Brooks, M. M.: Why play in the hospital? Nurs. Clin. N. Amer. **5**:431, 1970.

Bueker, K.: Adolescents need attention, Amer. J. Nurs. **60**:372, 1960.

Cohn, M. M.: The skin from infancy to old age, Amer. J. Nurs. **60**:993, 1960.

Daubenmire, M. J.: Pierce, L. M., and Weaver, B. R.: Adolescents in the hospital, Nurs. Outlook **8**:502, 1960.

Dawson, M., and Schultz, H. C.: Ministering to children in hospitals, Int. J. Relig. Educ. **32**:9, 1956.

Dittman, L. L.: A child's sense of trust, Amer. J. Nurs. **66**:91, 1966.

Drummond, E. E.: Communication and comfort for the dying patient, Nurs. Clin. N. Amer. **5**:55, 1970.

Errera, D. W.: Care of young urological patient, Hosp. Top. **69**:entire issue 1969.

Frenay, A. C.: Helping students work with the aging, Nurs. Outlook **16**:44, 1968.

Gaspard, N. J.: The family of the patient with long term illness, Nurs. Clin. N. Amer. **5**: 77, 1970.

Gillis, S. S., and Kagan, B. M.: Current pediatric therapy, ed. 4. Philadelphia, 1970, W. B. Saunders Co.

Glaser, B. J., and Strauss, A. L.: Awareness of dying, Chicago, 1965, Aldine Publishing Co.

Hamwi, G. J., Skillman, T. J., and May, C.: Nutrition in the aged, Geriatrics **15**:464, 1960.

Harris, R.: Advances in medical care of the elderly, Hosp. Progr. **50**:60, 1969.

Hess, E., Roth, R. B., Kaminsky, A. F., and McLaren, H., Jr.: Management of urologic problems in the aged, Geriatrics **15**:503, 1960.

Hott, J.: Rx: play PRN in pediatric nursing, Nurs. Forum **9**:288, 1970.

How confused is that elderly patient and why? Nurs. Update **1**:3, 1970.

Hymovich, D. P.: ABC's of pediatric safety, Amer. J. Nurs. **66**:1768, 1966.

Kangery, R. H.: Children's answers, Amer. J. Nurs. **60**:1748, 1960.

Lewis, C.: Nursing care of the neonate requiring surgery for congenital defects, Nurs. Clin. N. Amer. **5**:387, 1970.

Lowenberg, J. S.: The coping behaviors of fatally ill adolescents and their parents, Nurs. Forum **9**:269, 1970.

Ludick, E.: Nursing and the new pediatrics, Nurs. Clin. N. Amer. **1**:75, 1966.

Marlow, D. R.: Textbook of pediatric nursing, ed. 2, Philadelphia, 1965, W. B. Saunders Co.

Martin, S. E.: Party time in pediatrics, Amer. J. Nurs. **66**:1770, 1966.

Monroe, J. M., and Komorita, N. I.: Problems with nephrosis in adolescence, Amer. J. Nurs. **67**:336, 1967.

Moore, B.: When Johnny must go to the hospital, Amer. J. Nurs. **57**:178, 1957.

Moskowitz, E., and McCann, C. B.: Classification of disability in the chronically ill and aging, J. Chronic Dis. **5**:342, 1957.

Nash, B. E.: New dimensions in the care of the aging, Hosp. Progr. **51**:69, 1970.

Newton, K., and Anderson, H. C.: Geriatric nursing, ed. 4, St. Louis, 1966, The C. V. Mosby Co.

Norris, C.: The nurse and the crying patient, Amer. J. Nurs. **57**:323, 1957.

Pacyna, D.: Response to a dying child, Nurs. Clin. N. Amer. **5**:421, 1970.

Peszczynski, M.: Why old people fall, Amer. J. Nurs. **65**:86, 1965.

Prout, G. R.: Nursery nurses should be alert to urinary problems in children, Hosp. Top. **46**:88, 1968.

Robertson, J.: Young children in hospitals, New York, 1958, Basic Books, Inc.

Schlesinger, A. M.: Adolescence—time of weal or time of woe, Nurs. Outlook 8:496, 1960.

Schwartz, D.: Problems of self-care and travel among elderly, ambulatory patients, Amer. J. Nurs. 66:2678, 1966.

Scully, H. F., and Stevens, M. J.: Anesthetic management for geriatric patients, Amer. J. Nurs. 65:110, 1965.

Shafer, K. N., Sawyer, J. R., McCluskey, A. M., Beck, E. L., and Phipps, W. J.: Medical-surgical nursing, ed. 5, St. Louis, 1971, The C. V. Mosby Co.

Smolock, M. A.: The nurse's role in rehabilitation of the handicapped child, Nurs. Clin. N. Amer. 5:411, 1970.

Sorensen, G.: Dependency—a factor in nursing care, Amer. J. Nurs. 66:1762, 1966.

Stone, V.: Give the older person time, Amer. J. Nurs. 69:2124, 1969.

Tips in nursing management of the elderly patient, Nurs. Update 2:3, 1971.

Wallace, M., and Feinauer, V.: Understanding a sick child's behavior, Amer. J. Nurs. 48:517, 1948.

Webb, C.: Tactics to reduce a child's fear of pain, Amer. J. Nurs. 66:2698, 1966.

CHAPTER 6

Nursing functions in urologic diagnosis

Renal function is a prerequisite for life. It is therefore fortunate that with special tests and instruments available to the urologist, disorders of the urinary system can be diagnosed with an unusually high degree of accuracy. Some change from the normal pattern of micturition is commonly an initial symptom of urologic disorder. The nurse should urge anyone who indicates that he has any change in voiding pattern to seek urologic advice.

ABNORMAL PATTERNS OF MICTURITION INDICATING NEED
FOR UROLOGIC EXAMINATION

A decrease in the total daily urinary output to less than a pint (oliguria), unless accompanied by a sharp reduction in fluid intake or by excessive loss of body fluids by other routes, is a serious symptom. It is often indicative of renal failure; it may also indicate retention of urine in the bladder. It is therefore important for the nurse to assess the total situation and to report it to the doctor. The abdomen should be palpated to determine whether the bladder is distended or tender, and the patient should be observed for symptoms of dehydration. The fluid intake for the preceding several days should be reviewed and any unusual fluid loss by persistent vomiting, diarrhea, or excessive perspiration ascertained. If emptying of the bladder and hydration of the patient does not return the urinary output to normal, this should be reported to the doctor. Normally, liquid intake and urinary output are approximately the same. Unless the patient is being given diuretic drugs, a great excess in the ratio of urinary output to liquid intake (polyuria) is also abnormal.

Increase in frequency of voiding and a decrease in the amount of urine passed at each voiding or arising two or more times during the night to void (nocturia) is not normal. Difficulty in holding the urine for a period of time after becoming aware of the need to void (urgency) and involuntary and unexpected urination (incontinence) are indicative of urinary tract disorders.

Pain or a burning sensation in the urethra on urination (dysuria), painful spasms of the bladder after voiding (tenesmus), and difficulty starting the urinary stream (hesitancy) are common symptoms of urinary tract disease. Decrease in the size or force of the urinary stream and dribbling at the end of voiding are not normal.

Urine with an unusual appearance also indicates the need for medical attention. The discharge of blood from the urethra, before, during, or following micturition on even one occasion is abnormal. If this occurs in women, it must be ascertained that this is not menstrual flow. Phenazopyridine (Pyridium), a urinary analgesic, also gives urine a red color; occasionally, eating large amounts of beets will produce a similar color. Repeated output of deep yellow, cloudy, smoky, purulent, or malodorous urine is also abnormal.

It sometimes helps the doctor in making a diagnosis if the patient brings a sample of urine. Keeping a record of the *time* and *amount* of each voiding for 24 to 48 hours is also helpful. The patient can be instructed to do this himself. A calibrated measuring vessel, a watch, and paper and pencil are needed. If a suitable measuring vessel is unavailable, one can be made easily from a glass bottle by filling it with 1 ounce of water and placing a strip of adhesive tape or a crayon mark at the 1-ounce level, adding a second ounce and marking this point, and so forth. In follow-up urine examinations at home, Nitrazine paper to note the pH and Combistix to indicate the presence of sugar, blood, and protein are available. The patient should be instructed as to their use and recording of findings.

UROLOGIC EXAMINATION

The examinations and tests discussed in this chapter are commonly used in diagnosing many different urologic conditions. Examinations made in diagnosing specific disorders are discussed with the disorder.

Medical history and physical examination

The urologic examination usually begins with a complete medical history and physical examination, including pelvic and rectal examinations. Thorough examination is important because urinary symptoms may be secondary to disorders of other body systems. The nurse should explain to the patient the need for these procedures; she may do this as she prepares the patient for the examinations and as she assists the doctor.

It often reassures patients to know that medical information will be kept confidential. They should know that complete, frank answers to questions will help in determining the cause of any difficulty and in planning suitable treatment. Patients should be encouraged to discuss with the doctor any problems that may concern them but about which the doctor may fail to ask specifically. A woman should be prepared for questions she will be asked about her monthly periods, pregnancies, and deliveries. This gives her a chance to think through her answers under less pressure and thus give more accurate information.

The nurse should also assess the patient in as an objective manner as possible. Because this is usually a somewhat stressful time for patients, they do not always remember having been asked similar questions more than once. Through the nursing assessment, much can be ascertained that can make the hospital experience more palatable, lead to prevention of complications and discomfort, and provide an atmosphere for health teaching. Assessment of the patient should include an accurate description of the nurse's observations of the patient plus the patient's description of his feelings and complaints. Reviewing the patient's activities of daily living may reveal hygienic patterns that can be continued during hospitalization or, through teaching, improved during hospitalization. It is not unusual for the nurse to find patients practicing self-medication in addition to taking prescribed drugs. Such findings not only have implications in regard to the current reason for hospitalization but also for other family members and the time when the patient returns home. The patient's patterns of activity and or exercise should provide clues as to what might be expected of the patient when confined to bed or when limitations are imposed. An initial dietary history will allow for early planning and teaching, particularly when the patient is placed on a special or restricted diet. Facilities within the home may be found to be inadequate, such as toilet location and availability of water for cleansing and cooking.

Some patients will reveal more about themselves and their illness if they are provided with a basic list of questions to be answered at their leisure. Such an approach is less embarrassing for the patient who is reluctant to talk to strangers or who will provide only brief answers. If time permits such an approach, the history given by the patient can then act as a starting point for continued investigation into the patient's reason for seeking medical attention for the doctor, nurse, and other health workers coming in contact with the patient. It is not unusual to find the patient expressing more concern over financial, family, or other physical problems such as having their teeth pulled while hospitalized for urologic problems. The nurse must realize the patient's goals and reasons for hospitalization may differ from those of the doctor and the nurse, whose primary concern is the disease process. Planning with the patient and his family each aspect of his prescribed care is therefore a prerequisite in establishing rapport and working out as smooth a convalescence as possible.

The nurse should explain to the patient what the doctor will do during the examination and what he will expect the patient to do. It is important for a woman to know that a female nurse will be present during the examination and for a man to know that after the nurse has made the necessary preparation for his examination he will usually be left alone with the doctor. A male nurse may sometimes assist with the examination.

Both men and women often put off examinations that involve the genitourinary system because this type of examination usually arouses intense emotional reactions in both sexes. Fear, embarrassment, and cultural background play important roles in this emotional distress. In our culture, people are frequently afraid that their anxieties about cancer, venereal disease, or sterility will be verified. A person may also be fearful that some condition will be discovered that will require surgery or will result in sterility.

A calm, pleasant, interested, yet matter-of-fact manner often helps put patients at ease. The nurse should, however, appraise each patient and adjust her approach accordingly. Some patients, particularly girls who are very fearful, may need either a much more personalized or perhaps a more detached approach than usual.

Examination of female genitalia and rectum. The female genitalia is usually examined as part of a pelvic examination. However, only an external examination is done on children and teen-agers unless specific complaints are referred to the reproductive system.

The patient should be assured that her modesty will be maintained; while being examined she will be draped, the door will be kept closed, and a female nurse will be present. Ambulatory patients should always be told what clothing must be removed since panties or girdles interfere with the examination, waste time, and cause unnecessary embarrassment for both the patient and the doctor. The doctor should be consulted as to whether he wants the patient to void immediately prior to the examination. He usually will want this to be done since an empty bladder makes palpation easier, eliminates any possible distortion in the position of pelvic organs caused by a full bladder, and obviates the danger of incontinence during the examination. However, he may wish to have the patient void as part of the examination. Regardless of when the patient voids, the urine specimen should be saved. Usually this is a "clean catch" sample so that a culture of the specimen may be taken if desired. The empty bladder also permits the measurement of bladder residuum if indicated. In the practice of office urology the receptionist or nurse, when giving an appointment, should instruct the new patient to be prepared to furnish a urine sample. If it is known beforehand that a urethral discharge is present, the physician will want to examine the patient before she voids in order to collect specimens before the evidence is washed away.

Several positions may be used for examining the genitalia; the doctor will indicate the one in which he wishes the patient placed. The nurse

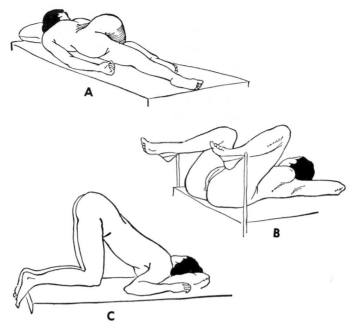

Fig. 6-1. A, Sims' (lateral) position. Note position of left arm and right leg. **B,** Lithotomy position. Note position of buttocks on edge of treatment table and support of feet. **C,** Knee-chest (genupectoral) position. Note placement of knees, shoulders, and head. (From Shafer, K. N., Sawyer, J. R., McCluskey, A. M., Beck, E. L., and Phipps, W. J.: Medical-surgical nursing, ed. 5, St. Louis, 1971, The C. V. Mosby Co.)

should determine whether the patient has arthritis or any other condition that would limit movement and prevent safe assumption of the desired position. Some of the positions used are uncomfortable and embarrassing for any patient, and the nurse should explain why the position is necessary for adequate examination.

When placing the patient in the *dorsal recumbent (lithotomy) position* (Fig. 6-1, *B*), the lower leaf of the examining table should be dropped before the patient gets onto the table. A footstool should be handy, and the patient should be guided to step up on the stool, turn, sit down on the edge of the table, and then lie back. It is better to place both legs in the stirrups at the same time. This must be done gently to prevent muscle strain; if the patient is anesthetized, this is essential. Metal stirrups are most satisfactory; however, if they are being used, the patient should wear her shoes because shoe heels help to hold the feet in the stirrups. When sling stirrups are used, care must be taken to see that there is no pressure on the legs since this can cause nerve damage. The buttocks are moved down so that they are even with the end of the table. The nurse should see that the pillow under the patient's head is pulled down at the same time to ensure comfort. The patient is then draped in such a manner that only the perineum is exposed. The triangular drape is most often used because it provides a flap that can be brought down for protection if a few moments should intervene between draping and examination.

If examination must be done in bed, the patient is placed across the bed with her feet resting on the seats of two straight chairs. This method can be used in the home if necessary. Or one or two pillows can be placed under the hips.

For *Sims' position* (Fig. 6-1, *A*) the patient is placed on her left side with her left arm and hand placed behind her; the left thigh should be at an acute angle with the body, and the right knee should be flexed upon the abdomen. She should be draped so as to expose the perineum. This position is also used for rectal examinations.

To place the patient in *knee-chest position* (Fig. 6-1, *C*), the lower end of the examining table is dropped and the patient gets on her hands and knees on the table. The buttocks will be uppermost, and the thighs should be at right angles to the trunk. The chest and the head rest on the table, and the head is turned to one side. The arms are raised over the head, and the knees should be apart. The feet should extend over the lower edge of the table to prevent pressure on the toes. The patient should be draped so as to expose only the perineum. If the examination must be done in bed, the patient should be placed crosswise on the bed.

Pelvic examination consists first of *inspection of the external genitalia* for signs of inflammation, bleeding, discharge, swelling, erosion, or other local skin changes. *Speculum examination* may be omitted if the patient is a virgin or a very small speculum may be used. Using the speculum, the doctor examines the vaginal walls and can see the cervix; thus it is possible to note any unusual signs such as alteration in the normal size or color, tears, erosion, or bleeding. The nurse should be sure that the light is adjusted so that the vaginal canal and cervix are well illuminated. An adjustable lamp gives the best illumination, but if such a lamp is unavailable, the nurse may hold a flashlight to provide suitable lighting. This is the time for the doctor to make a smear from the cervical secretion for microscopic examination and/or culture and for the semiannual Papanicolaou test for cancer. Two glass slides are used and dropped in a fixative solution of equal parts of alcohol and acetone before being sent to the laboratory. A *digital examination* then follows; for this the doctor will need gloves and lubricating jelly. Placing one or two fingers in the vagina, he palpates the abdomen with his other hand (bimanual examination). He concludes with a *rectal examination,* using one finger. By digital examination he can detect abnormalities in the placement, contour, motility, and tissue consistency of the base of the bladder and the uterus and its adjacent structures, including the ovaries, the fallopian tubes, and the rectum.

Responsibilities of the nurse during the examination include being present throughout the entire procedure for the protection of both the patient and the doctor, encouraging the patient to relax, and assisting the doctor as necessary. Additional equipment that may be needed should be available in the room so that the nurse will not have to leave the patient unattended; the equipment needed will depend upon the doctor and the patient.

Following the examination the nurse should quickly remove any lubricating jelly or discharge that may be on the patient's genitalia. Special perfumed cleansing pads are commercially available for this purpose. She should assist the patient from the table, taking both legs out of the stirrups simultaneously. In elderly patients, unnatural positions such as the knee-chest and lithotomy positions may alter the normal circulation of the blood sufficiently to cause faintness. Extreme care must be taken not to leave these patients sitting on the table; with the aid of a footstool, the nurse should assist them from the table and help them to a chair where they may wish to rest for a short time. If necessary, the nurse may help the patient to dress, and during this time or later she may explain any statements made by the doctor that are not clear to the patient.

Equipment should be rinsed with cold water, washed well with soap and water, rinsed, and sterilized. The linen on the table should be changed. The nurse should form the habit of washing her hands thoroughly after handling used equipment and should be especially careful to keep her contaminated hands away from her eyes and face to prevent infection with organisms such as gonococcus or tuberculosis.

Examination of male genitalia and rectum. Physical examination of the reproductive system of a man consists of careful inspection and palpation of the scrotum, noting skin, lesions, differences in size and contour of the scrotum, and any evidence of swelling. Transillumination of the scrotum is done to detect hydroceles and spermatoceles or any unusual enlargement of the structures contained within the scrotal sac. This must be carried out in a darkened room. Only cystic masses will allow the light to produce a red glow. By means of a rectal examination (Fig. 6-2) the doctor can detect enlargement and determine the symmetry and general consistency of the prostate gland and any nodules in it or the adjacent tissues. The penis, foreskin, glans, and meatus are inspected for signs of lesions or other abnormalities.

The nurse should see that the patient is draped and that he understands what the doctor will do and what will be expected of him, for example, giving a specimen of urine and breathing deeply to make palpation easier for the doctor. He should not empty his bladder immediately before examination because the doctor may wish to inspect the urethral meatus before signs of infection are washed away. Also, by watching the patient void, the doctor may be able to identify signs of possible urethral

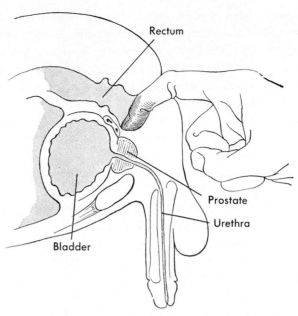

Fig. 6-2. Rectal examination to determine size and consistency of prostate gland. Note location of gland in relation to rectum. (From Shafer, K. N., Sawyer, J. R., McCluskey, A. M., Beck, E. L., and Phipps, W. J.: Medical-surgical nursing, ed. 5, St. Louis, 1971, The C. V. Mosby Co.)

obstruction. The female nurse prepares the necessary equipment and then leaves the patient alone with the doctor.

After the examination the male patient may have questions to ask the nurse. If he is to have special examinations or treatments later, the nurse is responsible for explaining the preparation and the procedure to him.

Examination of the newborn infant. There are times when the nurse may have the only opportunity to examine certain features of the newborn infant. She should thus be aware of the urologic conditions that require medical attention.

The nurse should always ascertain whether the baby is voiding, and she should observe the urinary stream and record this observation for future reference. Occlusion of the urethral meatus is an infrequent anomaly that, unless immediately corrected, causes death within a few weeks. Excretion of urine through an opening not at the tip of the penis in the male baby is indicative of a urethral anomaly. A male baby whose penis is curved should have medical attention, as should one whose foreskin does not readily retract. Male babies who do not have two testicles in the scrotum or who have any swelling of the scrotum should be referred to a doctor. Scrotal swelling such as hernias and hydroceles are not uncommon in young babies. The infant's abdominal musculature should be examined; protrusion of the abdomen may occur because of weak or congenitally absent abdominal muscles or umbilical hernias. This frequently leads to distention of portions of the urinary tract with resultant infection. Less than two umbilical arteries suggests the presence of genitourinary anomalies. A urachal opening may be present or the anterior bladder, abdominal wall, and genitalia may be absent (exstrophy).

Examination of urine. Urine specimens satisfactory for microscopic examination and for culture of bladder urine can be obtained from both men and women without catheterization. Unless catheterization is necessary for other diagnostic tests, the use of voided specimens has become a common procedure since the introduction of quantitative urine cultures. Bacterial infections of the urinary tract and the male reproductive tract rarely follow urethral intubation when it is properly performed in necessary circumstances.

A voided specimen or one obtained by catheterization of the bladder consists of urine that has passed through the kidneys, the ureters, and the bladder. If more definitive diagnosis is necessary, specimens may be collected from each kidney by ureteral catheterization during cystoscopic examination.

Uncontaminated urine specimens may also be obtained by needle aspiration of the bladder. This is rarely indicated.

VOIDED SPECIMENS. A specimen of urine is usually taken for *urinalysis* before other examinations are ordered. By urinalysis, abnormal constituents in the urine can be determined and these give important clues in diagnosis.

Sugar may indicate diabetes mellitus or a low renal threshold. Acetone may be found in the urine of patients with diabetes mellitus, but it may also be present in patients with ketosis resulting from other conditions such as starvation. The presence of acetone in the urine is common in infants and young children who have fever or who fail to eat for a day or two, because the glycogen reserve in children is lower than in adults. Plasma proteins in the urine such as albumin, globulin, or fibrinogen are suggestive of disorders involving the glomeruli. Because the size of the protein molecule determines the ease with which it passes through the damaged membrane, albumin, having the smallest molecule, is the protein found most often in the urine (albuminuria). Hemoglobin in the urine (hemoglobinuria) is caused by lysis of red blood cells; this may occur in the bladder because of strongly acid urine or it may begin prerenally in the circulatory system because of acute hemolytic anemia, a transfusion reaction from incompatible blood, or following exposure to cold. Red blood cells or gross blood in the urine (hematuria) is indicative of damage somewhere within the urinary system. Any abnormality in the specific gravity (below 1.003 or above 1.030) is usually due to inability of the renal tubules to be selective in resorption and excretion. For example, a marked decrease in specific gravity of the urine and an increase in the amount of urine is found in patients with diabetes insipidus and results from a deficiency of posterior pituitary hormone, which influences tubular water absorption.

A normal urine specimen does not necessarily indicate that there is no urinary tract infection or renal disease, nor does an abnormal one always indicate disease. For example, blood in a woman's specimen may be due to menstruation, albumin in a man's specimen may be due to prostatic fluid, and pus cells may have come from an adjacent area of infection such as the vulva or foreskin and not from the urinary tract. When a voided specimen from a female contains abnormal constituents, a *catheterized* specimen of urine is usually examined.

The specimen should be clean and should contain at least 75 to 100 ml. of urine. The external genitalia should be thoroughly washed prior to collection of the specimen. Preferably the patient should void directly into a clean specimen bottle; if another vessel is used to collect the urine, it should be thoroughly clean to prevent contamination of the specimen. First-voided morning specimens are preferable since they usually contain greater concentrations of abnormal constituents—one exception is in the check for orthostatic albuminuria. In this instance the first and second specimens must be compared.

When infection of the urinary system is suspected, a *urine culture* is ordered. A 5 to 10 ml. specimen of urine is collected in a sterile tube under aseptic conditions. This is sent to the laboratory where culture media are inoculated with the urine and any organisms present are allowed to grow. The organisms are then identified microscopically and their numbers estimated. This information guides the doctor not only in making the diagnosis but also in ordering drug therapy.

The culture tube should have a plastic top rather than a cotton or cork stopper since these could contaminate the specimen. The specimen should be labeled with the patient's name, the date, the cavity from which it was obtained, and whether it is a voided or catheterized specimen.

New screening devices for bacteriuria that can be carried out in a minimal amount of time are available commercially. Packages contain collection cups, pipettes, and culture plates from which the presence of infection can be confirmed, bacteria identified, and sensitivity to drugs determined.

To collect a *voided urine culture from a man*, the following procedure should be used. The prepuce is retracted and the penis thoroughly cleansed with a cotton pledget saturated with a mild antiseptic such as benzalkonium chloride (1:750); slight friction should be used and special attention should be given to the meatus. The patient is then asked to void about 15 ml., which is submitted for examination of the sediment. The patient then voids 10 ml. directly into the culture tube or the remainder into a small sterile pitcher (Fig. 6-3). If a pitcher is used, the urine is

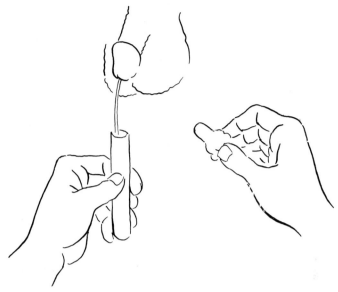

Fig. 6-3. Diagram of collection of voided urine culture from a man. Many times, wide-mouthed containers are used for collections. (Unpublished illustration of Dr. B. G. Clarke and Dr. L. Del Guercio.)

immediately poured into the culture tube or collection cup. This procedure is usually done by a male member of the nursing team or by the patient himself if he can collect the specimen with the necessary aseptic precautions after instructions. The second specimen is examined for albumin, sugar, acetone, casts, cells, and bacteria, and the pH is measured.

Voided specimens for cultures can often be collected *from small boys,* using the above method. An infant or uncooperative child may require the use of external drainage (described in discussion of collection of voided specimens from children). The tubing and collection bottle must be sterile. Commercially prepared, disposable units are also available for this purpose. They may be used for either male or female patients.

To collect a *voided urine specimen for culture from a woman,* the external genitalia should first be cleansed well with soap and water. Then, wearing a sterile glove, the nurse should separate the labia so that the urinary meatus is exposed and should cleanse this area as for catheterization. While the nurse (or the patient wearing a sterile glove) continues to hold the labia well separated, the patient voids. Some patients may be instructed to collect their own urine specimens successfully with the same technique. After the stream of urine has started, the sterile container is placed so as to collect a specimen. It is usually preferable to use a sterile pitcher and then immediately transfer the specimen to the culture tube or collection cup.

Voided specimens for cultures are extremely difficult to obtain *from very young girls,* but by applying a sterile Spicer urinal (Fig. 6-6) (described in discussion of collection of voided specimens from children), it is possible. Catheterization should be done when indicated.

The *two-glass test* provides separate specimens from a single voiding. This test is very helpful in determining whether the abnormality is below or above the bladder neck. Before the urine collection is attempted, the patient should be well hydrated and should have a full bladder. He is asked to void about 15 ml. into the first container; this gives the urethral "washing." Then he voids the rest into a second container; this gives the kidney and bladder "washings." If prostatic secretions are desired from a male patient, the best results are obtained by massage of the prostate gland via the rectum immediately after the second part of the voiding. This is collected on a slide or in a culture tube.

Urine specimens may be ordered to determine the presence of tubercle bacilli in the urinary tract. If a smear and culture for acid-fast (tubercle) bacilli are ordered, a specimen taken from the first voiding in the morning should be sent to the laboratory. The laboratory will usually supply the bottles for these urine samples, but if not, a sterile covered bottle should be used. The patient should void directly into the specimen bottle or into a sterile container, from which the urine is immediately emptied into the specimen bottle.

Urine may also be collected for *cytologic* or *Papanicolaou examination.* A first-voided morning specimen should be sent to the laboratory in a special bottle provided by the laboratory; this bottle usually contains 95% alcohol.

A *24-hour urine collection* is sometimes necessary. This may be analyzed for chemical content or it may be used as a culture for tubercle bacilli. The collection should be started at the appointed time by having the patient empty his bladder and this urine should be discarded. It should be completed by having the patient empty his bladder at the designated time and by including this urine in the specimen. It is important for the patient to understand that all urine must be saved during such a timed collection. He should be instructed to void into a separate receptacle before defecation lest part of the specimen be lost. Sometimes formaldehyde is used as a preservative. The specimen should be kept refrigerated. The nurse should always check to find out how much of the specimen the laboratory needs. If only a sample of the 24-hour urine output is needed, the total specimen should be mixed well before the sample is taken, and the total amount of urine voided in the allotted period should be recorded on the label.

When a test involves the collection of total urine output, it is important that the urine be collected from all available sources if more than the normal one exists. For instance, the patient may void normally yet have a nephrostomy tube from which urine drains. Specimens from each source should be collected in separate containers and marked as such since this may help determine the function of each kidney. Urine from a cystostomy tube and a urethral catheter may, however, be combined in the same specimen because both come from the bladder.

COLLECTING VOIDED SPECIMENS FROM CHILDREN. If the child is old enough to cooperate, adult techniques may be used. Infants and young children who are unable to use a potty require special techniques to collect voided urine specimens. Care must be taken to ensure that the apparatus used for collecting specimens from children provides for adequate and free drainage of urine and safety of the patient as well as for an accurate collection. Catheterization should be used as indicated. Regardless of what technique is used, several factors should be considered.

The genitalia should be cleansed with soap and water and rinsed thoroughly prior to the procedure. The collecting receptacle should be clean or sterile, depending on the kind of specimen the doctor wishes to be examined. Glass receptacles should have edges covered with adhesive to prevent cutting the tissues. The head of the bed should be slightly elevated so that gravity will aid the urine to run into the receptacle. The child should be restrained if necessary to prevent injury and/or contamination of the specimen. If the child is to be restrained for collection of a 24-hour specimen, restraints should be removed frequently and passive exercises given to the child if he cannot move himself. As little tape as possible should be used on the child's skin to prevent unnecessary irritation. The tape should be removed by pulling the skin away from the tape. Micropore paper tape is less irritating than adhesive tape. The child should be encouraged to take fluids. After the procedure the genitalia should be cleansed and dried.

One technique can be used to collect any type of voided specimen (single or 24-hour) from the male infant and from young boys. A finger cot or a finger of a soft rubber glove, adhesive tape, a large-bore connecting tube, drainage tubing, and a collection bottle are needed. Attach the open end of the glove finger or finger cot to the connecting tube by wrapping a strip of tape ½-inch wide, around it. Cut the tip from the glove finger or finger cot. Puncture it several times with a pin to allow air to escape when the child voids. Place the glove finger or finger cot over the penis and run a ½-inch wide strip of adhesive tape under the penis, bringing it around and crossing it over the lower part of the abdomen. The finger cot or glove finger should not be long enough to twist or constrict the penis. Attach the connecting tube to tubing and the collecting receptacle. Attach the drainage tubing to the bed to prevent the weight of it from pulling off the apparatus (Fig. 6-4).

For a single specimen an adequate size test tube may be used in place of the large-bore connecting tube. It is attached to the penis in the same man-

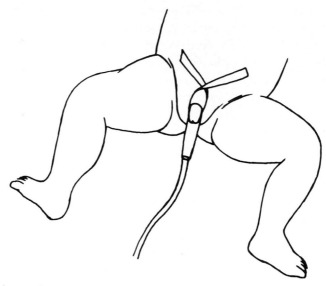

Fig. 6-4. Plastic sheath attached to baby boy's phallus to collect urine. Note tube that drains off urine into collecting receptacle.

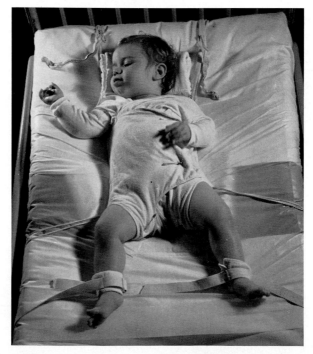

Fig. 6-5. Infant girl secured to bed prepared for collection of 24-hour urine specimen. Note well-padded ankle restraints. Flannel romper-type restraint with ties from back is used to support upper body and to prevent shifting of position. (From Geist, D. I.: Amer. J. Nurs. **60**:1301, 1960.)

A

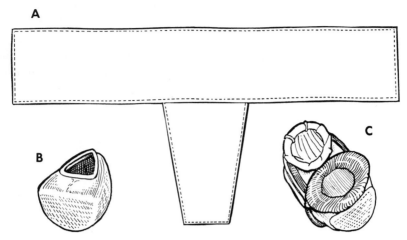

B

C

Fig. 6-6. Devices used to collect single urine specimen from an infant girl. **A,** ⊤ binder may be used to hold device in place. **B,** Birdcage feeder. **C,** Spicer urinal.

ner. An alternative attachment, when using the test tube, would be the use of a ⊤ binder. The test tube would then be inserted through the hole in the ⊤ binder, making sure that it fit snugly. The test tube would be placed over the penis and the ⊤ binder securely fastened. Depending on the age of the child, a mummy restraint (see Fig. 5-4), extremity restraints, clovehitch restraints, or a jacket restraint may be useful (Fig. 6-5). See a pediatric textbook for proper application of restraints.

To collect a single voided specimen from a female child, the Spicer infant urinal or a birdcage feeder may be used (Fig. 6-6). After cleansing the genitalia, spread the labia apart and place the receptacle over the urethra. The receptacle can be held in place by a tightly pinned ⊤ binder or a three-cornered diaper. If taping in place, strips of adhesive should run from the abdomen over the receptacle and under the buttocks. Restrain in the same manner as for a male child.

To collect a 24-hour specimen from a female child, a specimen halter that is attached to a plastic ring may be used. Plastic tubing attached to the ring is connected to a collecting receptacle.

Another method that may be improvised for small infants in an isolette utilizes a nylon sheet on which the infant lies. The sheet is anchored on rods and is suspended above a metal tray or similar receptacle. The infant lies uncovered on the sheet. Voided urine passes through the sheet, whereas feces are retained by it. The nylon sheet can be easily changed by slipping it off the rods and replacing it with a clean one. The infant's position can be changed frequently and his temperature maintained by controls on the isolette. Because the nylon sheet does not retain moisture, the skin is also protected.

Single or 24-hour urine specimens from male or female children may be collected with a commercial plastic urine collector, which is now available. The top is treated with adhesive-like material that sticks readily to the skin. This may be preferable to some of the techniques just mentioned since this adhesive seems to cause less skin irritation than adhesive tape and the same device can be used on either a male or female child. Either a single or 24-hour receptacle is available at a reasonable cost. Both types are disposable, eliminating any possible cross-contamination between children, as may occur when it is necessary to reuse equipment. If the commercially available plastic collectors are still inadequate, a pressure suction pump may be added. The plastic collector is modified by cutting the bottom and resealing to make a tent that lifts the bag from the skin and forms a dependent corner toward which the urine will flow. Two holes are made at the top of the bag, one through which a suction catheter is inserted, the point resting in the dependent corner of the bag. Through the other hole the air inflow tube is attached. The suction catheter is subsequently attached to a collection receptacle, which in turn is connected to the pump. Placing the infant in a slightly elevated position allows the urine to flow to the dependent corner, where it will be quickly removed via the suction. The air inlet will keep the skin dry and prevent excoriation of the skin. Tubing used in the system should have the same size lumens to maintain an even balance between air inflow and suction (Fig. 6-7).

DIAGNOSTIC PROCEDURES REQUIRING CATHETERIZATION. If a catheterized urine specimen for culture is ordered, the patient should be catheterized with care to avoid infection and trauma. After the catheter has been passed, a small amount of urine should be allowed to drain. Then, with care taken not to touch the rim or the inside of the culture tube or collection cup with the catheter or the hands, 5 to 10 ml. of urine should be collected directly into the tube.

Cultures are sometimes ordered of urine taken from the renal pelves during ureteral catheterization or when ureterostomy or nephrostomy tubes are in place. The ends of the tubes should be cleansed well with benzalkonium chloride (1:750) and the specimen taken directly into the culture tube or collection cup.

When collecting specimens from patients who have indwelling catheters, the system should not be disconnected, which allows introduction of bacteria. Most catheters are made of self-sealing latex, which can be punctured with a needle and urine withdrawn in a sterile syringe. Wipe the site of the catheter to be punctured with 70% alcohol, avoiding the lumen of the catheter that has been used to inflate the bag and in a three-way catheter the lumen used for input of irrigation fluid (Fig. 6-8).

The doctor may order a patient catheterized for *residual urine*. Normally, no urine remains in the bladder following voiding. If urine is re-

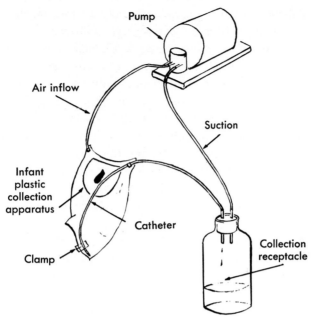

Fig. 6-7. System for collecting urine from infant plastic collection bag is shown. Note that air is forced into bag and fluid is suctioned from bag into collection bottle through the use of an attached pump.

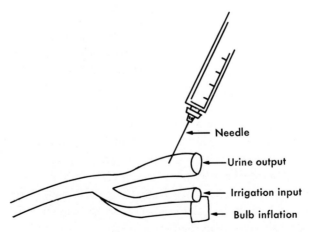

Fig. 6-8. When a three-way catheter is in use, urine may be aspirated from output limb of catheter by using a syringe and needle after washing outlet tubing with antiseptic. Urine may then be sent to the laboratory for culture and antibiotic sensitivity testing.

tained in the bladder, it stagnates and becomes a good medium for bacterial growth. It may also promote formation of bladder stones.

Immediately before a patient is catheterized for residual urine, he should empty his bladder. If there is a delay, additional urine will be excreted from the kidneys and an inaccurate result will be obtained. It is important to stress that the bladder be completely emptied because patients with urethral obstruction often tend to void only enough at a time to relieve the pressure. With additional effort, the patient may be able to empty the bladder completely. It is best to explain the procedure to the patient and then leave him alone for a few minutes. To evaluate the size and strength of the urinary stream and thereby estimate the amount of difficulty the patient has in voiding, the doctor may wish to observe the patient void. Since this observation is more meaningful if the patient does not know someone is watching, a basin rather than a urinal or bedpan may be provided and the screen or door left slightly ajar.

The nurse should check with the doctor before preparing for this type of catheterization because if he suspects a large quantity of residual urine he may wish the catheterization done with a Foley catheter, which can be left in the bladder. The amount of urine obtained should be measured and recorded and the urine saved in a sterile bottle to be used for specimens; this may prevent the need for additional catheterizations.

The doctor may wish to *calibrate the urethra* by passing catheters, bougies, or sounds of increasing sizes. This helps rule out significant strictures. The size of the calibration and dilatation should always be recorded.

Renal function tests

If anything in the general examination or the urinalysis is suggestive of renal damage, the doctor will probably order a number of renal function tests. Since the concentration of urea in the blood is regulated primarily by the rate at which the kidneys excrete this waste, the level of urea in the blood is an index of renal function. When renal function is impaired, there is an elevation of the blood urea level. Unfortunately, this also occurs when the patient is dehydrated since urea is resorbed through the tubules to a greater extent when the rate of urine flow is diminished. Either a *blood urea nitrogen* (BUN) or a *blood nonprotein nitrogen* (NPN) test may be used to determine this type of excretory function. Because it reflects impairment earlier, a *serum creatinine* test, which specifically detects glomerular malfunction, is more useful than the blood urea nitrogen test. A large portion of the renal mass may be destroyed before the blood urea nitrogen level exceeds normal.

It is important that the patient have no food contaminating protein for 6 hours before the blood is obtained for any of these tests. Since urea is an end product of protein metabolism, only a fasting blood specimen gives an accurate index of renal function. The normal blood urea nitrogen level is 8 to 15 mg. per 100 ml. of whole blood; the normal nonprotein nitrogen level is 25 to 30 mg. per 100 ml. of whole blood; and the normal serum creatinine level is 0.7 to 1.5 mg. per 100 ml. of blood plasma, depending on age and sex. (It is lower in children and women.) The nurse needs to note the blood urea or creatinine level of patients who have renal damage; if the level is high, the patient may have convulsions or may become confused or disoriented. Accidents and injury should be prevented by close observation and by having padded siderails and a mouth gag ready for immediate use.

Phenolsulfonphthalein test. Since phenolsulfonphthalein (a red dye) is a substance that the normal kidneys excrete completely, it is used to determine renal function. If the blood urea nitrogen level is normal, the phenolsulfonphthalein test (PSP) may be done to estimate the amount of obstruction below the kidney that may be delaying the emptying of the renal pelvis. Ninety-four percent of the dye is excreted through the tubules and 6% by glomerular filtration. It is helpful for the nurse to know how this test is done in the laboratory so that she will be more aware of the importance of obtaining proper specimens to prevent inaccurate results. Water is added to each specimen to reach a volume of 1000 ml.; the specimen is then alkalinized by adding sodium hydroxide since the dye is not visible in acid urine. In alkaline urine the dye turns pink. The color of each specimen is compared with a standard or a colorimeter to determine the amount of dye excreted in each specimen. Injection of more or less than 1 ml. (6 mg. of dye) will cause inaccuracies because 1 ml. of phenolsulfonphthalein is the basis for the color indicator. Blood in the urine will make the test inaccurate. Phenazopyridine, a urinary antiseptic that gives urine a red color, will also cause inaccuracies.

The patient voids, and this sample of urine is discarded after being inspected for any red discoloration. Then the patient is given an intravenous injection of exactly 1 ml. of phenolsulfonphthalein dye. Special care must be taken that the dye does not infiltrate the tissues; if it does, the test must be delayed for 24 hours, at which time another injection is made. The patient is urged to drink several glasses of water or other fluid before the dye is injected and during the test. He may eat if he wishes. Specimens consisting of all the urine the patient can void are collected exactly every 15 minutes for 1 hour. Sometimes the dye may be given intramuscularly. If so, the time intervals for collecting specimens are lengthened and the values for a normal test are reduced.

Occasionally the patient is unable to void at the desired time, but urination can usually be prompted by forcing fluids. If the patient is known to have residual urine in the bladder after voiding, a catheter may be passed before the dye is injected. If during the test the nurse becomes aware that the urinary output is inadequate in comparison to the fluid intake, the doctor may order the patient catheterized to ensure accurate results. Specimens are then obtained at the desired times by unclamping the catheter and draining the accumulated urine. Each specimen must be carefully labeled with the exact time of collection. The label on the first specimen should indicate the time the dye was injected. Normally the dye will begin to appear in the bladder 3 to 6 minutes after intravenous injection, with approximately 20% to 25% of it appearing in the first specimen and 65% to 75% being excreted within 1 hour.

The patient who is not acutely ill can usually collect his own specimens for a phenolsulfonphthalein test if he is given a watch, properly labeled bottles, and careful instructions. The nurse must make certain that he does this correctly and that he will send for her if he is unable to collect any one of the specimens at the appointed time.

Urea clearance test. The urea clearance test measures the efficiency of the glomerular filtration of plasma. Normally, 55 to 75 ml. of plasma are cleared of urea per minute. Since some urea is resorbed, it is important that the total specimen of urine be sent to the laboratory so the rate of urine flow can be determined. If an accurate result is to be obtained in the laboratory, the urine flow must be at least 2 ml. per minute. Therefore most laboratories ask that the patient drink two glasses of water when the discard specimen is obtained and two more after voiding for the first timed urine specimen. The patient should fast until after the blood sample is taken. One hour after the discard specimen is obtained, the patient is asked to void again, emptying his bladder completely. This entire voiding is collected and labeled as the first specimen. The exact time at which the discard specimen and this specimen are collected should be indicated. Then a blood sample is taken for blood urea nitrogen determination. An hour later, a second urine specimen is obtained, and all the specimens, carefully identified, are sent to the laboratory. If the patient is unable to void normally and to empty his bladder completely, catheterized specimens should be collected. If the test has been accurate, the urea in the blood will be elevated and the urea in the urine decreased in patients with poor renal function, whereas the reverse will be true if there is no disease. The two urine specimens should give comparable results.

Creatinine clearance test. A creatinine clearance test may be used instead of a urea clearance test; it is a more accurate measure of the glomerular filtration of plasma and does not depend on urine flow rate. For this test, urine is collected over a 24-hour period, beginning and ending in the morning. Abbreviated tests of 15 minutes and 1 hour are less reliable. At the completion of the period of urine collection a blood sample is drawn for serum creatinine determinations; the patient should be fasting. The normal amount of creatinine excreted in the urine during a 24-hour period varies with age; a 5-year-old child will excrete approximately 0.36 gm.; a 17-year-old young adult, approximately 1.5 gm.; an adult, 1.2 to 1.7 gm. The test values are recorded as milliliters per minute, hour, or day.

Concentration and dilution tests. If there is any indication of glomerular malfunction, urine concentration and dilution tests for tubular function are ordered. When excretion of body wastes is normal and fluids are restricted for a relatively long period of time or large amounts of body fluids are lost by perspiration, respiration, diarrhea, vomiting, or hemorrhage, larger than normal amounts of the plasma fluid will be resorbed through the tubules, causing a concentrated urine. When large amounts of fluid are taken into the body, the normal kidneys will excrete larger amounts, causing the urine to be more diluted than usual.

When renal damage has occurred, one of the first functions to be lost is the ability of the renal tubules to concentrate and to dilute urine. When renal damage is severe, the specific gravity of the urine is said to be "fixed," meaning that no matter what the fluid intake is, the specific gravity of the urine will be that of the plasma without its protein (that part filtered through the glomeruli into the tubules) or about 1.008 to 1.012. A fixed low specific gravity therefore is indicative of serious renal disease. The ability of the kidneys to concentrate urine can be measured by several tests.

FISHBERG CONCENTRATION TEST. The Fishberg concentration test is commonly used. The patient eats his usual evening meal and is instructed to take no more food or fluids until after completion of the test the next morning, when urine specimens are collected at 6, 7, and 8 A.M. Morning specimens are collected because normal kidneys concentrate urine during the night at approximately twice the rate they do during the waking hours. The finding of specific gravities of any of the three morning specimens below 1.024 is considered evidence of renal impairment.

ADDIS CONCENTRATION TEST. The Addis concentration test is much more vigorous in the dehydration of the patient. It gives a more sensitive measurement, but if the patient's nonprotein nitrogen determination is high or if he is a child under 5 years of age, it is used with caution because of the danger of precipitating a serious electrolytic imbalance. Fluids are markedly restricted for 24 hours; the amount allowed varies with the laboratory making the test. During the last 12 hours of the test all urine is saved and analyzed for the number of different cells and casts and the total amount of protein present. There should be no more than 650,000 white cells, 300,000 red cells, 2000 casts, or 60 mg. of protein per 24 hours.

DILUTION TEST. The dilution test is used to determine the ability of the kidney to dilute urine. It may be done at any time of day, but the patient should remain inactive during the test. He should completely empty the bladder at the beginning of the test and then is usually asked to drink

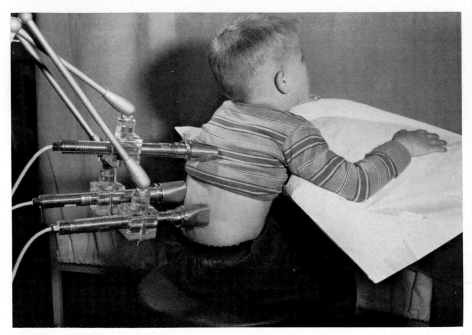

Fig. 6-9. Pediatric patient having renogram made. Note probe over each kidney and additional probe over chest used to monitor blood disappearance rate of isotope-labeled test agent.

1200 ml. of fluid within a half hour (the doctor should be consulted as to the amount to give children). Urine specimens are then collected every half hour for 3 hours. A person with normal hydration and normal renal function will excrete almost the total 1200 ml. in the 3-hour period, and the urine will have a specific gravity of about 1.002. Since most patients have difficulty in drinking 1200 ml. of fluid in a half-hour period, it sometimes helps if the water is mixed with fruit juice to make a weak fruit ade. Each specimen should include all urine voided and should be sent to the laboratory; the label on the specimen should include the exact time of each voiding and the initial amount of fluid drunk.

Radioisotope renography. As a renal function test, the radioisotope renogram aids in evaluating renal vascularity, function, and ability to evacuate urine. It is most useful in determining obstruction of the upper urinary tract, detecting unilateral renal disease in hypertensive patients, and discovering acute renal failure of less than 48 hours' duration. It has practical value in the follow-up of the patient with a medically or surgically treated renal disorder for evaluating treatment and prognosis. In addition, the renogram is of value in judging function of transplanted kidneys and for early detection of rejection of the graft.

There are no special restrictions, physical or dietary, for the patient prior to the examination. After the procedure, safety precautions, because

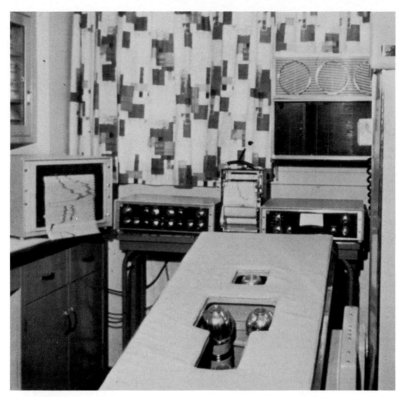

Fig. 6-10. Table and equipment used for radioisotope renography. Note that there are four scintillation probes beneath table, two of which are in apposition to kidneys. The lower probe is under bladder region, while cephalad probe is under chest and monitors the blood level of radioactivity. Dual overlapping pen recorder on left shows tracings obtained for each kidney. Recorders are connected to scintillation probes through electronic discriminators shown in background.

of injection of a radioactive substance, are unnecessary since only trace doses are used. Safety precautions must be taken, however, by the individuals handling the radioactive material. The patient should be told what will be expected of him during the procedure. He will be placed in a supine or upright position. Scintillation probes are positioned under the posterior aspects of each kidney and a third counter may be located over a highly vascular area of the chest to monitor the disappearance of the isotope from the blood (Figs. 6-9 to 6-11). The probes are connected through rate meters to recorders (Fig. 6-12). A compound such as iodohippurate sodium (Hippuran) tagged with I^{131} or I^{125} is injected intravenously in a minute amount. Following the radioisotope renogram a uroflometry and bladder residual test may be performed by placing the scintillation probe over the posterior bladder area and having the patient void. Thus maximum as well as average flow rates can be recorded and computed in addition to the determination of residual urine in the bladder. The test lasts only a few

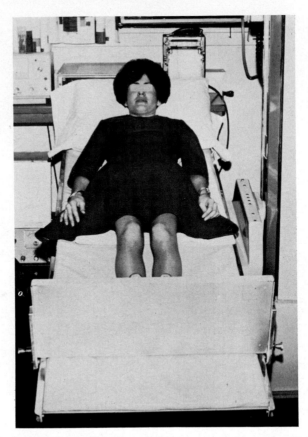

Fig. 6-11. Patient is shown having radioisotope renogram made. Note that testing equipment is all external to body, thus avoiding trauma or discomfort.

minutes and there is no limitation to the number of tests the patient may have.

Renal scintillation scanning (photoscanning). An outline of functioning renal tissue may be obtained by injecting chlormerodrin labeled with Hg^{203} and Hg^{197} intravenously (Fig. 6-13). This material stays in the renal tubular cells for several weeks. A scintillation probe passing back and forth over the kidney detects the radiation from the kidney and it is recorded on paper or x-ray film. Nonviable areas of the kidney produced by infarcts, cysts, or tumors will show as "cold spots," that is, no recording of radioactivity. The test is not specific for the type of disease and does not show small areas of disease (less than 1 inch in diameter). Iodohippurate I^{131} can be used also but passes through the kidney so rapidly that it is less convenient for routine testing.

SCINTILLATION PHOTOGRAPHY. The test agents mentioned with regard to scanning are used for this test, except that iodohippurate I^{131} or I^{125} is preferable. Instead of a moving probe, a large stationary scintillation

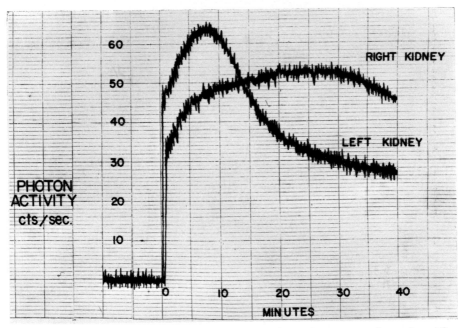

Fig. 6-12. Example of normal left radioisotope renogram showing initial vascular spike, secondary functional rise, and final excretory drop in tracing. Right tracing is characteristic of renal dysfunction due to stenosis of renal artery. Note that vascular spike and functional segments are decreased, while excretory phase is prolonged. Renogram is invaluable in cross-comparison of renal status.

crystal, backed by a battery of multiplier phototubes, receives the renal radiation signals. Through an ingenious electronic device the signals are recorded on photographic film in proportion to the radioenergy in each area of the kidney. The results are recorded more quickly than with a scan, and a series of time-lapse films may be made to demonstrate the dynamics of renal function.

The *positron camera* is a more modern version of the scintillation camera. Recording equipment is placed both in front and behind the kidney and, through subtraction, the mathematical product is photographed. A different isotope (positron emitter) must be used. The technique for such renal testing has not yet been perfected.

Intravenous pyelography. An intravenous pyelogram (IVP) is the most commonly ordered test when renal disease is suspected. In this series of roentgenograms the absence, presence, location, size, and configuration of each kidney as well as the filling of the renal pelves and outlines of the ureters can be determined. Some idea of the lower urinary tract is also obtained. The taking of different radiographic views allows irregularities, opacities, and other defects to be studied and compared. Several types of radiopaque preparations such as diatrizoate sodium (Hypaque) or meglumin diatrizoate (Renografin) are used. Before the test is performed, an

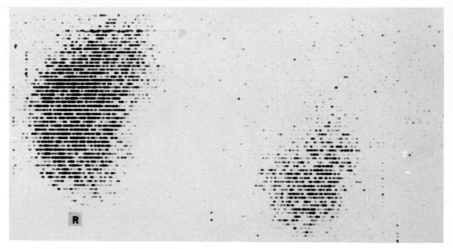

Fig. 6-13. Example of a renal scintiscan. Note absence of radioactivity in upper pole of left kidney due to renal tumor.

attempt is often made to determine the sensitivity of the patient to the test agent. However, a negative reaction to a sensitivity test does not guarantee that the patient will not have a severe reaction. It is generally believed that such testing is highly unreliable and it is done more for legal than for medical reasons. When allergic reactions are evident, a retrograde pyelographic study may be chosen.

The patient should be initiated into this examination by an explanation of the procedure, its purpose, and the reasons for the physical preparation. It is often done on an outpatient basis, and written as well as verbal instruction should then be given. The patient is usually instructed to omit food and fluids from 12 o'clock the night before until after the examination is completed because this produces a better concentration of the radiopaque medium in the urinary tract and a clearer roentgenogram. Food and fluid are usually withheld 6 to 8 hours if the patient is an infant or a child under 7 years of age, but a specific order should be obtained for each child. The test is contraindicated in patients with multiple myeloma.

Since the kidneys lie retroperitoneally, it is important that the bowel be empty of gas and fecal material that may cause shadows on the film.

Many physicians order 60 ml. (2 ounces) of castor oil or 10 ml. of cascara to be given about 8 P.M. the evening prior to the day of the test. These are adult dosages; the nurse should consult a pharmacology book for determining the appropriate dosage for children of various ages. Castor oil is made more palatable if it is mixed with a citrus fruit juice and if a few milliliters of sodium bicarbonate are stirred in immediately before it is offered to the patient. Some patients prefer to suck on a section of orange or lemon immediately after taking castor oil. Tasteless castor oil is also now available. Bisacodyl (Dulcolax), a bowel irritant, may be used. This cathartic should be taken by mouth ½ hour following the evening meal. Usually four tablets are ordered for an adult. If the patient is suspected of having an acute inflammation of the abdominal viscera, peptic ulcers, or colitis or if he has a colostomy, a ureterosigmoidal transplant, or is extremely debilitated, all of these relatively vigorous cathartics are contraindicated. Therefore, before giving the medication, the nurse should know something about the physical condition of the patient and should bring to the doctor's attention anything about the patient that makes her suspect the cathartic might be contraindicated.

Infants and children under 7 years of age often are given no bowel preparation. Before the radiopaque substance is injected, a roentgenogram (scout film) of the abdomen is taken to determine the amount of gas in the bowel overlying the kidneys. If there is too much gas, the infant may be given 8 to 10 ounces of formula since the air he swallows with this may push down on the gas-filled bowel and leave the renal field free. Young children may be given carbonated beverages for this same purpose. If a cathartic is used, the child should be carefully watched for signs of dehydration since not only is he being purged but also fluids are being withheld for an excessively long time.

The patient who has received a cathartic should not be given sedation to induce sleep, and he should be told where to find the call light and the bathroom or bedpan. If he is elderly or debilitated, he must be urged to call for the assistance of the nurse to go to the bathroom. Patients can become quite weak from drastic catharsis, and this may lead to accidents.

The nurse should determine and record the effectiveness of efforts to evacuate the bowel and she should report ineffective results to the doctor. Occasionally, if the cathartic has been ineffectual or if it is contraindicated for some reason, enemas may be given. The enema must be given early in the morning to allow time for excretion of the fluid absorbed during the enema and for expulsion of feces and flatus. The very elderly patient usually has difficulty emptying the bowel completely following an enema; for this reason enemas are sometimes ordered for the evening before the urogram. A rectal suppository such as bisacodyl may be preferable to an enema.

If the patient has received barium prior to intravenous pyelography, the bowel must be emptied especially well because any residual barium may obscure the renal picture. Usually, however, this problem can be prevented by careful scheduling of the tests so those for renal function precede barium swallows, gastrointestinal series, or barium enemas.

For the test the patient is placed on a full-length x-ray table in the supine position. A roentgenogram of the abdominal area (a plain film, or KUB, the designation for kidney-ureter-bladder) is taken first. This gives information as to the size, shape, and position of the kidneys and reveals the presence of various stonelike shadows, parts of the skeleton, soft tissue masses, fluid, and fecal accumulation.

The radiopaque preparation is injected by a physician or under his observation. The patient should know that he may have a feeling of warmth, flushing of the face, and a salty taste in his mouth as the doctor slowly injects the drug intravenously. This usually lasts only a few minutes and is often relieved by taking deep breaths. The nurse should then watch for signs of respiratory difficulty, sudden diaphoresis and clamminess, or urticaria, any of which may indicate an untoward reaction to the contrast medium. If the patient complains of numbness or tingling of any part of the body, of palpitation of the heart, or of any other unusual sensation, he must be attended constantly and the doctor must be immediately summoned. Tripelennamine hydrochloride (Pyribenzamine), diphenhydramine hydrochloride (Benadryl), epinephrine (Adrenalin), methylprednisolone sodium (Solu-Medrol), and oxygen should be available for immediate use if necessary.

Roentgenograms are usually taken 2, 5, 10, and 15 minutes after the drug is injected (Fig. 6-14). If delayed renal function caused by obstruction is suspected, roentgenograms may also be taken 1 and 2 hours later. Often a double dose (60 ml.) or high infusion (150 ml.) is given to obtain better delineation of the urinary system. When delayed roentgenograms are necessary, the patient must either be returned to his bed or protected from discomfort on the table. If he is left on the table, a soft bath blanket should be placed under him and he should be assisted in changing position at 15-minute intervals.

The patient should be allowed prompt access to fluids following this dehydration period.

Cystoscopy and retrograde studies

Cystoscopy is the examination of the inside of the bladder through a metal instrument called a *cystoscope* (see Figs. 3-7 and 3-8). The instrument is constructed with illumination, which enables the examiner to see the interior of the bladder with remarkable magnification and clarity. Small cystoscopes are available for use with children and even infants.

A *cystoscopic examination* is indicated for all patients who have or have had hematuria because, although blood in the urine may be due to other causes, it is one of the earliest signs of malignant growths anywhere along the urinary system. The examination may be done as part of an intensive diagnostic study or it may be done as an emergency diagnostic measure. By doing an immediate cystoscopic examination the doctor may locate a point of hemorrhage in the prostate gland, the bladder, or the upper urinary tract that might otherwise escape detection since such hemorrhages fre-

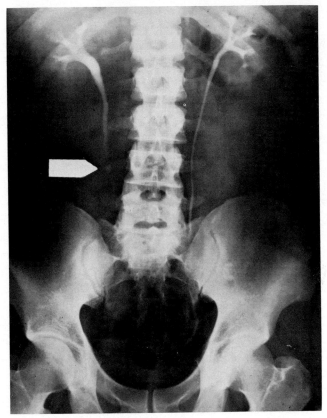

Fig. 6-14. Excretory urogram outlines calyces, pelvis, and ureters. Note stone in mid-portion of the right ureter (arrow).

quently stop spontaneously for a time. Examination of the urethra and prostate gland are possible also.

Nursing attention before and during a cystoscopic examination can contribute greatly to its success and to lessening the patient's discomfort. The nurse should be especially aware of her function as an intermediary between the patient and the urologist since the patient is often reluctant to discuss with the specialist matters that he would mention freely to his family doctor. The patient should know just what he will experience in the cystoscopy room; he may not have any idea of what to expect and may be reluctant to ask the doctor. The nurse should give thorough explanations before the procedure is begun and she should remain with the patient during the procedure, giving him reassurance and encouragement. This helps him to relax and decreases discomfort, much of which is caused by contraction or spasm of the urethral sphincters. Some hospitals require a signed permit before this procedure is done.

If the patient is emotionally prepared and relatively comfortable, he should be able to relax enough so that the cystoscope can be passed with little discomfort, provided there is no obstruction in the urethra. Deep breathing will sometimes help the patient relax. The passing of the instrument will be accompanied by a desire to void. During the examination the bladder is gradually filled with distilled water to distend its wall and to make visualization more effective. This intensifies the urge to void. At this point the capacity of the bladder, an important physiologic measurement, is noted. Some of the fluid is then drained from the bladder to relieve discomfort.

Fluids are usually forced for several hours before the patient goes to the cystoscopy room. This ensures a continuous flow of urine in case urine specimens are to be collected from the kidneys. If an anesthetic is to be given, fluids may be administered intravenously.

A sedative such as secobarbital and a narcotic such as morphine or meperidine may be given about a half hour prior to the examination. A local anesthetic such as lidocaine (usually 0.5% to 2%) may be instilled into the urethra 10 minutes prior to insertion of the cystoscope. If the patient is a child or an extremely apprehensive adult or if much manipulation is anticipated, a general anesthetic may be necessary to prevent sudden, vigorous movement during the examination, which might cause trauma to the urethra or even perforation of the bladder.

Clothing from the waist down must be removed and often a hospital gown is worn. The patient is placed in the lithotomy position on the cystoscopy table and is draped in such a manner that only the genitalia and perineum are exposed. In placing the patient in position, care must be taken that pressure is not exerted upon the popliteal spaces since such pressure might cause circulatory embarrassment and lead to thrombosis in blood vessels. Because of arthritis and related disorders, some elderly patients are unable to rest comfortably in the stirrups; it may be necessary to use slings in place of the stirrups and to place extra pillows under the patient's head and shoulders. If prolonged time on the table is necessary, the patient's legs should be removed from the stirrups at intervals and flexed and extended a few times.

Ureteral catheters (nylon, radiopaque, calibrated, sizes 4 to 6 Fr. or smaller for children) may be passed through the cystoscope and inserted into the ureteral opening in the bladder, up the ureter, and into the renal pelvis. This procedure is known as *ureteral catheterization* and may involve one or both of the ureters. Specimens obtained directly from the kidneys are examined microscopically and for concentration of creatinine (Fig. 6-15). Urine obtained in this manner may be cultured and studied for tubercle bacilli, cancer cells, and other abnormal constituents.

Renal function tests may be carried out by injecting indigo carmine (a blue dye) or phenolsulfonphthalein (a red dye) intravenously and timing

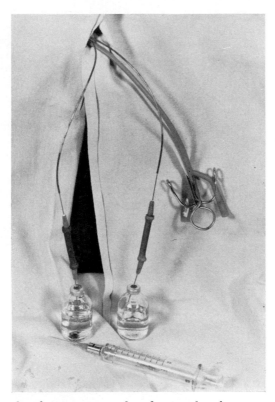

Fig. 6-15. Patient has been cystoscoped and ureteral catheters passed to each renal pelvis. Urine is being collected in vacuum bottles to avoid leakage around catheters. Divided renal function tests to be performed include rate of urine flow per minute and creatinine and sodium concentrations. Indigo carmine or phenolsulfonphthalein may be given to note initial appearance time as well as relative concentrations. Syringe is used to renew vacuum in bottles. Foley catheter is used to check for leakage of urine into bladder.

the appearance of the dye from each kidney. If function is normal, the dye will appear from each side in 3 to 6 minutes.

Ureteral catheters may be inserted and left in place even though the cystoscope is withdrawn. They are frequently left in place prior to gynecologic or extensive pelvic surgery in which there may be danger of accidentally injuring an unrecognized ureter. They may also be left in place to provide better drainage of the kidney in certain conditions; for example, when a stone is lodged in the ureter.

A sharp roentgenographic outline of the renal pelves and the ureters is obtained by injecting 3 to 6 ml. of radiopaque substance such as methiodal sodium (Skiodan) gently up each ureteral catheter after urine specimens have been collected. While the solution is being injected, the patient may feel slight discomfort in the kidney region, but pain should not be experienced unless too much of the solution has been injected, causing over-

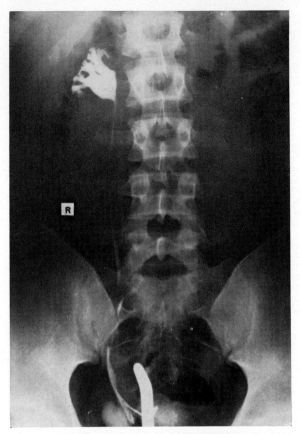

Fig. 6-16. Retrograde pyelography. After ureteral catheter is passed by means of cystoscopy, contrast material is injected to make right retrograde pyeloureterogram.

distention of the renal pelvis. Air is sometimes injected to outline non-opaque calculi. As the doctor withdraws the catheters and the cystoscope, he again injects the contrast medium (1 to 2 ml.), which fills the ureters, and another roentgenogram that will show the outline of the ureters is made immediately. This examination is known as *retrograde pyelography and ureterography* (Fig. 6-16).

Care should be taken that the patient, especially an elderly one, does not stand or walk alone immediately after the procedure since blood that has drained from the legs while he was in the lithotomy position flows back into the vessels of the feet and legs as he stands up. Accidents due to dizziness and fainting can occur from the sudden change in distribution of blood, which reduces the blood supply to the brain.

Cystoscopic examinations of the urinary system are often done on an ambulatory basis, either in a clinic or in a doctor's office. Even though a period of rest in the clinic is encouraged, the outpatient should be advised to bring someone with him who can be certain that he gets home safely. If food has been withheld before the examination, the patient should have something to eat before leaving for home. He or his relatives should be given printed instructions for care at the conclusion of the tests. These should be used as a supplement to verbal instructions since the latter must often be given as the patient is preparing to leave the clinic and after he has had sedation and therefore may not be remembered accurately.

After any cystoscopic procedure the patient's urinary output should be observed. The urine may sometimes normally be pink-tinged, but more extensive bleeding should be reported to the doctor. If dyes have been used, the patient should be told that the urine may be an unusual color. The patient may have a "full" sensation and a feeling of burning in the bladder; he may also have pain in the lower back. Mild analgesics such as acetylsalicylic acid and codeine sulfate may be prescribed to relieve discomfort, but usually the greatest relief is obtained from warm tub baths, which produce relaxation and relieve muscle tension. If the patient feels chilly, a heating pad or hot-water bottle applied over the bladder region or to the lower back may be used. Fluids should be forced to dilute the urine and thereby lessen irritation to the mucous membrane lining of the urinary tract. Fluids should be offered at hourly intervals for at least 4 hours.

Sharp abdominal pain after cystoscopy should be reported to the doctor, and analgesic drugs should be withheld until he has examined the patient because the bladder or ureters may have been accidentally perforated, causing peritonitis. Chills and marked elevation of temperature may follow cystoscopic procedures. These are thought to be caused by a general systemic reaction to the foreign substances introduced, possible bacteremia, the instrumentation, and the pain. The patient should remain in bed for a few hours following these procedures and should be asked to notify the nurse or doctor if he has any sensation of chilling or if he voids blood clots. Chilling and elevation of temperature usually respond within a short time to extra warmth and to warm fluids by mouth. Blood cultures may need to be started or antibiotics given.

The nurse in the cystoscopic unit is responsible for preparation and aftercare of equipment needed during cystoscopic examinations. (See discussions of the nurse in the operating room, the sterilization of equipment, and the care of catheters and cystoscopic equipment.) The cystoscope is connected to a flask of distilled water that must be sterile and must be kept covered and filled. (Sterile disposable flasks of water and tubing are commercially available.) It is also connected to a battery from which the current for the light comes; this should be serviced at regular intervals to ensure efficiency and safety. Extra cords and light bulbs for the cystoscopes should always be available. Fiberoptic lighted instruments are gradually replacing battery-energized bulbs.

Other roentgenographic studies

Cystography. Cystography is an x-ray study of the bladder made by injecting a radiopaque substance such as methiodal sodium or 5% sodium iodide through a urethral catheter into the bladder; sometimes air is injected as the contrast medium. The roentgenogram taken following the injection will show irregularities in the size and shape of the bladder. Bladder diverticula as well as traumatic rupture can be visualized. Areas of the bladder filled by a stone or tumor mass will also be delineated. Vesicoureteral reflux may be demonstrated (see Fig. 2-5). After the pictures are taken, the patient is often asked to empty his bladder and then a final film is taken. This is another method of measuring residual urine. Serial films may be taken as he voids to delineate the urethra. No special preparation of the patient is necessary.

Urethrography. When the doctor wishes to study the contour of the urethra (especially to detect strictures or diverticula), a urethrogram may be ordered. There is no special preparation. A radiopaque substance of jelly-like consistency is injected into the urethra and a roentgenogram is taken (retrograde urethrogram). The patient is then asked to void to expel the remaining jelly (voiding or antegrade urethrogram). A less viscous agent is used in females.

Vena cavography. Renal mass lesions or periaortic masses involving the renal veins or vena cava may be demonstrated by injecting contrast material into the vena cava via the femoral vein (Fig. 6-17). Usually 60 ml. of 50% diatrizoate is used, and several films or a cineradiography study will show deformities or obstruction of the vena cava. Compression is placed over the puncture site after the test, and hemorrhage is rarely a problem. The nurse should observe the inguinal region for this complication.

Retroperitoneal pneumography. When adrenal or retroperitoneal tumors are suspected and cannot be demonstrated by plain radiography, they may be outlined by gas-contrast methods. A presacral injection of carbon dioxide or oxygen is made into the retroperitoneal connective tissues. The patient is usually prepared as for intravenous pyelography, but a sedative such as soluble phenobarbital may be given before the examination because there is some discomfort—abdominal pain, cramping, nausea, vomiting, and faintness are common. The nurse should remain with the patient during the procedure.

A needle, similar to that used for spinal puncture, is inserted just anterior to the coccyx into the deeper presacral areolar tissues. The doctor usually keeps one finger in the rectum during the insertion to guide the needle. After insertion, 400 to 800 ml. of the gas being used is injected on one or both sides. If the kidney area is to be delineated, the patient is usually seated since gas rises. He may be turned from side to side if both kidneys are to be delineated. The roentgenograms are then taken.

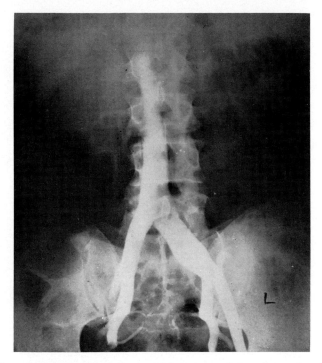

Fig. 6-17. Vena cavogram. Contrast material is injected into femoral vein to outline the ileac vessels and vena cava. If obstruction is present, compression of vena cava as well as collateral circulation will appear. This is used to outline lymph node enlargement and tumor masses impinging on vena cava.

There is some danger of air embolism when oxygen is used in this procedure. The patient should remain in bed for several hours after the procedure; he should be placed on his left side so any gas in the heart will rise and be trapped in the right atrium. Meanwhile the patient should be kept absolutely quiet and equipment for oxygen administration should be prepared. The incidence of complications appears to be lowest when carbon dioxide is used for this test, but the best pictures are obtained with oxygen, which is not dissipated as rapidly as carbon dioxide.

Tomography. A small tumor in the parenchyma of the kidney may not be apparent in a routine pyelogram; therefore special techniques that give pictures of sections of the kidney may be used. A *tomogram (laminagram, planigram, stratigram, body-section radiogram)* is a plain roentgenogram of a section of the body (kidney region in this instance) taken with a rotating x-ray tube. The films delineate tissues at the level at which the tube radiates.

A *nephrotomogram* is a tomogram taken after intravenous injection of a radiopaque agent. For this examination the patient is placed on an x-ray table and a radiopaque material such as acetrizoate sodium is then given intravenously. Physical preparation of the patient is the same as for intra-

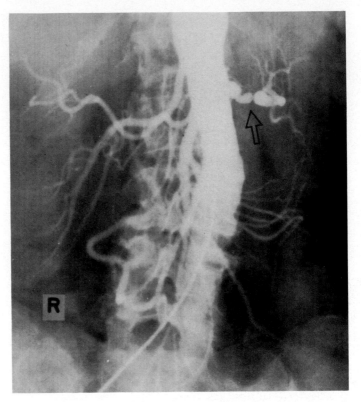

Fig. 6-18. Arrow points to multiple stenotic lesions of left renal artery demonstrated by transfemoral aortogram.

venous pyelography. He should be instructed to expect the same sensations when the material is given, and he should be observed for the same drug reactions. Since regulation of the time interval is dependent upon the patient's cooperation, the nurse should carefully explain the procedure so the patient will understand his role.

Renal angiography. For this roentgenogram a concentrated organic iodide contrast material such as 50% to 75% diatrizoate is injected intra-arterially into the aorta not far from the renal vessels. This type of study clearly outlines the renal blood supply and is particularly indicated in cases of hypertension of suspected renal origin (Fig. 6-18). It may also be used to demonstrate large renal neoplasms, aberrant renal blood vessels, and the absence of a kidney. It is sometimes used postoperatively to study the remaining renal tissue or to demonstrate vessels torn from trauma.

Regardless of the route of injection to be used, physical preparation of the patient is usually the same as for intravenous pyelography and the same precautions against drug reaction should be taken. Care must be taken to prevent extravasation of the drug into tissues because it is extremely irritating; phlebitis may occur. A syringe filled with physiologic solution of sodium chloride should be used while determining placement of the needle and the syringe containing the contrast medium connected only after the needle is in the vessel. Tight bandages are applied over femoral injection sites immediately after removal of needles to prevent any hemorrhage.

When the contrast medium is injected intravenously, the examination is called *intravenous abdominal aortography*. First, circulation time from the injection site to the tongue is determined to guide the timing of the films; dehydrocholate sodium is also added to the radiopaque material as a further guide. (See discussion on tomography.) The radiopaque material, divided into two syringes, is injected simultaneously into a large vein in each arm with large-caliber (12-gauge) needles; cutdowns on the veins may be necessary. To prevent obstruction of the subclavian veins by the first ribs, the arms should be lifted and the shoulders relaxed during the injections. The patient is instructed to hold his breath 2 or 3 seconds before the film is to be taken. Since he will be holding his breath at the time he needs to indicate tasting the dehydrocholate sodium, he is told to indicate this by making tasting motions. An intravenous pyelogram series is usually taken in conjunction with this test.

When the contrast medium is injected intra-arterially, the examination is known as *aortography*. There are two types of aortography: translumbar and femoral percutaneous. For a *translumbar aortogram*, the radiopaque material is injected into the aorta near the origin of both renal arteries by puncturing the aorta with a long needle inserted through a translumbar route. The patient may be given a general anesthetic for the procedure, but local anesthesia is equally popular. If *femoral percutaneous aortography* is done, the skin and subcutaneous tissue over the femoral artery (the inguinal area) to be used is infiltrated with a local anesthetic. A small arterial catheter is then inserted into the femoral artery and threaded retrogradely into the aorta or directly into the renal artery and the radiopaque substance is injected. If a renal parenchymal lesion is under study, *selective renal arteriography* is ideal. The catheter is manipulated directly into the main or accessory renal artery in order to get better definition of the tissue being examined. In the past some danger was inherent in these procedures because of the toxicity of the test agents. Today, when the tests are performed by experienced personnel, complications are rare.

Roentgenograms to detect metastasis. To determine whether there is any evidence of a carcinoma having spread to other parts of the body, a metastatic x-ray series may be ordered. This involves x-raying the chest, skull, spine, and long bones; these are common sites of metastatic lesions. There is no special preparation of the patient for these studies, but since they take considerable time, the debilitated or elderly patient may need to rest following the procedure.

LYMPHANGIOGRAPHY. Since many tumors metastasize by lymphatic channels, there is some merit in attempting to define such events by injecting regional lymphatics with contrast solutions. This is done in the foot and is a tedious and time-consuming procedure. Some risk is involved in that the oily substance used may lodge in the lungs, causing pneumonitis or embolization. Tumors of the testes, bladder, and prostate are the urologic neoplasms most commonly studied by this method. The nurse should observe the patient for coughing, dyspnea, cyanosis, or shock.

QUESTIONS

1. List some abnormal patterns of micturition.
2. How would you instruct a patient to keep a record of urinary output?
3. How would you instruct a patient to keep a record of urinary pH?
4. How would you instruct a patient to keep a record of the presence of sugar, blood, or protein in the urine?
5. How may a nurse assist in obtaining the patient's past medical and related history?
6. Describe three positions for female pelvic and rectal examinations.
7. Why are regular rectal examinations in the adult male so important?
8. How may a urine specimen be obtained in the male infant?
9. How may a urine specimen be obtained in the female infant?
10. How is a urine specimen usually obtained in the adult female?
11. How is a routine urine specimen obtained in the adult male?
12. What is the significance of obtaining a two-glass urine specimen in a male?
13. What is a Papanicolaou examination?
14. How is the urethra calibrated?
15. Name several renal function tests and describe one in detail.
16. What is the principle of a radioactive kidney test?
17. Name some radioisotopes used in renal function testing.
18. What is the difference between a renogram and a scintiscan and scintiphotograph?
19. What is the principle of the intravenous pyelogram?
20. In what patient is an intravenous pyelogram contraindicated?
21. What is the usual preparation of a patient for an intravenous pyelogram?
22. What is the instrument called that is used to examine the interior of the bladder?
23. What is the difference between a retrograde pyelogram and an intravenous pyelogram?
24. What information is gained from a cystogram?
25. Name five different urologic roentgenographic procedures.
26. What is the difference between an abdominal aortogram and a selective arteriogram?
27. What x-ray procedure is used to detect retroperitoneal lymph node metastasis from a tumor?

REFERENCES

Brody, L. H., Salladay, J. R., and Armbruster, K.: Urinalysis and the urinary sediment, Med. Clin. N. Amer. **55**:243, 1971.

Ensor, R. D., Anderson, E. E., and Robinson, R. R.: Drip infusion urography in patients with renal disease, J. Urol. **103**:267, 1970.

Geist, D. I.: Round-the-clock specimens, Amer.J. Nurs. **60**:1300, 1960.

Kelly, A. E., and Gensini, G. G.: Renal arteriography, Amer. J. Nurs. **64**:97, 1964.

Lindan, R., and Keane, A. T.: The catheter team, Amer. J. Nurs. **64**:128, 1964.

MacKinnon, H. A.: Urinary drainage: the problem of asepsis, Amer. J. Nurs. **65**:112, 1965.

Mainwaring, C.: Clean voided specimens for mass screening, Amer. J. Nurs. **63**:96, 1963.

McLeod, J. W., Mason, J. M., and Pilley, A. A.: Prophylactic control of infection of the urinary tract consequent on catheterization, Lancet **1**:292, 1963.

Mohammed, M. F. B.: Urinalysis, Amer. J. Nurs. **64**:87, 1964.

O'Flynn, J. D.: Advances in urology, Practitioner **197**:5034, 1966.

Pillay, V. K. G.: Clinical testing of renal function, Med. Clin. N. Amer. **55**:231, 1971.

Rennie, I. D.: Proteinuria, Med. Clin. N. Amer. **55**:213, 1971.

Rowson, L.: The lateral position in catheterization, Nurs. Clin. N. Amer. **5**:189, 1970.

Sato, F. F.: New devices for continuous urine collection in pediatrics, Amer. J. Nurs. **69**:804, 1969.

Tests of renal function (laboratory review), Nurs. Clin. N. Amer. **2**:800, 1967.

Winter, C. C.: Radioisotope renography, Baltimore, 1963, The Williams & Wilkins Co.

Winter, C. C.: Radioisotope uroflometry and bladder residual test, J. Urol. **91**:103, 1964.

Winter, C. C.: Radioisotope urologic tests. In Ney, C., and Freidenburg, R. M., editors: Radiographic atlas of the genitourinary system, Philadelphia, 1966, J. B. Lippincott Co., pp. 712-718.

Winter, C. C.: Pediatric urological tests using radioisotopes, J. Urol. **95**:584, 1966.

Winter, C. C.: Application of the scintillation camera in urology, J. Urol. **97**:766, 1967.

Winter, C. C.: Practical urology, St. Louis, 1969, The C. V. Mosby Co.

Winter, C. C.: The genitourinary system. In Cole, W. H., and Zollinger, R. M., editors: Textbook of surgery, New York, 1970, Appleton-Century-Crofts.

CHAPTER 7

Renal parenchymal diseases

This chapter deals with those diseases peculiar to the kidneys other than obstruction, calculi, infection, or tumors. The treatment is therefore medical rather than surgical. The urologist is often called upon to carry out diagnostic measures in patients with such diseases because disorders requiring surgical intervention must be distinguished and the various renal disorders often have similar initial symptoms and findings.

In pediatric patients the most common medical renal disorder is acute glomerulonephritis. Toxic nephritis caused by overdoses of aspirin and other poisonings is common. Congenital anomalies account for most of the surgical renal disorders in children.

Subacute and chronic nephritis are more often seen in the adult patient with concomitant hypertension and renal failure, but they may occur at any age.

ACUTE RENAL FAILURE

A common cause of acute renal failure is shock due to serious accidents with blood loss and hypotension and periods of low pressure during sergery. Toxic agents such as mercury bichloride, other poisons, endotoxins from bacteria, and a number of antibiotics can destroy tubular cells. Certain allergic phenomena are capable of producing temporary renal shutdown. When the kidney is unable to eliminate body wastes, electrolytes, and fluids, the patient develops azotemia (elevation of blood urea nitrogen, creatinine, and uric acid levels), and if this continues unabated, a clinical syndrome known as uremia sets in.

The first sign of impending acute renal failure is a marked decrease of the urinary output. If the output is below 500 ml. per 24 hours, the condition is known as oliguria. If the output is less than 300 ml. per 24 hours, the condition is called anuria. The patient gradually becomes lethargic and anorexic, and as the blood electrolyte levels become unbalanced, the patient may become irritable and even psychotic. If the intake of fluids is not restrained, the patient develops swelling of the subcutaneous tissues, and pulmonary edema may occur. Since the failing kidneys are unable to excrete potassium, an excessive rise in the serum level of this ion may cause the heart to stop abruptly. The blood pressure tends to be elevated mildly and this is noted particularly when the patient gains weight because of increasing fluid retention. Moderate anemia may develop, with the patient exhibiting pallor. The urine characteristically has a fixed specific gravity in the range of 1.010. In the late stages of uremia the patient becomes acidotic and his breath acquires a characteristic odor. Respirations may become labored and a frost may appear on the skin. This is usually accompanied by pruritus (itching of the skin). Headaches, visual disturbances, nausea, and vomiting are other symptoms. With the rise of serum urea and creatinine levels, the blood calcium drops and the patient may exhibit tetany or even convulsions. Finally, the patient may bleed from the intestinal tract, further contributing to the anemia, which may become severe in the advanced state of uremia.

The microscopic findings in the kidney show that the basement membrane of the tubules or even the tubular cells themselves are destroyed. The glomeruli appear to be intact but filter blood at a decreased rate. The filtrate is allowed to pass back into the circulation since there is no viable tubular mechanisms to control resorption.

One of the first considerations of the urologist is to rule out obstructive uropathy caused by stones, tumors, or compression upon the ureters that could reduce the urine outflow. If the blood urea nitrogen level is not markedly elevated, an excretory urogram using a double dose or high infusion of contrast material may be feasible. Usually, however, a cystoscopic examination and intubation of at least one ureter is necessary to rule out obstruction. This carries an increased hazard in comparison with routine cystoscopy and retrograde pyelography when the urine output is normal. Approximately 50% of patients with acute renal failure recover with conservative management. Daily fluid intake is restricted to an amount equal to 500 ml. plus the volume of urinary output for 24 hours. A strict nonprotein and nonpotassium diet is essential. The former reduces the work load of the kidneys, which are already unable to eliminate nitrogenous products. Patients become restless and agitated; depression is often exhibited. Oral hygiene and skin care are important considerations. Intensive nursing care is paramount. A few additional patients are salvaged by the use of peritoneal dialysis or the artificial kidney. Recovery usually commences sometime between the seventh and twentieth day. The danger is not automatically over in the recovery phase since the patient will eliminate huge quantities of fluids and electrolytes and is subject to electrolyte imbalances.

The emphasis today is on preventing acute renal failure by correcting shock as soon as possible when it is encountered, preventing hypotension during surgery, and keeping toxic and poisonous materials out of the reach of small children. Patients with urinary infection are particularly prone to develop gram-negative septicemia with endotoxic shock. Careful management of urinary infections with appropriate antibiotics is most important. Closed-space infections such as hydronephrosis must be drained.

Treatment and nursing care

A primary objective in the management of patients with acute renal failure is to maintain a good fluid and electrolyte balance until the renal cells can recover and the course of the disease is reversed. Careful measurement of intake and output on an hourly basis is absolutely essential. The patient is weighed daily and ideally there is a slight but continuous loss of weight. An increase in weight portends congestive failure. Fluid intake is limited to an amount equal to 500 ml. plus the urinary output volume for 24 hours. All potassium must be removed from the diet and none must be given intravenously. The patient's caloric intake cannot be maintained at a normal level, but every effort should be made to give as many calories as possible in the form of hard candy, butter balls, and intravenous glucose. A 10% glucose solution can be given if the intravenous tubing extends into the vena cava. This also affords the opportunity to monitor the central venous pressure, an excellent index of cardiac and vascular efficiency.

Nausea and vomiting may make it more practical to give all the fluid and calories intravenously. The patient must remain in bed to minimize using endogenous calories and breaking down tissue into waste products to be excreted by the kidneys. He must move from side to side at regular intervals or rest upon an air or other type of antidecubitus mattress to avoid the development of pressure ulcers. Protein in the diet is undesirable and it must be sharply limited or deleted since the catabolic products of protein metabolism contribute to the work load of the kidneys and raise the urea nitrogen level in the blood. Mouth care is essential since the patient's mucous membranes become dried and he will frequently have a bad taste. There is a predisposition for inflammation of the salivary glands, which carries a grave prognosis. Ginger ale may obviate mouth dryness and is often permitted. Norethandrolone (Nilevar) or other anabolic drugs should be given to prevent the breakdown of endogenous protein. Infections should be controlled with appropriate antibiotics. Infections are more prone to get out of hand in such seriously ill patients.

It is desirable that the patient be in a private room with special nurses or in an intensive care unit so that attention may be given to his many needs and the rigid management schedule may be carried out. If potas-

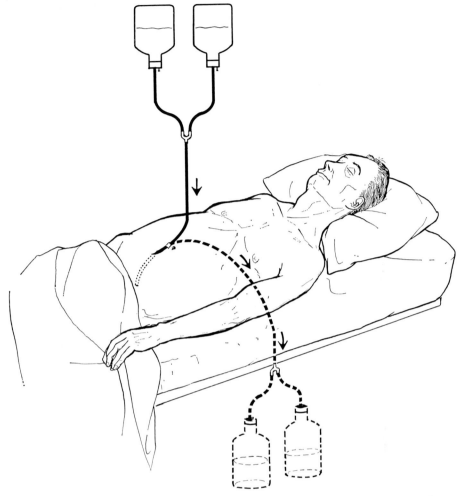

Fig. 7-1. Intraperitoneal dialysis. Two liters of dialyzing fluid are being infused into peritoneal cavity. Later, the same bottles will be placed on floor to allow syphon drainage of cavity (dotted lines). Note indication of position of catheter in peritoneal cavity.

sium intoxication occurs, insulin may be added to the intravenous glucose; this helps remove the potassium from the bloodstream. If exchange resins are used, they may be given orally through a nasogastric tube or in enemas to remove potassium from the bloodstream. The resins absorb the potassium and carry it out of the body. Cathartics and enemas are generally not desirable or as efficient in removing potassium as the exchange resins.

Peritoneal dialysis may be necessary if the patient's condition deteriorates or if he develops excessive edema or too high a level of potassium (Fig. 7-1). If the patient has had abdominal injury or surgery, peritoneal dialysis is contraindicated and use of the artificial kidney is the method

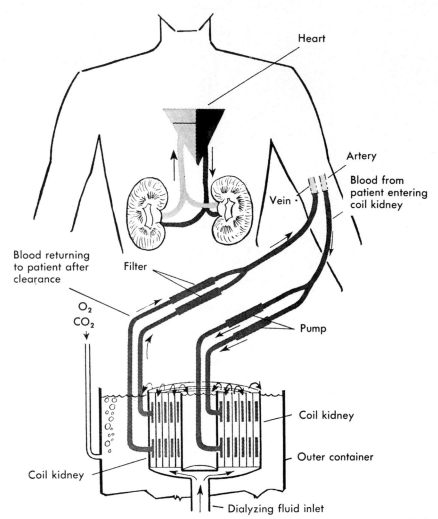

Fig. 7-2. Extracorporeal dialysis. Blood runs from cannulated artery to artificial kidney and then returns into cannulated vein. (From Earle, H.: Today's Health 39:52, 1961.)

of choice. There are a number of types of artificial kidneys available, but they all have in common the principle of dialyzing the patient's blood, which is removed through a cannula in the radial or other main artery. After the excessive fluid and waste products or toxins in the blood are removed, it is returned to one of the larger veins in the body (Fig. 7-2). Most artificial kidneys must be primed with fresh blood that has been heparinized to prevent clotting, thus increasing the danger of the patient hemorrhaging, which he is already prone to because of the uremia. A trained team of nurses, doctors, and laboratory technicians are needed to carry out both peritoneal dialysis and hemodialysis (Fig. 7-3). The

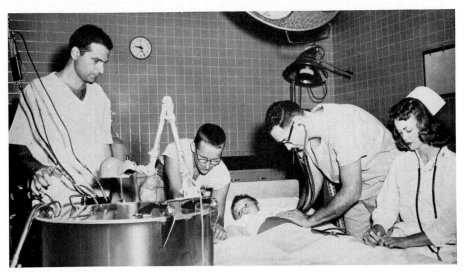

Fig. 7-3. Child attached to artificial kidney. Nurse stays by his bedside. (From Earle, H.: Today's Health 39:52, 1961.)

blood must be monitored by chemical analysis of its various constituents and the patient's weight and blood count carefully checked.

Visitors must be carefully screened; anyone with upper respiratory infection or other infectious disease is not allowed to come into contact with the patient. Most patients with advanced renal failure have indwelling bladder catheters so that hourly urine output can be measured. When the catheter has been in place for several days, a low-grade infection invariably occurs and may be a source of generalized complications. As mentioned earlier, antibiotics should be used judiciously. The urinary tract must be sterilized upon removal of the catheter. Therefore periodic urinalysis, cultures, and antibiotic sensitivity tests are necessary throughout the treatment and follow-up period of acute renal failure. Cardiac failure, pulmonary edema, and septic shock are the three most feared complications of acute renal failure. Pulmonary edema is caused by overhydration, and the nurse and aides must be alert for signs of shortness of breath, respiratory wheezing, and excessive coughing. Occasionally these acute symptoms will be preceded by dependent edema. Moist rales may be heard in the lungs through a stethoscope. If pulmonary edema or hyperkalemia (elevated serum potassium level) or a combination occur, the heart may fail. The pulse becomes very rapid, weak, or irregular and the patient's blood pressure may drop to shock levels. The electrocardiogram will exhibit abnormalities. The doctor must institute emergency measures such as placing tourniquets on the arms, immediately removing some of the blood, or instituting hemodialysis.

Patients that exhibit mental aberrations should be managed using sedatives or tranquilizers and bodily restraint as needed. Noise should be kept to a minimum to provide a calm, quiet environment. Siderails may be required to keep the patient from falling out of bed. The patient will not be helped by arguments, prolonged attempts at verbal persuasion, or bodily force.

The patient's recovery will be heralded by an increased outflow of urine (diuresis). This may be gradual but is usually accelerated. This is one of the dangerous periods since the patient may lose an excessive amount of fluid and electrolytes and careful replacement must be made. The patient will be very weak and is still subject to serious infections. Care must be taken not to become complacent during the period of recovery.

CHRONIC RENAL FAILURE

The patient in the end stages of irreversible renal disease will have anorexia, weight loss, general malaise, and possibly edema. He is always anemic due to depressed bone marrow production of red cells and loss of blood due to intestinal bleeding. An elevated blood pressure may be a concomitant problem, particularly with chronic glomerulonephritis. The chief approach will be fluid, electrolyte, and diet management. Fluid intake is usually normal or, if no edema is present, slightly increased since the kidneys are unable to concentrate the urine and therefore there is a slower excretion of waste products. An accurate record of urinary output must be charted. The doctor may order a low-salt diet since the renal tubular system has a decreased ability to resorb sodium. Salt substitutes are available and one may be chosen that the patient finds palatable. In many patients, potassium must be reduced because of the inability of the kidneys to eliminate it. A variable protein content in the diet is ordered. If the patient is suffering from severe anorexia, the dietician may be helpful in suggesting flavoring such as vinegar, lemon, brown sugar, minced barley, mint, rum, cloves, cinnamon, or salt-free tomato juice to increase the food intake. The patient may have better luck in tolerating carbonated beverages than solid foods. The family can be consulted as to the patient's likes and dislikes in home cooking. If gastrointestinal hemorrhage is encountered, bland foods or a liquid diet may be necessary.

Special attention must be given to the care of the skin and mucous membranes in the extremely ill patient, as described in the previous section.

The patient's anemia will not respond to iron or hematinic drugs and he must usually learn to live with a low blood count. Occasionally, blood transfusions will be necessary to boost the patient's general condition. However, the transfused blood cells do not survive as long as in nonuremic patients. If the patient becomes acidotic, hyperventilation may develop.

In the severe uremic syndrome the patient's breath has a urinary odor. Sodium bicarbonate and calcium gluconate are frequently given in oral or intravenous solutions to counteract acidosis. Phosphate absorption from the gastrointestinal tract may be decreased by giving aluminum hydroxide gel by mouth; this binds the phosphates and allows them to be eliminated by the bowel. Bowel care, as in all hospitalized patients, must be carefully monitored. Stool softeners and scheduled laxatives prevent abdominal distress and fecal impaction.

The pruritus frequently encountered is due to the elimination of urea and sodium by way of the skin and may be counteracted with weak vinegar solutions to dissolve the urea crystals (2 tablespoonfuls to 1 pint of water). Antipruritic drugs are also available. Since the disease is irreversible, it is not prudent to submit most patients to peritoneal dialysis or hemodialysis.

In younger individuals who do not have degenerative and other systemic diseases, renal transplantation has been found applicable. Generally, the patient's diseased kidneys are removed and he may then be maintained on dialysis until a suitable donor kidney is available. The donor kidney may come from an identical twin, close relative, or normal person with a matching blood type. Another popular donor source is a normal kidney removed from an accident victim who dies of head injuries. Occasionally a normal kidney may be removed from a patient for various reasons and this "free kidney" is a most fortuitous gift. After kidney transplantation the patient may have to be maintained on azathioprine (Imuran) or it may be given only when a rejection episode occurs. Likewise, steroids are useful in suppressing the rejection phenomenon. Great care must be taken to prevent infection or to treat it vigorously if it occurs since patients with transplanted kidneys are particularly susceptible to infections. This may be due to the fact that in many such patients the white blood count or white blood cell–forming organs are suppressed by the drugs or irradiation if used. Adequate explanations to both the patient and his relatives and a confident and reassuring manner on the part of the nursing staff as well as efficient and courteous care of the patient's needs help greatly. When a patient feels safe and secure, many emotional situations are stabilized and many symptoms will disappear that are emotional in origin. These same features of good medical and psychiatric bedside care are of tremendous help to the family of a dying patient. If the patient or his relatives desire religious support, the appropriate minister, priest, or rabbi should be in attendance.

GLOMERULONEPHRITIS
Acute glomerulonephritis

Acute glomerulonephritis strikes young children most frequently between the ages of 2 and 12 years of age and males twice as often as females. The etiology is attributed to an antigen-antibody reaction to a streptococcus infection such as laryngitis, tonsillitis, sinusitis, scarlet fever, and chickenpox or any of the respiratory-type infections. The urine is not infected and organisms cannot be cultured from the renal system. Because of the disabling nature of this disease, it is of utmost importance that all upper respiratory infections be viewed with respect and all streptococcal infections be treated vigorously with appropriate antibiotics such as penicillin, sulfonamides, tetracycline, or the current drug of choice as indicated by the physician. The onset may be sudden, with the patient exhibiting weakness, anorexia, pallor, edema, increased blood pressure, headaches, and gross or microscopic hematuria. Nausea, vomiting, and a low-grade fever are not unusual. Visual acuity may be decreased because of retinal edema. The course of the disease may be fulminating and the patient may rapidly progress to the uremic state and ultimate death. More often recovery begins within 10 to 14 days.

Many times the onset is insidious, with the patient developing weakness, lethargy, and anorexia, and the physician discovers microscopic hematuria and urinary casts with proteinuria and anemia. The blood pressure may be normal or only minimally elevated.

The laboratory tests, while varying considerably, usually show albuminuria, granular and hyaline casts (cylindruria), and the presence of red cells and perhaps a few white cells in the urine. Red blood cells are not seen under normal conditions, although up to three or four white cells per high-power field is within normal limits. Since the kidney function is impaired, the serum creatinine and blood urea nitrogen levels may be slightly elevated. Likewise, the phenolsulfonphthalein (PSP) or creatinine clearance tests may show decreased excretion in the urine specimens. The kidneys may be unable to concentrate urine to as high a specific gravity as normally and the amount of protein may vary from small to huge amounts in the urine.

General supportive measures include bed rest, the avoidance of intercurrent infections, particularly of the upper respiratory tract, and good nursing care. An adequate explanation must be given to the patient because the period of bed rest and inactivity may be considerable. Children must be occupied without undue tiring by a scheduled regimen. The patient's course is usually monitored by the sedimentation rate, the blood pressure level, the blood count, blood antistreptolysin O (ASO) titers, and urinalysis. Dietary management varies greatly, but the physician must decide on the basis of the state of edema, the degree of proteinuria, and blood electrolytes as to the degree of salt and protein allowances. A high-carbohydrate diet is often prescribed. In the edematous patient the nurse should be alert for complications such as pulmonary edema, cardiac failure, and increased intracranial pressure. The former will be manifested by wheezing and shortness of breath and the latter by severe headaches and visual disturbances, or the patient may have convulsions or become very irritable or comatose. A precipitous elevation of blood pressure should alert the nurse to notify the physician.

Spontaneous recovery from acute glomerulonephritis within a few weeks to a year or more is the rule. Normally about 5% of the patients die from the acute disease and many times this number eventually succumb from complications. Some of the patients who recover continue to have evidence of renal disease in a subacute or chronic form. They may show proteinuria, hematuria, or hypertension for many years. The kidneys may remain stationary in their functional capacity or there may be a gradual decrease in their ability.

Subacute and latent glomerulonephritis

If the patient has not recovered from the acute phase within 6 to 8 weeks, the disease is then termed subacute. Recurrent streptococcal infections may produce acute exacerbations; there must be a continual vigilance and appropriate measures must be taken to prevent and treat such an occurrence. When symptoms extend beyond a year, the disease is termed chronic. The asymptomatic patient with only albuminuria and cylindruria is one who has latent nephritis. Patients with chronic nephritis must be careful not to overexert themselves. They must obtain sufficient amounts of rest and watch their diets and fluid intake to prevent undue stress on the kidneys. These patients must be seen at regular intervals by their physician to see if there is any change in the status of the disease and to receive any new instructions concerning general health care.

Chronic glomerulonephritis

Many patients are discovered to have chronic glomerulonephritis without exhibiting the acute phase. The discovery may be heralded by edema, hypertension, visual disturbances, and nocturia since the patient's ability to concentrate urine is decreased. General weakness, lassitude, and weight loss are not unusual. The diagnosis is generally made by examination of the urine, which will show proteinuria, casts, and microscopic hematuria. Since the latter may also be caused by stones or tumors, an excretory urogram and cystoscopic examination are usually necessary to rule out such disorders. The kidney function may be slightly to greatly diminished, according to the severity of the disease. Serum proteins may be depressed, with a reversal of the albumin-globulin (A/G) ratio. The course of the disease will be unpredictable at first, but after a period of observation the physician will gain some insight as to the future course. Some patients will linger in this state for many years, while others will gradually or suddenly develop renal failure. The dietary recommendations will include a definite protein intake regulated according to the degree of proteinuria and level of serum proteins. Salt restriction may be indicated in the hypertensive patient, and antihypertensive medications are prescribed. Pregnancy should be avoided since women with this disease are more susceptible to toxemia and abortion. Any long-term illness or disability such as chronic glomerulonephritis requires adequate explanation to the patient's relatives and emphasis on the fact that the management schedule must be followed carefully if optimal results are to be achieved.

NEPHROSIS

Nephrosis is a renal disease that occurs in the young age group, particularly in children between 1 and 6 years of age. The cause is unknown. It is frequently associated with or confused with glomerulonephritis. The onset may be insidious or introduced with the striking finding of generalized edema that will cause the face to appear puffy, the eyelids to become distended, the abdomen to become bloated, and the lower extremities to appear swollen (Fig. 7-4). The skin may have a waxy pallor because of the edema rather than the anemia. The child will be listless but at times irritable. The urine will show high levels of protein and the serum albumin level will be low. The total proteins are depressed, with a reversed A/G ratio. The serum cholesterol will conversely be elevated. Renal function tests indicate normalcy early in the disease, although urine output may vary to the point of oliguria. The treatment is of a general supportive nature, with special attention to the prevention and control of infections, which are one of the chief causes of death. These children are unusually susceptible to pneumonia, skin ulcerations, and other infections. The dietary management includes a low-protein diet and often a low-salt intake. Fats and carbohydrates are usually unrestricted. A vitamin supplement is given. Certain diuretics may be ordered and often the administration of ACTH or cortisone may cause a remission. Many other medications such as ion exchange resins have been used and their application will depend upon the physician's evaluation of the status of the patient. Rarely abdominal paracentesis is necessary because of incapacitating ascites (intraperitoneal fluid).

RENAL HYPERTENSION

Many renal diseases are associated with or are the cause of elevated blood pressure. Hypertension is found with glomerulonephritis, polycystic renal disease, bilateral chronic pyelonephritis, and occasionally with renal neoplasm, cyst, or hydronephrosis. Other than the last three entities, hypertension associated with these renal diseases is not correctable. Approximately 3% of the population of the United States have elevated blood pressures. About 5% of these people have a potentially correctable form

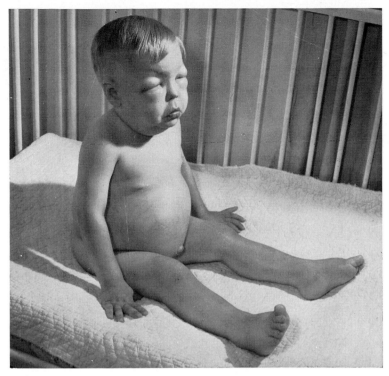

Fig. 7-4. Child with nephrosis. Note edema of face, eyelids, abdomen, and lower extremities. (From Benz, G. S.: Pediatric nursing, ed. 5, St. Louis, 1964, The C. V. Mosby Co.; University of Minnesota Photographic Laboratory.)

of renal hypertension. The kidney tissue is ischemic because of constriction of the main renal artery or one of its branches or because of unilateral or segmental pyelonephritis. The constricting lesions are usually fibromuscular arteritis in younger individuals, especially females, or atherosclerosis in older individuals. Any extrinsic mass compressing the renal artery can likewise produce hypotension within the renal parenchyma. The decreased blood pressure or pulse pressure (the exact factor remains to be determined) causes a reaction within the juxtaglomerular apparatus, resulting in renin production. Renin is an enzyme that acts upon a polypeptide substrate formed in the liver to produce angiotensin I. This is an inactive decapeptide. A converting enzyme further acts upon angiotensin I, splitting off two peptides, histadyl and leucine, and forming a powerful vasoconstrictor, angiotensin II. This is a stable, heat-resistant substance that has been produced synthetically. The removal of a kidney or a segment of a kidney producing renin will cure half of such hypertensive individuals. The operations vary from complete or partial nephrectomy to revascularization of the kidney by correcting the constriction in the renal artery. The lesion may be excised or the lumen may be enlarged with a patch or bypassed with a vascular or synthetic graft from the aorta. In children the splenic artery may be used as a shunt attached to the renal artery distal to the constricting lesion. In many patients a characteristic bruit produced by the renal artery lesion is heard in the epigastrium or back. The diseases that are correctable by surgery occur at any age, but most of the lesions are the result of atherosclerosis and therefore are found after the age of 40 years.

Any patient with hypertension of unknown etiology, regardless of the history, should be given a battery of tests to detect correctable renal hypertension. The survey consists of (1) assay of the blood for renin activity, (2) a radioisotope renogram, which depicts the vascularity, function, and excretion of the individual kidney (see Fig. 6-12), (3) an excretory urogram, which outlines the internal architecture of the kidney as well as the appearance time and concentration of the contrast material (see Fig. 6-14), and (4) a renal arteriogram, which outlines the arteries to the kidneys (Fig. 6-18). The latter is indispensable since it serves not only as a diagnostic test but also as a guide to the surgeon wishing to revascularize the kidney. Other preoperative investigations include standard divided renal function tests which are performed by cystoscopy and catheterization of each ureter (Fig. 6-15). Urine is collected from each kidney for several timed periods to note the urine flow rate as well as the concentration of sodium and creatinine or other solutes that may be infused intravenously (for example, para-aminohippurate). In the typical example of unilateral renal disease causing hypertension the affected kidney will show a 50% or more reduction in urine flow rate and a 15% or more reduction in sodium concentration but a twofold or more increase in the creatinine or hippurate concentration as compared with its mate. Since lesions or disease can occur segmentally or bilaterally, the differential tests occasionally are misleading. It is better to depend upon a battery of renal tests than upon any one screening maneuver.

Renal biopsy (needle or open operation) has been advocated by some to ascertain the juxtaglomerular apparatus changes in the affected kidney and its otherwise normal microscopic appearance. Likewise, biopsy of the unaffected kidney should show normal renal architecture if a reasonable outcome from surgery is to be expected.

Bioassay of venous blood samples for angiotensin (indirect measurement of renin activity) has been used extensively. An elevated angiotensin level in the peripheral blood is usually indicative of renal hypertension. The source of renin may be further isolated if each renal vein is catheterized and its blood analyzed. The prepared plasma is injected into a rat and the blood pressure response noted. The presence of angiotensin will elevate the rat's blood pressure (Fig. 7-5). Immunoassays and radioisotopic methods are now being introduced.

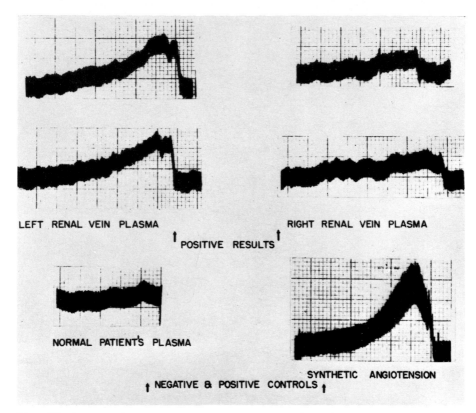

LEFT RENAL VEIN PLASMA   RIGHT RENAL VEIN PLASMA

POSITIVE RESULTS

NORMAL PATIENT'S PLASMA

SYNTHETIC ANGIOTENSION

NEGATIVE & POSITIVE CONTROLS

Fig. 7-5. Bioassay for angiotensin is performed by processing patient's plasma and injecting small sample into vascular system of rat. If angiotensin is present, rat's blood pressure will rise as seen in examples. Normal patient's processed plasma is used for negative control, and synthetic angiotensin is infused as positive control. Either peripheral venous blood or individual renal venous blood samples may be used.

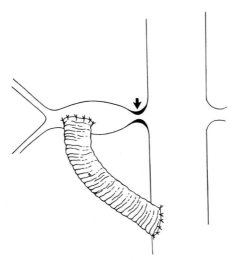

Fig. 7-6. Example of synthetic graft used to bypass stenosis of renal artery.

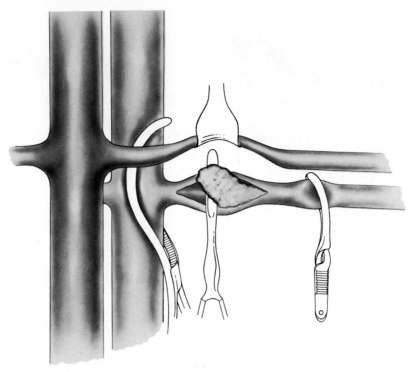

Fig. 7-7. Illustrating technique of performing an endarterectomy of left renal artery. Note that left renal vein must be retracted away from artery since it lies anterior to this vessel.

Even if the patient's blood pressure is not completely corrected after renal surgery, it may be reduced to a tolerable level or the patient may be more amenable to drug therapy.

Following nephrectomy the patient is kept in bed without oral intake of food or fluids for 1 day and is maintained on intravenous feedings. Following this he is placed on a graduated diet and allowed to ambulate. The blood pressure is monitored several times a day to note its return to normal or any evidence of persistent elevation. The angiotensin assay is repeated to note if it has returned to a normal level.

After a revascularization operation has taken place (Figs. 7-6 and 7-7), the patient's blood pressure is likewise monitored and careful fluid intake and output records kept. Since the renal artery may have been clamped for a period of time during surgery or the patient may have had an episode of hypotension, unilateral or bilateral renal shutdown is possible postoperatively. Intravenous mannitol is usually given during and after such surgery to offset the possibility of acute renal failure. The blood pressure may drop precipitously to normal while the patient is on the operating table or it may come down gradually over a period of hours, days, or weeks. The renal function can be monitored with renograms, excretory urograms, or a scintillation camera. Long-term follow-up blood pressure monitoring is required as well as renal function tests. These patients are prone to develop a recurrence of the hypertension.

RENAL TRANSPLANTATION

Pediatric or young adult patients with severe renal failure are candidates for renal transplantation. They must not have malignancies, other serious disorders, or degenerative diseases; there must be an excellent chance for survival. An identical twin remains the best donor of a kidney. Since the patients are often minors, parental and sometimes judical consent must be obtained. The legal implications, let alone the moral and social factors involved in using live donors, have not been completely resolved. The emotional impact on all concerned calls for the utmost reassurance and support by the "transplantation team." Nevertheless, surprisingly little difficulty along these lines has been encountered. Close relatives and people with nearly the same blood types comprise the next most suitable live donors. Because of the scarcity of live donors and free grafts (normal kidneys removed for other surgical reasons), cadaver kidneys are now receiving great attention and are being used in increasing numbers. These donors are usually young accident victims in prime health before death. The ticklish problems of determining the time of death, gaining consent for donation, and preserving the kidney for transplant pose difficult but not insurmountable problems. Dual transplants are possible in some instances. Preservation of the graft prior to anastomosis is enhanced by special perfusion and cooling techniques. The technical details of renal vascular and ureterovesical anastomosis have been worked out quite well and do not pose serious difficulties. The usual method is to place the donor's left kidney into the recipient's right iliac fossa, anastomosing the renal artery to the hypogastric or external iliac artery and the renal vein to the external iliac vein. The critical phase of transplantation is still the rejection phenomenon (antigen-antibody reaction). This is thought to be centered in the white blood cells, and the development of antiserum is one of the latest advances in this field. Other methods of combating rejection of the graft are splenectomy, thymectomy, irradiation of the transplanted kidney, irradiation of white cells, hydrocortisone administration, azathioprine therapy, and antilymphocyte globulin. Special attention is given to the prevention and treatment of infections since the recipient's resistance is lowered by immunosuppressive measures and infection is a chief cause of rejection and death.

Occasionally the patient will need dialysis to carry him through periods of crisis, and many patients are maintained on periodic dialysis prior to transplantation. The recipient's kidneys are usually removed at the time of transplantation or later since they often cause hypertension (produce renin because of ischemia) or easily develop pyelonephritis.

Nursing care

The nurse caring for patients with transplants discovers that one of her major roles is that of teacher, in addition to giving expert nursing care. At the time of diagnosis and continually throughout postoperative periods, teaching the patient and his family is an individualized process. The better the understanding of both the patient and his family, the more likely postoperative complications will be avoided. The patient must be well versed in what to expect after transplantation as to rejection symptoms, medication, fluid intake-output, signs of infection, diet, and activities of daily living. It is important that all the staff caring for the patient agree on the plan for each patient and consistently provide him with guidance and information that does not conflict.

Since patients' symptoms may vary, the alert nurse will anticipate all possibilities and prepare for them. Dietary regimes may necessitate changes in the patient's usual pattern. Because of the importance of diet, all efforts should be made to tailor changes in diet therapy to the patient's likes and dislikes, with emphasis on the reasons for the specific diet regime. An understanding of fluid balance in relation to kidney function will be necessary for patients if they are expected to cooperate in their care and assist in management of intake and output. Hygienic care is a major area of concern due to the patient's low resistance to infection. Cleanliness and frequent good mouth care will help alleviate symptoms of dry skin and a sore mouth. Patients should expect dizziness and visual changes. If the patient is to be maintained on hemodialysis until a donor is available, instruction as to the limitations of this procedure must be repeatedly covered.

General postoperative care will be similar to that for any surgical patient. In some centers the patient may go directly from surgery to an intensive care unit and may or may not be placed in reverse isolation. Wherever the patient resides, personnel with upper respiratory infections should not come in contact with the patient, the aim being to protect the patient from unnecessary sources of infection. The patient will need intensive care for 3 to 4 days. Immediately after surgery, vital signs will be taken every 15 minutes until stable, every 30 minutes for 4 hours, and then hourly. The temperature will be monitored every 4 hours. The patient will be on oral intake and will receive fluids intravenously, the amount based on the urinary output. Hourly urine output is measured in milliliters and its specific gravity recorded. A nasal gastric tube connected to low suction may need to be irrigated hourly with 30 ml. of saline solution. Although the patient is to lie flat, his head may be elevated on pillows. Antibiotic therapy such as streptomycin and methicillin sodium (Staphcillin) and immunosuppressive agents such as azathioprine, ALG, and prednisolone are the usual drugs given. Laboratory determinations of Na, K, Cl, CO_2, BUN, creatinine, blood cell count, and platelets are performed daily. Urine is also checked daily for Na, K, Cl, creatinine, urea, sugar, and protein. Weekly chest films and determination of the total protein, Ca, K, alkaline phosphatase, fasting blood sugar, SGOT, SGPT, and bilirubin are required plus stool, urine, throat, and sputum cultures. The patient will have a urethral catheter and a reddish urine that should clear within 48 hours may be expected.

Because infection is the most important complication, scrupulous catheter care is essential. Coughing and deep breathing, strict aseptic techniques used in caring for the wound, frequent good mouth care, and general hygienic care will all assist in its prevention.

Symptoms and signs of rejection of the kidney should be watched for constantly. These are fever, hypertension, elevation of blood urea nitrogen, gain in weight, decreased urine output, lowered creatinine clearance, swelling, tenderness, and redness at the kidney site, and a general increase in tiredness, irritability, anxiousness, restlessness, and lethargy.

Acute rejection may take place within minutes of the vascular anastomosis or within the first postoperative week. Dosages of immunosuppressive agents are usually increased, and depending on the severity of rejection, the diet is restricted in protein, potassium, and sodium. If intensive treatment does not reverse rejection, the transplanted kidney will be removed; the patient then must await another donor. It is important that the patient and his family have been prepared emotionally for this situation. The goal of the patient, family, and staff has been to return the patient to a normal life. Teaching prior to surgery regarding prevention of infection, diet, drug therapy, symptoms of rejection, and urinary output will now need reemphasis. If self-care has been stressed throughout the patient's hospitalization, independence and responsibility for periodic follow-up can be effectively accomplished. The nurse's role does not end with the patient's discharge from the hospital. Seeing the patient in follow-up visits or in his own home environment will provide a better opportunity to understand the patient facing renal transplantation, the importance of family relationships, and the comprehensive nursing care required. The nurse interested in care of the renal transplant patient is urged to consult the latest articles on nursing techniques and care since there is continual change.

QUESTIONS

1. List some common causes of acute renal failure.
2. What is the chief sign of acute renal failure?
3. Acute renal failure must be differentiated from what other urologic entity?

4. What is the primary objective in managing acute renal failure?
5. What are the chief dangers to the patient in acute renal failure?
6. What are some complications of chronic renal failure?
7. What is the usual age of patients developing acute glomerulonephritis?
8. What is the etiology of acute glomerulonephritis?
9. How is the course of acute glomerulonephritis monitored?
10. What is the usual outcome of acute glomerulonephritis?
11. What is the definition of subacute glomerulonephritis?
12. Why should pregnancy be avoided in a patient with chronic glomerulonephritis?
13. What is the difference between nephrosis and glomerulonephritis?
14. What renal abnormalities may cause hypertension?
15. What percent of the hypertensive population have a correctable form of renal hypertension?
16. How is angiotensin II produced?
17. What is the juxtaglomerular apparatus?
18. List some of the tests used to detect correctable renal hypertension.
19. From what sources may blood be obtained for the performance of bioassay of angiotensin (renin)?
20. What types of operations may be performed to correct renal hypertension?
21. What type of patients are candidates for renal transplantation?
22. Where may kidneys be obtained for a renal transplantation?
23. What are three causes of failure of renal transplantation?
24. How is the patient monitored following renal transplantation?
25. What are some of the symptoms and signs of renal rejection?

REFERENCES

Arneil, G. C.: Nephritis. I. Acute hemorrhagic nephritis, Nurs. Times 57:586, 1961.
Arneil, G. C.: Nephritis. II. The nephrotic syndrome, Nurs. Times 57:622, 1961.
Breakey, B. A., Woodruff, M. W., and Reus, W. F., Jr.: The adaptability of the Kolff twin coil artificial kidney for dialysis in infancy, J. Urol. 86:304, 1961.
Burns, R. O., Henderson, R. W., and Hager, E. B.: Peritoneal dialysis, New Eng. J. Med. 267:1060, 1962.
Downing, S. R.: Nursing support in early renal failure, Amer. J. Nurs. 69:1212, 1969.
Fried, W.: Anemia of renal failure, Med. Clin. N. Amer. 55:3, 1971.
Hedger, R. W.: The conservative management of acute oliguric renal failure, Med. Clin. N. Amer. 55:121, 1971.
Lippman, R. W.: Urine and the urinary sediment; a practical manual and atlas, ed. 2, Springfield, Ill., 1957, Charles C Thomas, Publisher.
McDonald, H. P., Jr., and Waterhouse, R. K.: Chronic renal failure from urological diseases: treatment by sodium balancing and low-protein diet of high biological value, J. Urol. 103:262, 1970.
Monroe, J. M., and Komorita, I.: Problems with nephrosis in adolescence, Amer. J. Nurs. 67:336, 1967.
Oyamo, J. H.: Diagnosis and treatment of lupus nephritis, Med. Clin. N. Amer. 55:71, 1971.
Schlesinger, E. R., Sultz, H. A., Mosher, W. E., and Feldman, G.: The nephrotic syndrome. Its incidence and implications for the community, Amer. J. Dis. Child. 116:623, 1968.
Schweitz, L.: Hypertension and renal disease in pregnancy, Med. Clin. N. Amer. 55:47, 1971.
Shebelski, D. I.: Nursing patients who have renal homotransplants, Amer. J. Nurs. 66:2425, 1966.
Starzl, T. E.: Experience in renal transplantation, Philadelphia, 1964, W. B. Saunders Co.

Stewart, B. H., Dustan, H. P., Kiser, W. S., Meaney, T. F., Straffon, R. A., and Mc-Cormack, L. J.: Correlation of angiography and natural history in evaluation of patients with renovascular hypertension, J. Urol. **104**:231, 1970.

Strauss, M. B., and Welt, G.: Diseases of the kidney, Boston, 1963, Little, Brown & Co.

Swinney, J.: Conservative surgery of the kidney, Nurs. Mirror **126**:33, 1968.

Watson, I.: Nursing care of patient with glomerulonephritis, Canad. Nurse **62**:48, 1966.

Winter, C. C.: Correctable renal hypertension, Philadelphia, 1964, Lea & Febiger.

Winter, C. C.: The performance of divided renal function tests in renal hypertension; a practical method, J. Urol. **91**:203, 1964.

Winter, C. C.: Renogram and other radioisotope tests in the diagnosis of renal hypertension, Amer. J. Surg. **107**:43, 1964.

Winter, C. C.: Three angiotensin tests in the investigation of renal hypertension: bioassay, infusion, renogram, J. Urol. **96**:858, 1964.

Winter, C. C.: Practical urology, St. Louis, 1969, The C. V. Mosby Co.

CHAPTER 8

Obstructive uropathy

Obstruction of the urinary tract is a common entity. It not only compromises the function of structures proximal to the point of obstruction but the attendant stasis promotes infection and stone formation. The newborn male infant may have posterior urethral valves. The female child may have a stricture of the urethral meatus (Fig. 8-1). Bladder neck contracture is occasionally seen; more often, obstruction of the ureterovesical junction or of the ureteropelvic (UP) junction is encountered. As the male ages, hyperplasia or neoplastic enlargement of the prostate frequently occurs. If the obstruction occurs in the urethra or bladder neck, the bladder may show evidence of decompensation as manifested by trabeculations, cellules, saccules, or diverticula (Fig. 8-2). The ureterovesical valves may become incompetent and the ureters may exhibit dilatation, kinking, or tortuosity, and the kidneys may show hydronephrosis and diminished thickness of the parenchyma.

STRICTURES

Strictures in the urethra may be congenital or acquired. In the male the latter are by far the most common and usually follow infection from gonococci or other bacteria or they may be caused by trauma or the passage of catheters or instruments. Females of all ages frequently have urethral meatal stenosis.

Urethral strictures are most commonly treated by dilatation with sounds, filiform-followers (see Fig. 3-4), or gradually by the use of a series of catheters of increasing sizes. The stricture may be incised by internal urethrotomy (using a urethrotome) or by an open operation (urethroplasty) (Fig. 8-3). Many patients have chronic strictures, requiring many treatments or operations. Rarely, the urine must be diverted. The nurse must help the patient in overcoming discouragement and depression caused by long, drawn-out treatment.

244

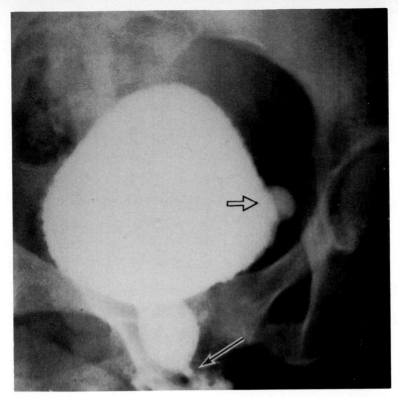

Fig. 8-1. Voiding cystourethrogram shows severe stenosis of urethral meatus in female patient (large arrow). Urethra proximal to stenosis is markedly dilated. There is trabeculation of bladder wall and at least one diverticulum is demonstrated (small arrow).

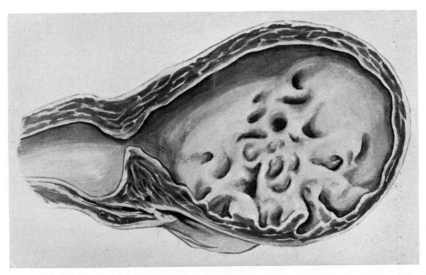

Fig. 8-2. Sagittal view of prostatic fossa, bladder neck, and bladder. Note elevated posterior lip of bladder neck, which represents median bar formation causing bladder neck contracture. As a result, bladder has become heavily trabeculated with cellules, saccules, and possible diverticula (these openings are to be seen). The prostate itself is not enlarged.

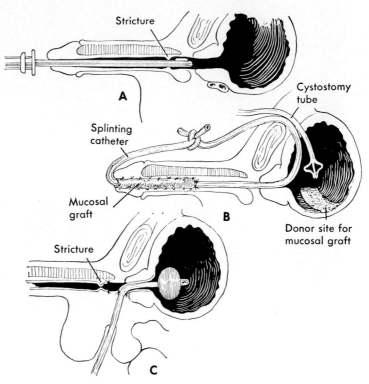

Fig. 8-3. A, Schematic drawing showing passage of urethrotome in treatment of stricture of male urethra (internal urethrotomy). **B,** Schematic drawing of plastic reconstruction of urethra. Note splinting catheter and cystostomy tube; urine should drain only through cystostomy tube. Note donor site in bladder; this is a bladder mucosal graft. **C,** Schematic drawing of placement of urethral catheter following perineal (external) urethrotomy. Note urethral stricture below external urethral sphincter. (From Shafer, K. N., Sawyer, J. R., McCluskey, A. M., and Beck, E. L.: Medical-surgical nursing, ed. 4, St. Louis, 1967, The C. V. Mosby Co.)

BLADDER NECK CONTRACTURE

Bladder neck contracture is most often encountered after the age of 40 years and is secondary to chronic prostatitis, which causes shrinkage of the prostate and contracture at the bladder neck.

DIVERTICULUM

Diverticula of the bladder may be congenital or they may develop because of bladder neck, prostate, or urethral obstruction (Fig. 8-4). They occur most often adjacent to the ureteral orifice and especially in the upper motor neuron neurogenic bladder. They cause residual urine and predispose to cystitis. If large, they are best treated by excision, either alone or in conjunction with surgical relief of bladder outlet obstruction.

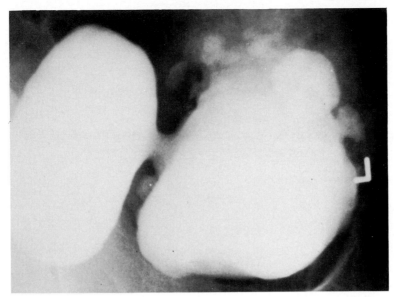

Fig. 8-4. Cystogram shows many vesical diverticula. Note narrow neck of diverticulum on right side of bladder.

BENIGN PROSTATIC ENLARGEMENT

A common form of bladder neck obstruction is caused by benign enlargement of the prostate in older males. The symptom complex of slowing of the urinary stream with increased frequency of urination and nocturia is known as prostatism. Prostatism may be due to malignant enlargement of the prostate. This is the fifth most common male malignancy, but it is also the type that causes the most deaths due to neoplasms in males. This disease will be discussed under tumors of the urologic system in Chapter 11.

Benign prostatic hypertrophy is treated by enucleation of the prostate through an open operation if it is more than 75 to 100 grams in weight; transurethral resection is the treatment of choice if it is of a smaller size. The enlargement may be primarily in the lateral lobes, or a median lobe may be present. For transurethral resection a resectoscope is used and the tissue is trimmed away with a wire loop to which electric current is applied (Fig. 8-5). The current can be varied so that pure cutting, fulguration, or a blend of the two can be applied to the tissue. A cold punch resectoscope is sometimes used (Thompson resectoscope). It removes tissue in small pieces by a guillotine action upon tissue that is pressed into the fenestra of its operating element. Bleeding points are then coagulated with an electrode.

The open operations, which enucleate the benign adenomas but leave

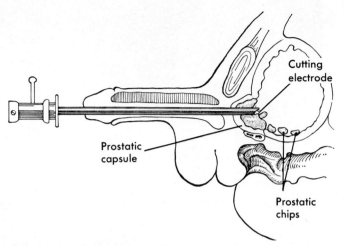

Fig. 8-5. Diagram of transurethral resection of prostate gland. Resectoscope is inserted through urethra. Note cutting and cauterizing loop of instrument and tiny pieces of prostatic tissue that have been cut away. (From Shafer, K. N., Sawyer, J. R., Mc-Cluskey, A. M., Beck, E. L., and Phipps, W. J.: Medical-surgical nursing, ed. 5, St. Louis, 1971, The C. V. Mosby Co.)

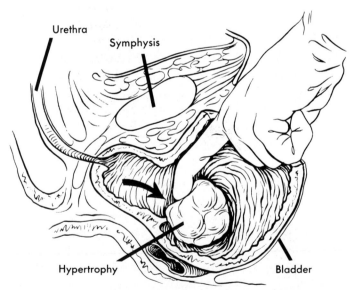

Fig. 8-6. Suprapubic prostatectomy is performed by opening bladder and enucleating prostate with finger inserted into prostatic urethra as shown here. Rim of normal prostatic tissue compressed by enlarging adenoma forms false or surgical capsule. Prostatic fossa will reepithelize to form new posterior urethra and will be smaller than cavity left behind at time of surgery.

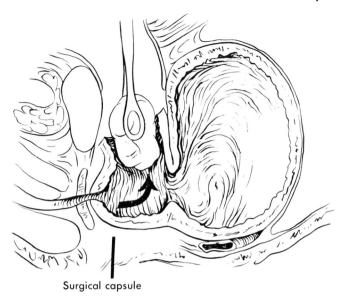

Surgical capsule

Fig. 8-7. Retropubic prostatectomy is performed through incision in lower abdomen and opening the anterior prostatic fossa to enucleate hypertrophied prostate.

the true capsule and a thinned-out portion of the normal tissue known as the false capsule, may be carried out through the suprapubic route (Fig. 8-6), the retropubic approach (Fig. 8-7), the transsacral route, or the perineal approach (Fig. 8-8). In the latter operation the patient is placed in the extreme lithotomy position and an incision is made in the perineum similar to some of the old lithotomy operations (see Fig. 11-10). Care must be taken to avoid entering the rectum since a rectal fistula may be catastrophic. The posterior capsule of the prostate is opened and the gland enucleated. This procedure is less shocking than other types of prostatectomy and is most suitable for the large gland in older males in whom sexual desire and ability have waned. This operation, because it interferes with the nerve supply to the prostate, usually makes the patient impotent. There is about a 5% incidence of incontinence also. It is the most difficult of the prostatectomies to master. The suprapubic prostatectomy is carried out through an incision in the lower abdomen, and an extraperitoneal approach to the bladder is made. The bladder is opened, and a finger is used to enucleate the gland from within the prostatic urethra. It is a blind operation and control of bleeding may be difficult. A pack is occasionally left in the prostatic fossa for a day or two. The retropubic operation for a large gland uses the same skin and fascia incision as the suprapubic procedure. However, the bladder and prostate are pulled superiorly and an incision is made in the anterior prostatic fossa. The gland is enucleated similar to the perineal method. It

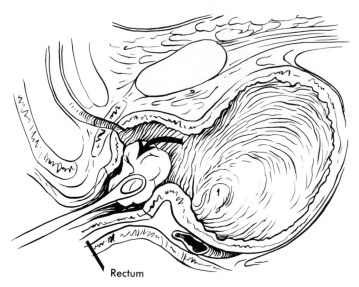

Rectum

Fig. 8-8. Perineal prostatectomy is performed by approach just anterior to rectum and by incising posterior prostatic fossa. It is a mirror image of retropubic prostatectomy.

is easier to see bleeding points, which can be fulgurated or sutured. An indwelling catheter is usually left for 2 or 3 days after transurethral resection, but it must be left longer following the open operations. If operative hemorrhage is a problem, a suprapubic tube may be placed in addition to a urethral catheter for purposes of continuous irrigations and to act as a safety valve in case clots plug the urethral catheter. In the open operation a wedge of the posterior bladder neck or a Y-V bladder neck plasty may be carried out to ensure a good result. Contracture of the bladder neck is possible after all types of prostatectomy, but more so after a transurethral resection.

Prostatectomy for benign disease does not act as a prophylaxis against cancer, which may occur later since a remnant of prostatic tissue is left in the false capsule. The posterior lamella is the site of origin in 75% of the cases of prostatic cancer. Total prostatectomy (including the capsule) is usually limited to the curable stages of cancer of the prostate or to cases in which there is an intractable and symptomatic infection of the prostate. Prostatic stones are not uncommon and usually are located in the periphery of the gland. Such stones make it impossible to eradicate infection by massage or drugs.

After a prostatectomy, catheters must be checked repeatedly, especially if the drainage is bloody, to ensure that the tubes are patent. If gentle irrigation does not establish free drainage, the doctor should be notified. He may employ traction on the catheter for short periods of time to control venous ooze. A full bladder or one distended with clots is painful; this may be noted visually or by palpation of the lower abdomen. The patient often has bladder spasms, and it should be explained to him that these are caused by the presence of the catheter. The dressings applied after open prostatectomy are usually saturated and must be changed as often as necessary to keep the patient dry. A tissue drain will be present and care must be taken not to dislodge it. Montgomery straps are useful for dressings that require frequent changing. After the catheter is removed, the times and amounts of micturition should be recorded, or the doctor may wish the first few specimens saved for inspection. The patient may have poor sphincter control during the first 24 hours. He may pass blood intermittently for 2 to 4 weeks. He may still have difficulty in voiding temporarily, especially after transurethral surgery.

URETERAL OBSTRUCTION

Strictures can occur at any site in the ureter, but they are most commonly located where the ureter normally narrows—at the ureterovesical junction (Fig. 8-9) where the ureter crosses the iliac vessels and at the ureteropelvic junction. Strictures may be caused by infection such as tuberculosis or by the passage of stones or instruments, or they may occur postoperatively.

The lower ureter may be obstructed by a ureterocele, which is a distention of the intramural ureter that causes its mucosa to bulge into the bladder lumen (see Fig. 2-4). Rarely, a ureterocele may obstruct the bladder neck or even protrude from the female urethral meatus. Ureteroceles occur commonly with complete duplications of the ureter and usually involve the distal ureter (from the upper pole). If a ureterocele is excised, reimplantation of the ureter may be necessary to prevent vesicoureteral reflux. The ureter that is obstructed without a ureterocele may also be managed by reimplantation into the bladder (ureteroneocystostomy) using an antireflux technique (Fig. 8-10).

Obstruction at the ureteropelvic junction (Fig. 8-11) is corrected by a pyeloplasty if the kidney is worth salvaging. There are many types of pyeloplasties that may be utilized, depending on the type of ureteral obstruction and the anatomy of the renal pelvis. Aberrant or accessory renal arteries are a common cause of obstruction of the ureteropelvic junction (Fig. 8-12). Operative correction merely involves moving the vessels away from the ureteropelvic junction; they are not ligated since this would cause infarction of a portion of the kidney (the arteries do not intercommunicate). A pyeloplasty is not always necessary in such a situation, but lysis of adhesions and careful calibration of the ureteropelvic junction are in order (Fig. 8-13). A kidney that is badly damaged by hydronephrosis may be removed if the mate has nearly normal function.

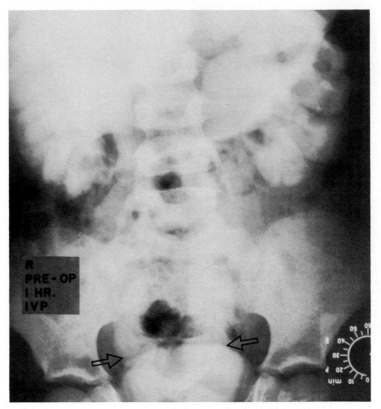

Fig. 8-9. Excretory urogram of young girl. At 1 hour, both kidneys show hydronephrosis and both ureters are markedly dilated down to the bladder level. Note thinness of renal parenchyma. Partial obstruction of both ureterovesical junctions (arrows) was found to be the etiology.

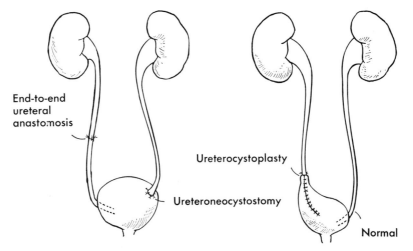

Fig. 8-10. Plastic repairs of ureter. (Adapted from unpublished illustration of Dr. B. G. Clarke and Dr. L. Del Guercio.)

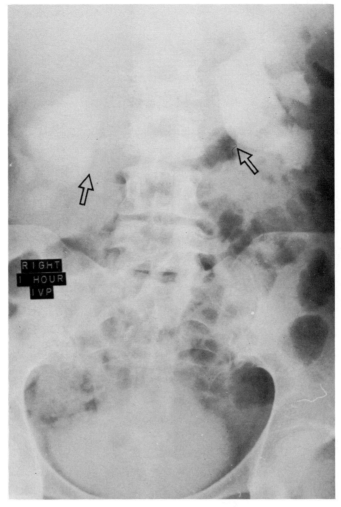

Fig. 8-11. Excretory urogram shows bilateral hydronephrosis represented by dilatation of both renal pelves and calyces. Obstruction at both ureteropelvic junctions (arrows) is the cause.

However, many obstructions of the ureteropelvic junction are bilateral, with one side developing a greater degree of disability than the contralateral kidney. In some obstructive situations a loop of the ureter may be brought to the flank as a temporary cutaneous loop ureterostomy. This is quite useful in the pediatric age group when there is hope of reinstituting the lower urinary system. When this is not feasible, the ureter may be brought directly to the skin as a cutaneous ureterostomy. This works best if the ureter is dilated. Both ureters may be so handled if bilateral obstruction is found, or one ureter may be anastomosed to its mate (transureteroureterostomy) and only one ureter brought to the skin, allowing

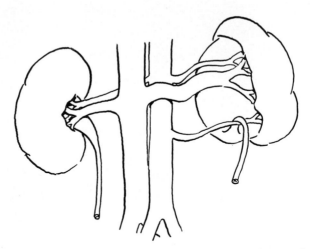

Fig. 8-12. Diagram of aberrant vessel to left kidney. Note kink caused in ureter and hydronephrotic renal pelvis. Right kidney is normal. (Unpublished illustration by Dr. B. G. Clarke and Dr. L. Del Guercio.)

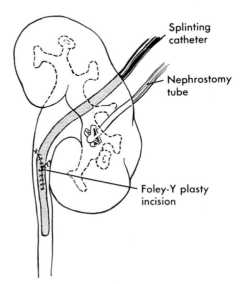

Fig. 8-13. Schematic drawing showing placement of splinting catheter after Foley-Y plasty incision of ureter. Note nephrostomy tube used to drain urine. (From Shafer, K. N., Sawyer, J. R., McCluskey, A. M., Beck, E. L., and Phipps, W. J.: Medical-surgical nursing, ed. 5, St. Louis, 1971, The C. V. Mosby Co.)

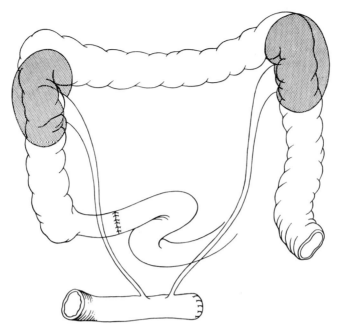

Fig. 8-14. Sketch of Bricker procedure (bilateral ureteroileocutaneous anastomosis). Note that ileal segment acts as conduit rather than as reservoir for urine coming from ureters.

a single urinary outlet. If the ureters are of normal caliber, the cutaneous ends are apt to constrict; in an effort to obviate this, omentum may be wrapped around the distal ends to act as a buffer between the skin and ureter.

A popular form of urinary diversion when disease of the bladder or urethra is intractable is the Bricker procedure (Fig. 8-14). This innovation, introduced in 1948, utilizes an isolated short segment of small bowel to act as a conduit between the ureters and the skin. The ureters are anastomosed to the proximal end of the ileal segment by end-to-side anastomoses, and the distal end of the ileal segment is brought to an opening in the abdomen, usually in the lower right quadrant. An isolated segment of colon may be substituted for ileum and presumably has strongly peristaltic emptying force. Also, it lends itself to location of the stoma in the left lower quadrant. Conversely, the colonic contents are infested and an attempt must be made to sterilize the rectum and large bowel before the operation; in contrast, no preparation is necessary when ileum is used. Collecting bags or devices must be worn for all types of urinary ostomies.

RETROPERITONEAL FIBROSIS

Rarely, the midureters become encased in fibrous tissue, causing unilateral or bilateral hydronephrosis. Anemia, weight loss, low backache, and fever are common findings. Pyelograms show the typical location of the ureteral stricture. The cause is unknown in most instances, but patients taking ergot or methysergide maleate (vasoconstricting drugs) are known to develop this condition. Withdrawal of the drugs will usually cause resolution of the fibrosis and hydronephrosis. Other patients require ureteral exploration to rule out tumor and stone and ureterolysis or ureteral resection for relief of hydronephrosis and backache and/or azotemia due to the obstruction. A good outcome is usually to be expected unless retroperitoneal neoplasm is found as the cause of ureteral obstruction. Strictures of the lower ureters in females are commonly related to gynecologic disease or pelvic surgery. Nursing care is the same as for any patient with hydronephrosis or ureteral surgery.

NEPHROPTOSIS

The right kidney is more mobile than its mate and in women especially it may descend several inches in the upright position. Usually there is no discomfort or other problems. Rarely, such a "floating kidney" will become obstructed at the ureteropelvic junction, and severe pain and temporary hydronephrosis will occur (Dietl's crisis). The relief of pain by assuming the supine position or the demonstration of intermittent hydronephrosis during the attack may warrant surgically suturing the kidney into its normal anatomic site (nephropexy). The operation also is usually performed with most pyeloplasties.

QUESTIONS

1. List some common sites and types of obstruction of the urinary system.
2. What is the usual management of urethral strictures?
3. What is the most frequent type of urethral obstruction in the female?
4. Bladder neck contracture is most commonly associated with what other disease?
5. The fifth most common malignancy in the male other than skin cancer is of what organ?
6. What is a diverticulum?
7. What are the different approaches used for removing the prostate gland?
8. What is a ureterocele?
9. What operative procedure is performed to correct vesicoureteral reflux?
10. What operative procedure is used to correct obstruction at the ureteropelvic junction?
11. What is the Bricker procedure?
12. Retroperitoneal fibrosis commonly affects which portion of the ureter?
13. What drug can cause retroperitoneal fibrosis?
14. A "floating kidney" is more common in which sex and on which side?
15. What is nephroptosis and a nephropexy?

REFERENCES

Ceccarelli, F. E., and Smith, P. C.: Studies on fluid and electrolyte alterations during transurethral prostatectomy, J. Urol. 86:434, 1961.
Higham, A. R. C.: Prostatic obstruction, Nurs. Times 57:447, 1961.
Hudson, P. B.: An atlas of prostatic surgery, Philadelphia, 1962, W. B. Saunders Co.

Kasselman, M. J.: Nursing care of the patient with B.P.H., Amer. J. Nurs. **66**:1026, 1966.

Lyon, R. P., and Tanagho, E. A.: Distal urethral stenosis in little girls, J. Urol. **93**:379, 1965.

Maloney, J. D., and Smith, J. P.: Temporary cutaneous loop ureterostomy, J. Urol. **103**:790, 1970.

Rubin, E.: Types of prostatectomy discussed; good nursing service essential, Hosp. Top. **43**:110, 1965.

9

CHAPTER

Infections

Urinary infections may involve any part of the urologic system and may be localized or generalized. They commonly migrate from one part of the genitourinary system to another (for example, bladder to kidney, prostate to epididymis).

CYSTITIS

The most common site of urinary infections is the bladder, and this infection is known as cystitis. It affects females much more often than males and particularly in their most active sexual years. This is thought to be due to the fact that the urethra is traumatized and easily contaminated from the vaginal tract, the rectum, or the male partner. The female urethra is short, and bacteria may enter much more readily than in the male, who has a long, pendulous urethra. Male cystitis most commonly arises from infection in the urethra or prostate. The male may become infected from sexual contact, beginning with a urethritis that may be non-specific, viral, or gonorrheal in type and ending with a chronic prostatic infection. Cystitis causes the bladder to be irritable so that the patient has the urge to void more often (urgency), and increased frequency may occur both day and night (nocturia). The act of urination causes burning (dysuria), and bladder cramps or spasms (tenesmus) occur often. Frequently the inflammation causes the bladder wall to bleed, and gross hematuria may be exhibited. In such cases the infection is known as hemorrhagic cystitis. Bacteria that split urea into ammonia will produce an alkaline urine that will foster the precipitation of calcium and stone formation. Calcium ammonium phosphate stones therefore are the most common type in infected urine. The first attack of cystitis, which is usually superficial, is readily cleared by sulfonamides or broad-spectrum antibiotics, but the causative organism should be ascertained by urine culture and antibiotic sensitivity tests should be carried out. The urine sediment characteristically will show bacteria and an increased number of white cells, many of which may clump. The former can be seen on a wet smear or by staining the urine with methylene blue or Gram's stain. Obtaining a clean, midstream voided specimen is a reliable method of collecting urine from the male for examination. It is more difficult to obtain a midstream, clean specimen from the female, and any voided urine showing evidence of infection must make the examiner wary of a contaminant from the vaginal canal. Therefore, when bacterial growth or pyuria is found in the urine specimen of a female, a catheterized specimen should be obtained to verify the presence of infection. A bacterial colony count of over 10,000 per milliliter is also highly indicative of true infection rather than contamination. The residual urine should be checked after voiding since stagnant urine fosters infection and makes it much more difficult to eradicate. In addition to antibacterial therapy, corrective measures to reduce residual urine should be carried out.

Interstitial cystitis almost always occurs in females (95%) between the ages of 25 and 60 years. The patient will have episodes of increased frequency of urination, dysuria, tenesmus, and nocturia, and the bladder capacity is reduced. Gross and microscopic hematuria may be present. Remissions occur only to be followed by reappearance of the disease. Characteristically, no bacteria can be cultured and the etiology remains obscure. Many urologists believe this type of cystitis represents a psychosomatic illness. Treatment varies a great deal, but much relief is obtained by overdistention of the bladder under anesthesia or fulgurating the bleeding ulcers (Hunner's ulcers). Rarely is it necessary to resort to indwelling catheters, intestinocystoplasty, or urinary diversion. The nurse will find these patients very demanding of attention as well as of narcotics for relief of pain. The nurse must be patient and firm in her care.

Infection may ascend from the bladder to the kidneys by means of vesicoureteral *reflux*. Reflux usually is the result of a congenital malformation of the intramural ureter in that the length and obliquity are insufficient. Or reflux may be secondary to cystitis, with edema and fixation of the intramural ureter causing it to lose its mobility and valvelike action. Reflux in the latter situations will often disappear upon eradication of the infection. Reflux also produces a residual urine problem. When structural and functional changes in the upper urinary system begin to appear, reflux should be corrected by surgical intervention.

PYELONEPHRITIS

Pyelonephritis may be caused by a blood-borne organism, but more commonly an ascending infection from the lower urinary system by means of vesicoureteral reflux is the etiologic mechanism. The disease is manifested in its acute phase by flank pain, fever, chills, and occasionally nausea, vomiting, anorexia, malaise, and symptoms of general urinary tract infection such as dysuria and increased frequency of urination. The urine must be examined and cultured and appropriate antibiotic therapy instituted. An adequate course of therapy must be administered; usually this means 10 to 30 days of treatment with careful follow-up urine examinations to ensure that the infection has been eradicated and remains so. Pyelonephritis is a serious disease, and if it becomes chronic, the kidneys gradually may be destroyed. The patient then becomes uremic and x-ray films show the kidneys have become contracted and perhaps irregular in outline.

Occasionally a yeast (fungus) infection prevails and the urine is strongly acid in pH reaction. Alkalinization to eradicate the yeast is tried. Parenteral amphotericin B therapy is effective, but the toxic reactions are considered too hazardous for general use and the drug is reserved for life-threatening situations.

TUBERCULOSIS OF THE URINARY SYSTEM

Tuberculosis of the urinary system usually begins in the kidneys, with the organisms originating from the lungs or gastrointestinal tract. The renal infection may start as a small cortical abscess that eventually erodes into a calyx and then involves the pelvis and the rest of the kidney. The kidney may gradually shrink. The pyelographic appearance is that of "moth-eaten" calyces (Fig. 9-1), and in the late stages the kidney may become calcified and is known as a "putty kidney." Then, of course, all function is lost. Tuberculosis descends via the ureters to the bladder and causes generalized cystitis and urethritis. There is a tendency for the ureter to undergo fibrosis and stricture formation in its lower third. The bladder that sustains a long-term tuberculous infection will contract so that the patient must urinate every few minutes day and night with considerable discomfort. Gross hematuria will then occur intermittently. The urinary findings are those of pyuria without visible bacteriuria by ordinary microscopy. Tuberculosis must be suspected and smears (Ziehl-Neelsen stain) and cultures made. The skin test for tuberculosis is virtually always positive but is not the definitive diagnostic test. A negative test lessens the possibility that the diagnosis is tuberculosis. The treatment of tuberculosis is specific and includes isoniazid, para-aminosalicylic acid, and streptomycin. Other drugs that have been used with success include ethionamide, cycloserine, viomycin, and kanamycin. Treatment must be carried out from 6 months to 2 years, depending on the urine cultures and appearance of the pyelograms. Bed rest at first is desirable, but later the patient may not need to be hospitalized. Tuberculosis of the urinary system is not very contagious, but the patient should take precautions during the treatment period to avoid transfer of the disease through sexual contact;

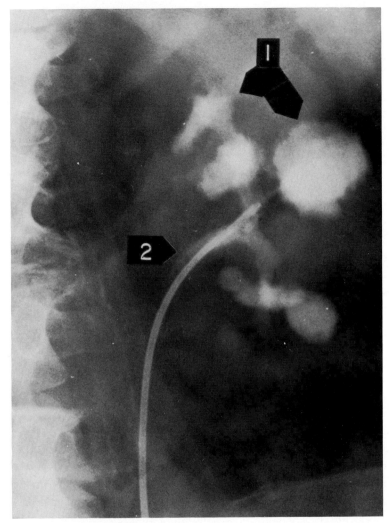

Fig. 9-1. Retrograde pyelogram of left kidney demonstrates "moth-eaten" and dilated calyces, **1**, and narrowing of infundibular-pelvic structure within kidney, **2**. This is due to tuberculosis.

the male should use a condom. Surgery is occasionally indicated for a closed infection or abscess of the kidney. Partial or total nephrectomy may be necessary. If the total kidney is removed, it is advisable to remove the entire ureter also. Ureteral strictures can be repaired and contracted bladders can be enlarged by intestinocystoplasty (a rarely performed operation).

As in other chronic diseases, occupational therapy, social services, and occasionally psychiatric therapy are useful adjuvants to medicine and surgery. The patient is often worried about finances and "home fires."

Tuberculosis societies and special tuberculosis hospitals are available for patients in special need.

PERINEPHRITIC ABSCESS

Infection in the fat-filled space around the kidney may be caused by blood-borne organisms, but it is most commonly a complication of pyelonephritis with or without calculus disease or trauma. A dull flank ache with tenderness and bending toward the affected flank is common. Chills and fever are suggestive of the infection and a flank mass may be indicative of the abscess. The psoas shadow is lost on the plain roentgenogram of the abdomen on the affected side. Pyelographic and urinary studies are useful in the diagnosis. Incision and drainage confirm the diagnosis and are also the treatment. Nephrectomy at a subsequent date may be indicated. Appropriate antibiotic therapy is necessary to prevent complications such as septicemia and chronic pyelonephritis and cystitis.

The nurse must use sterile technique in changing dressings, and the patient may be isolated. Care must be taken not to contaminate other patients.

URETHRITIS, URETHRAL DIVERTICULA, AND PROSTATITIS

Urethritis in the male is usually sexual in origin. It may be nonspecific in that no definite organism can be seen or cultured, or it may be a specific infection such as gonorrhea. Sulfonamides, penicillin, and broad-spectrum antibiotics are generally effective in combating urethritis. The disease may be manifested by a urethral discharge that may be yellow or white and stains the undergarments. Protective pads may be necessary, and the nurse and associates should protect themselves as with any other disease that is contagious by direct contact. Occasionally, protozoa such as *Trichomonas* or fungi such as *Monilia* cause urethritis or prostatitis. Urethritis commonly occurs in association with prostatitis, or the latter may be a sequela of urethritis.

Urethral diverticula occur in both sexes, producing a urethral discharge or simulating incontinence. Urethral glands that become infected or catheter pressure in the male is frequently the cause. Symptoms are similar to urethritis and the diagnosis is made by palpation of a periurethral cystic mass and by a urethrogram. The diverticula are usually excised. If untreated, they cause continuous infection and may develop into a fistula.

Prostatitis is much more difficult to eradicate than simple urethritis and in the *acute* form should be treated with drugs, heat, and sexual abstinence. *Chronic* prostatitis responds usually to a series of prostatic massages with or without chemotherapy or antibiotics. The presence or absence of prostatic stones must be ascertained by obtaining an x-ray film.

Prostatic massage will be of no avail if stones are present. In contrast to the acute phase, sexual activity is beneficial in the chronic stage. Antibiotics will be the chief form of therapy, and occasionally a prostatectomy may be necessary. Urethral strictures and bladder neck contracture are common sequelae of urethritis and prostatitis. Rarely, *urethral fistulas* will form, with one or more channels opening into the scrotum, perineum, or penile shaft. (Multiple openings are described as a "waterpot" perineum.) Fistulas are common in paraplegic or quadriplegic patients who have indwelling urethral catheters over a long period of time. Pressure necrosis usually occurs at the penile-scrotal junction. Such fistulas are very difficult to close and keep sealed.

Prostatic abscesses occur rarely. The patient has chills, fever, and rectal pain. He may have difficulty in voiding. The urine will be infected. The diagnosis is confirmed by digital examination of the prostate; a bulging, fluctuant mass is palpated. The abscess should be drained. This is performed transurethrally, either with a sound or a resectoscope. Some urologists prefer to expose the abscess through the perineal route. A drain is left in the wound for a few days. Later sitz baths are prescribed. Antibiotics are always used.

EPIDIDYMITIS

One of the most common infections of the male reproductive system, epididymitis may be caused by any pyogenic organism. Usually the organism is gram negative and originates in an infected prostate or the lower urinary tract. The bacteria may reflux from the urethra or prostate by way of the vasa deferentia, or as some believe, microbes may travel through the lymphatics. This is why some urologists perform a bilateral vasectomy as a prophylactic measure against epididymitis prior to a prostatectomy. Less commonly, the bacteria arrive from some distant site of infection by way of the bloodstream. The disease may also be a complication of gonorrhea or of tuberculosis of the urinary system. The patient usually complains of severe tenderness, pain, and swelling within the scrotum, which may be hot to the touch. His temperature may be markedly elevated, and he is likely to have general malaise and to feel very ill. He often walks with a characteristic "duck waddle" in an attempt to protect the affected part. It is by this sign that the observant nurse may first detect difficulty in the patient who is too embarrassed to describe his trouble. The patient with a tuberculous infection frequently develops a scrotal fistula (an opening draining pus from the interior of the scrotal sac to the outside skin).

The patient with epididymitis should be put to bed and the scrotum may be elevated either on towel rolls or with adhesive strapping (Fig. 9-2). An ice bag can be used to help reduce the swelling and to relieve the pain and discomfort. Application of heat locally is usually contraindi-

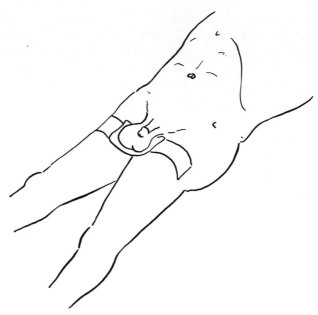

Fig. 9-2. Bellevue bridge; elevation of scrotum on adhesive strip. (Unpublished illustration of Dr. B. G. Clarke and Dr. L. Del Guercio.)

cated because the normal temperature of the scrotal contents is below normal body temperature and excessive exposure to heat may be detrimental to the germinal cells. If an ice cap is used, it should be removed for short intervals every hour to prevent skin necrosis. Antibiotics are usually given. The doctor also usually wants the patient to drink at least 2000 ml. of fluid daily since an associated urinary infection is common. When the patient is allowed out of bed, the physician frequently has him wear a scrotal support or suspensory.

The differential diagnosis includes torsion of the spermatic cord, torsion of the appendix of the epididymis or testis, and tumors. These are not accompanied by signs of infection and tumors are rarely tender. Torsion causes the testicle to be elevated and further manual elevation does not relieve the pain (Pregn's sign).

Patients with tuberculous epididymitis, although they may have scrotal swelling and a fistula, rarely have pain. Their care is similar to that for a patient with renal tuberculosis. If they have a draining fistula, contamination of others by the drainage must be prevented. The patient and all personnel should be taught to wash their hands scrupulously if they become contaminated with the drainage. The patient is usually asked to use a bathroom not shared by others. If this type of facility is not available, he must bathe at his bedside and use a urinal and bedpan rather than the toilet. All equipment used for personal care as well as that used for changing the dressings must be scrubbed well and sterilized before being used by others. Linen should be handled as "isolated"; the isolation procedure varies in different hospitals. In the home, contaminated linen should be submerged in a pail or large pan of water and boiled for 20 minutes. It may then be washed with the clothes of others.

Since bilateral epididymitis usually causes sterility, special attention is given to the prevention of this infection. Untreated epididymitis leads rather rapidly to orchitis and necrosis of testicular tissue, septicemia, or both. An indwelling urethral catheter predisposes to epididymitis. For this reason, men in whom a catheter would be necessary for bladder drainage over a long period of time often have a cystostomy performed to obviate the necessity for a catheter in the prostatic urethra.

An elderly patient who must have surgery of the prostate gland that will require leaving a urethral catheter indwelling for a long time may be advised to have a bilateral vasectomy before or during the prostatectomy to prevent any infection from migrating via the vasa deferentia to the epididymides. Since this procedure sterilizes the patient, it is not usually done on a young man. Permission must be granted by the patient. The vasectomies are done through two very small incisions in the scrotum or in the groin. After the vas deferens is divided, each free end is tied with a suture. Often the operation is done prior to any urethral manipulation in preparation for surgery. Local anesthesia is used. Postoperatively the patient should still be watched for symptoms of epididymitis since the organisms may have invaded the epididymis prior to vasectomy.

ORCHITIS

Infection of the testicle is known as orchitis. It is usually of bacterial origin but may be a complication of the mumps virus, especially when mumps are contracted after puberty. Although orchitis following mumps occurs in a relatively small percentage of patients, it usually causes testicular atrophy and, if bilateral, causes sterility. Any boy after puberty or any man who has not had mumps and is exposed to this disease should consult his doctor; gamma globulin is often given immediately. If there is any doubt as to whether the person has had mumps, the globulin is usually given. Although the globulin may not prevent mumps, the disease is likely to be less severe and less likely to cause complications. The use of mumps vaccine is now a practical measure of prevention.

The symptoms and the treatment of orchitis are similar to those of epididymitis. Stilbestrol, cortisone, and antibiotics may be given. If response to medical treatment is not prompt, the tunica albuginea may have to be opened surgically to improve the circulation to the testis since swelling constricts the spermatic vessels and predisposes to atrophy of the organ.

INFECTIONS OF THE EXTERNAL GENITALIA

Any lesion on the external genitalia requires medical attention, and no ulcer of the genitalia should be treated by the patient before he sees a doctor lest the diagnosis be obscured. Although lesions are present in association with a wide variety of conditions, they should always be considered infectious until proved otherwise because each of the venereal diseases, with the exception of gonorrhea, produces a genital lesion or ulceration.

Chancroid

Chancroid is a venereal disease that occurs in both men and women and is caused by *Haemophilus ducreyi* (Ducrey's bacillus). It is characterized by a raised lesion on the external genital 1 to 5 days after contact. This lesion becomes a pustule and then develops into a painful ulcer with extensive local inflammation and spread. It is treated locally with sulfathiazole powder and systemically with chloramphenicol or chlortetracycline.

Granuloma inguinale

Granuloma inguinale is a genital infection. It is seen most often in Negroes, and it is not uncommon in the southern United States. There is a gradual superficial painless ulceration and granulation of the vulva in women and of the glans penis in men. This ulceration extends to the inguinal region in both men and women. The diagnosis is made by finding Donovan bodies in stained smears of the lesions. It may be treated with streptomycin, chloramphenicol, stibophen, or antimony preparations.

Lymphogranuloma venereum

Lymphogranuloma venereum is a venereal disease caused by a filtrable virus that spreads via the lymphatic vessels. It is diagnosed by a positive Frei test (blood test). At any time from 6 to 60 days after contact the inguinal nodes become very swollen and tender. These are called "buboes" and they may ulcerate. In women, perirectal inflammation and scar formation are characteristic. Rectal strictures and fistulas as well as urethral strictures develop. There may be complete destruction of the bladder or bowel sphincter muscles, with resultant incontinence. If there is interference with lymph channels, elephantiasis, a hard lymphatic swelling of the lower trunk and legs that completely distorts their size and shape, may also develop. This may make walking almost impossible. Until the advent of chlortetracycline, there was no satisfactory treatment.

Chancre of syphilis

A chancre is a painless indurated ulcer frequently found on the glans penis; however, it may be found elsewhere in the genital area and on the

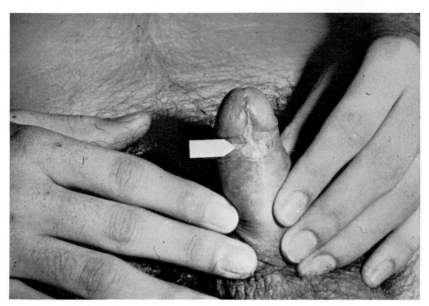

Fig. 9-3. Arrow indicates chancre (initial lesion of syphilis).

lips, mouth, or nipples. It is the initial lesion of syphilis (Fig. 9-3) and appears at the end of the incubation period (10 days to 10 weeks). It is caused by the spirochete *Treponema pallidum.*

During the early course of the chancre the serologic blood test is often negative because insufficient reagin has been produced to render it positive. The chancre is, however, teaming with live spirochetes, and fluid obtained from the lesion will reveal them easily under a dark-field microscope. It is unfortunate if the patient is given penicillin prior to this test because this antibiotic causes disappearance of the spirochetes within 24 hours and the opportunity to make a definite diagnosis by observation of the living organisms is thus lost. Diagnosis must then be made by means of a serologic test, which must be delayed for weeks and is subject to the hazards of false-negative reactions that will cloud the clinical picture. The patient may then remain inadequately treated and develop complications of latent syphilis. Even if not treated, the chancre heals spontaneously within 3 to 8 weeks; however, by this time, systemic syphilis is firmly established.

The patient with a chancre is rarely hospitalized; diagnosis and treatment of both the lesion and the underlying disease are carried out in the doctor's office, in the hospital clinic, or in a community clinic. The nurse working with these patients must refrain from passing moral judgment but should show genuine professional concern. This is important in encouraging patients to get medical care for potentially infected sexual partners, in keeping the patient himself under medical care and follow-up, and in preventing him from further infecting others. There is a statutory law that this disease and other major venereal diseases be reported to the local health office.

Syphilis is currently treated with penicillin, although some other antibiotics are equally effective. The ideal dosage and distribution of dosage has not been conclusively established, but 2.4 to 6 million units of penicillin are given in a period of 1 to 3 weeks, depending on the stage of the disease. This effects a cure in 90% of all patients with early syphilis. Patients in whom the diagnosis is made and adequate treatment started in the early chancre stage fortunately will never experience the signs and symptoms of untreated syphilis. It is established, almost beyond doubt, that biologic cure can be effected by adequate treatment in the early stages of the disease. Reinfection is possible, and it is rather frequent in those treated for early infectious syphilis. (For a more complete discussion of syphilis see a medical nursing textbook.)

A lesion of viral origin often confused with the serious venereal diseases is *condylomata accuminata* (venereal warts). They occur upon the external genitalia of both sexes and within the urethra as well as perianally. Small warts may be treated with podophyllin applications, while larger and more extensive collections are more expeditiously removed by scalpel or cautery.

SEPTICEMIA

Gram-negative septicemia is common in urologic patients and most frequently follows instrumentation or surgery. Thus entrance into the bloodstream is provided for the urinary bacteria. As the bacteria proliferate in the choice culture medium of blood, they produce an endotoxin that constricts the capillaries, produces a pooling of plasma, and reduces venous return to the heart, and shock ensues. Fifty percent of the patients developing gram-negative septic shock die. It is one of the most common causes of hospital deaths in urologic patients. Treatment is prophylactic, employing vigorous antibiotic therapy for urinary infection and as much avoidance of trauma to the uroepithelium as possible. In early shock, large doses of methylprednisolone and isoproterenol should be administered along with massive antibacterial therapy. Central venous pressure, pulse, temperature, and arterial blood pressure must be carefully monitored. Occasionally, vasopressors are used. Cardiac failure and/or renal shutdown may occur (see Chapter 7) and careful intake and output of fluids must be charted. Special duty nurses or intensive care units should be utilized.

QUESTIONS

1. What is the most common urinary tract infection in females?
2. What is the usual origin of cystitis in the female?
3. What are the symptoms of cystitis?

4. How can the colony count be used to differentiate contamination from actual urinary tract infection?
5. What is the difference between interstitial cystitis and ordinary cystitis?
6. How does infection usually get into the kidney from the bladder?
7. How can one differentiate pyelonephritis from cystitis when the urine is infected?
8. How is a yeast infection of the urinary system managed?
9. What is the sequence of events in tuberculosis of the urinary tract?
10. How is a positive diagnosis of tuberculosis of the kidney made?
11. What drugs are used in the treatment of urinary tuberculosis?
12. What is the origin of a pyelonephritic abscess?
13. What is the etiology of male urethritis?
14. What organisms commonly cause male urethritis?
15. What is the chief sign of a urethral diverticulum?
16. What is the treatment of acute prostatitis?
17. What is the treatment of chronic prostatitis?
18. How is a prostatic abscess diagnosed?
19. What is the treatment of a prostatic abscess?
20. What is the usual origin of epididymitis?
21. How does one differentiate epididymitis from torsion of the spermatic cord?
22. What operation of the scrotum is used to produce sterility?
23. What common childhood disease causes orchitis?
24. Name four types of venereal disease affecting the genital system.
25. How are these differentiated?
26. What is the current treatment of syphilis in the acute stage?
27. What is the most common cause of death in a urologic patient?
28. What are some of the consequences of septicemia?

REFERENCES

Conger, K. B.: Gonorrhea and nonspecific urethritis, Med. Clin. N. Amer. **48**:767, 1964.
Cooper, H. G.: Transmission of M. tuberculosis via genital tract, J. Urol. **104**:914, 1970.
Craig, I.: Collecting specimens of urine. The nurse holds the key to diagnosis of infections, Nurs. Times **62**:531, 1966.
Cromwell, G. E.: The teenager and venereal disease, Amer. J. Nurs. **59**:1738, 1959.
Doolittle, K. H., and Taylor, J. N.: Renal abscess in the differential diagnosis of mass in kidney, J. Urol. **89**:649, 1963.
Ehrlich, R. M., and Lattimer, J. K.: Urogenital tuberculosis in children, J. Urol. **105**: 461, 1971.
Gow, G. W.: Genitourinary tuberculosis, Lancet **2**:261, 1963.
Howard, F. S.: Estrogen treatment of chronic urethritis in the female, Calif. Med. **66**: 352, 1947.
Jewett, H. J., and Colston, J. A. C., Jr.: Urethritis, cystitis, and prostatitis: diagnosis and treatment, Med. Clin. N. Amer. **45**:1547, 1961.
Lattimer, J. K., Reilly, R. J., and Segawa, A.: Significance of isolated positive urine culture in genitourinary tuberculosis, J. Urol. **102**:610, 1969.
Lattimer, J. K., Wechsler, H., Ehrlich, R. M., and Fukushima, K.: Current treatment for renal tuberculosis, J. Urol. **102**:2, 1969.
Levi, D. E., and Evans, A. T.: Positive urine cultures in pediatric medicine, J. Urol. **104**:944, 1970.
Lyon, R. P., and Marshall, S.: Urinary tract infections and difficult urination in girls: long-term followup, J. Urol. **105**:314, 1971.
Nourse, M. H.: Pyelonephritis and the urologist, J. Urol. **85**:211, 1961.
Rehm, R. A., and Fishman, A.: The value of the urine smear in detecting bacteriuria, J. Urol. **89**:930, 1963.
Rodman, M. J.: Combating urinary tract infections, RN **31**:59, 1968.
Santora, D.: Preventing hospital-acquired urinary infection, Amer. J. Nurs. **66**:790, 1966.

Shapira, H. E.: Studies on metronidazole (Flagyl) in the therapy of urogenital trichomoniasis in the male patient, J. Urol. **93**:303, 1965.

Smith, D. R.: Psychosomatic "cystitis," J. Urol. **87**:359, 1962.

Smith, J. V., and Boyce, W. H.: Allopurinol and urolithiasis, J. Urol. **102**:750, 1969.

Smith, L. H., and Martin, W. J.: Infections of the urinary tract, Med. Clin. N. Amer. **50**:1127, 1966.

Smith, R. D., and Aquino, J.: Viruses and the kidney, Med. Clin. N. Amer. **55**:89, 1971.

Weil, M. H., Shubin, H., and Biddle, M.: Shock caused by gram negative micro-organisms, Ann. Intern. Med. **60**:384, 1964.

Wilson, F. M., Shumaker, E. J., Fentress, V., and Lerner, A. M.: Epidemiologic aspects of postoperative sepsis in urologic practice (with note concerning antibacterial prophylaxis), J. Urol. **105**:295, 1971.

Winter, C. C.: Vesicourethral reflux and it's management, New York, 1969, Appleton-Century-Crofts.

Youmans, J. B.: Syphilis and other venereal diseases, Med. Clin. N. Amer. **48**:573, 1964.

Zufall, R.: Treatment of the urethral syndrome in women, J.A.M.A. **184**:894, 1963.

CHAPTER 10

Urinary calculi

TYPES AND CAUSES

Although the causes of urinary calculi are not completely understood, stasis of urine is known to predispose to stone formation. This is especially true if there is associated infection. Urea-splitting organisms such as *Escherichia coli, Proteus, Staphylococcus,* and *Streptococcus* make the urine markedly alkaline, and calcium phosphate, a common constituent in urinary stones, is relatively insoluble in an alkaline medium. In contrast, some elements such as cystine and uric acid are insoluble in acid urine. In order for stones to form, crystals must coalesce or there must be some nucleus about which the stone-forming materials collect; this may be pus, blood, devitalized tissue, crystals, tumors, or a foreign body such as a catheter.

Patients who require intubation of any part of the urinary tract for extended periods of time are prime candidates for stone formation. Preventive therapy such as maintenance of good drainage, forcing of fluids, and dietary regimens that reduce the amount of inorganic materials commonly found in stones or change the pH of the urine may decrease the incidence of stone formation. Irrigating the intubated cavity with 0.25% acetic acid solution or 10% Renacidin may decrease the alkalinity of urine and dissolve calcium or phosphate deposits. Acid-ash diets or ingestion of ascorbic acid to acidify the urine may be in order to prevent catheter encrustation.

Patients with fractures or bedridden patients who cannot move about freely are prone to stone formation. This probably is due to the excessive amount of calcium released from the bones in such patients and to stasis of urine in the dependent calyces of the kidneys resulting from the horizontal position of the body. As a prophylactic measure, the doctor encourages mobilization of these patients at the earliest possible time. They

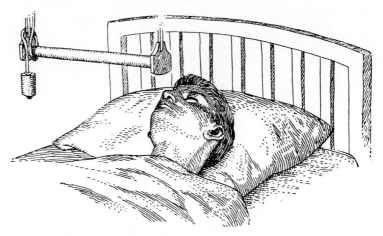

Fig. 10-1. Bedridden patients such as those suffering from paraplegia or quadriplegia are especially vulnerable to stone formation. Moreover, early signs of kidney or ureteral stone such as pain are often unrecognized in paralyzed patients. Note trapeze available for use by paraplegic patient to help him move and exercise, which is helpful in preventing stone formation.

should at least be turned from side to side in bed every 1 to 2 hours. If a patient is unable to walk, he sometimes can be placed in a wheelchair or, if necessary, on a stretcher twice a day for an hour or two. Tilt tables, rocking beds, and oscillating beds are helpful. If the patient's legs are immobilized, he should be encouraged to exercise his arms. Use of a bed trapeze does more than just help the patient move himself; it also helps to prevent formation of renal calculi and decubiti (Fig. 10-1).

Hyperparathyroidism and gout are diseases that result in hyperexcretion in the urine of calcium and uric acid, respectively. The former is the cause of no more than 5% of calcium stones. A diet that is deficient in vitamin A also predisposes to stones; this deficiency, however, is rare among persons in the United States. Patients with abnormal cysteine metabolism may develop cystine stones.

The patient with urinary calculi usually seeks medical care because of symptoms of pain caused by obstruction and/or infection (Fig. 10-2). Excruciating pain in the flank and abdomen is a common symptom of ureteral calculi. Differentiation from other causes of acute abdominal pain may be difficult. There may be gross hematuria caused by trauma from a jagged stone moving down the ureter, although hematuria from stones is more often microscopic. Sometimes the patient complains of increased frequency and urgency of urination, symptoms of cystitis or bladder stones. Often a stone is "silent," causing no symptoms for years; this is especially true of large stones in the kidney. Small, nonobstructing renal calculi may be responsible for a dull ache or discomfort in the kidney area.

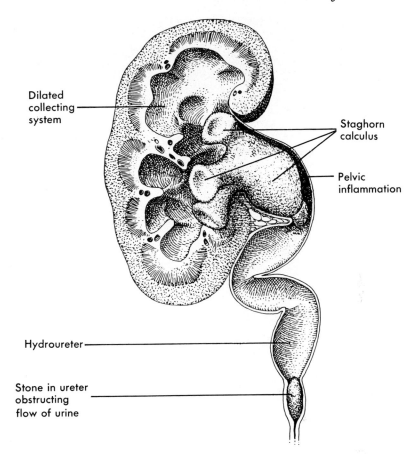

Dilated
collecting
system

Staghorn
calculus

Pelvic
inflammation

Hydroureter

Stone in ureter
obstructing
flow of urine

Fig. 10-2. Sketch of dilated kidney and ureter due to staghorn calculus in renal pelvis and stone obstructing midureter.

Diagnostic procedures

The diagnosis of ureteral calculi is often suggested from the history. Most urinary calculi are found by plain roentgenography and by intravenous urography. (See Fig. 6-14 for roentgenogram of ureteral calculus.) Sometimes a cystoscopic examination is performed, and a ureteral catheter may be passed. This procedure is carried out if there is any uncertainty about a density being in the ureter or if a tumor is suspected rather than a stone. Oblique films must be included in the study.

Eighty-five percent of urinary stones contain calcium and are opaque to x-rays. The remaining 15% are chiefly uric acid stones that cannot be seen by roentgenography. A few are cystine stones, and these are usually opaque. Rarely, nonopaque stones such as xanthine or matrix calculi are encountered.

If it is impossible to pass a catheter beyond the stone and a retrograde

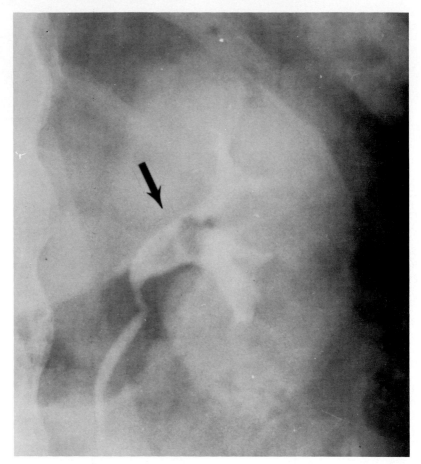

Fig. 10-3. Retrograde pyelogram demonstrates radiolucent filling defects within renal pelvis (arrow). These defects are caused by nonopaque calculi of uric acid variety.

pyelogram is needed, a ureteral catheter with a cone tip may be placed in the ureteral orifice to block the ureter. The contrast material is forced up the ureter and often beyond the stone. Air pyeloureterography is useful for demonstrating nonopaque calculi (Fig. 10-3).

Since there is a very high incidence of recurrence of renal calculi, not only must the immediate problem be treated but also the reason for stone formation must be discovered, if possible, and treated. Therefore intensive diagnostic studies may be done after the removal of stones. Stones are usually subjected to laboratory analysis to determine their mineral composition. The results serve as a guide to the doctor in his search for the cause of stone formation and as an aid in planning suitable prophylactic treatment.

After appropriate diets for several days, 24-hour urine specimens may be analyzed for their calcium and phosphorus content. The Sulkowitch test to determine the qualitative calcium content in the urine (a single specimen) may be ordered, but it is a crude test of questionable value. Calcium and phosphorus levels in the blood should be determined.

If hyperparathyroidism is more strongly suspected following these tests, a parathyroid screening test may be ordered. This test takes several days. For 2 days the patient is given a diet containing 150 mg. of calcium. On the third day, blood for calcium, phosphorus, creatinine, and total protein determinations is drawn and a 24-hour urine collection completed. On such a regimen the urine of a patient with hyperparathyroidism will usually contain more than 175 mg. of calcium in 24 hours, the serum calcium will be more than 11 mg.% , and the serum phosphorus will often be less than 2.5 mg.% in patients with normal serum creatinine levels. Patients with decreased renal function will have distorted values for these blood constituents. The "free calcium" is important in stone formation, and since the protein binds a portion of the serum calcium, the protein level must be taken into account in the interpretation of serum levels of calcium.

If the screening test suggests parathyroid disease, a calcium tolerance test may be indicated. This test is done in the same manner as the screening test until the third day. On this day, 15 mg. of calcium gluconate per kilogram of body weight is given intravenously over a 4-hour period. Blood for calcium and phosphorus studies is collected 30 minutes after completion of the injection. If there is a normal response to the increased serum calcium, the serum phosphorus will show more than a 1 mg.% rise from preinfusion levels. Urinary phosphorus and creatinine ratios are also monitored, and failure of this value to fall is compatible with hyperparathyroidism.

If gout is suspected, the blood uric acid level is determined. This level is also elevated in leukemic patients undergoing therapy that have a large breakdown of nucleic acids.

A careful search by clinical, bacteriologic, and radiographic methods is always made in patients with infections and obstructive lesions that may predispose to stone formation. A familial history of stones is common in those who form cystine stones.

NEPHROCALCINOSIS

This disease differs from renal calculus disease and medullary sponge kidneys (stone deposited in collection ducts of papillae) in that the calcium deposits are within the renal parenchyma rather than in the calyces or pelvis. This makes the renal situation more serious and subject to progressive deterioration without any possibility of removal of the deposits and often little relief of general symptoms. Hyperparathyroidism is one of the causes of hypercalcemia and hypercalciuria, which are often associated with this disorder. The patient may develop renal tubular acidosis with elevation of the serum chloride level and depression of the carbon dioxide–combining power. The urine tends to be alkaline, and tubular function is decreased. The patient is often asymptomatic or suffers from the symptoms of disturbed metabolism. He may have microscopic hematuria and pass casts and occasionally gravel. The diagnosis requires x-ray verification of stone deposits in the renal parenchyma. Treatment and nursing management are the same as for renal failure, renal infection, or the metabolic disturbance that is present. The patient is generally placed on a low-calcium diet; mobilization is encouraged as well as a good fluid intake.

Medical and nursing care

Of all renal calculi, 90% pass out through the ureter, bladder, and urethra spontaneously. All patients with relatively small stones therefore should have all the urine strained. Urine can be strained easily by fastening two opened gauze sponges (4 by 4 inches) over a funnel or by using a tea strainer. It is necessary to watch closely for the stone because it may be no larger than the head of a pin and the patient may not realize it has passed. Stones larger than 1 cm. in diameter are not often passed.

If there is no infection, if there is not complete obstruction, and if the stone is of a size likely to pass, it may be left in the ureter for weeks or months. The patient is allowed to continue work and encouraged to be active unless he is employed in a job such as piloting an airplane; in such a case an episode of severe colic might endanger the lives of people on the plane. The stone is observed periodically by radiographic examination for size and location. Periodic radioisotope renography is a convenient method for following the renal function and ability to evacuate urine. This test spares the patient the radiation exposure from frequent excretory urograms. Fluids should be taken freely because this may help the stone to move along the urinary tract. Patients frequently have two or three attacks of acute pain (ureteric colic) before the stone passes. This is probably because the stone gets lodged at a narrow point in the ureter, causing temporary obstruction (see Chapter 2).

Ureteral colic. The patient with ureteral colic is acutely ill. He has excruciating pain in the flank if the stone is high in the upper ureter, or it usually radiates to the genital region if the stone is in the lower ureter (Fig. 10-4). He frequently is nauseated and vomits. Although he is acutely ill, he may be so uncomfortable that he cannot remain in bed until the pain has been relieved and he may walk about or be doubled-up in agony. Narcotics and antispasmodic drugs are usually ordered. After narcotics have been given, the patient must be protected from injury resulting from dizziness if he is still ambulatory. As the pain eases, the patient

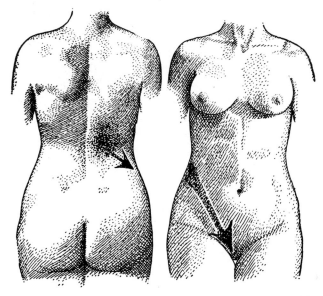

Fig. 10-4. Kidney pain is referred to region directly over kidney, while ureteral pain, depending upon level of obstruction, will be referred down toward genital region.

can usually be made relatively comfortable in bed, and when the nausea subsides, fluids and food may be given.

After the acute attack is over, the patient is encouraged to be up and actively about. He should be given pain medication to control attacks of colic.

Ureteral dilatation and drainage. If the stone fails to pass, the doctor may pass one or two ureteral catheters through a cystoscope up the ureter and past the stones. Pain will be relieved by draining the kidney. The catheters are usually left in place for 24 hours. They dilate the intramural ureter, and when they are removed, they may pull the stone down into the bladder, or the stone thereafter may pass spontaneously. A little mineral oil instilled into the ureter may help the stone to pass.

Ureteral catheters may be most effectively attached to drainage equipment without encroaching on the catheter lumen by punching a small hole in the rubber top of a medicine dropper and threading the catheter through it. To make the hole, use a large red-hot needle or a pin; hot metal permanently perforates rubber. The medicine dropper top is then attached to the glass connector of the drainage tubing (see Chapter 3). Needles make poor adapters since they reduce the lumen size, tend to puncture the catheter, and easily obstruct. If there is a catheter in each ureter, the catheters should be labeled "right" and "left" with adhesive tape. Ureteral catheters must be checked frequently to ensure that they are draining. If the urine is purulent or sanguineous, the catheters may become obstructed. The orders should be checked for irrigation instructions. If patency cannot be reestablished by irrigation, the doctor should be notified. Ureteral catheters may be irrigated with a special ureteral syringe and adapter, the tip of which fits over the catheter, or with a syringe and blunt needle. No more than 5 ml. or irrigating solution (sterile physiologic solution of sodium chloride) should be instilled, and the solution should be allowed to drain by gravity. Patients with ureteral catheters should be kept in bed. An indwelling bladder catheter is attached to the ureteral catheter(s) to prevent dislodgment. The patient should be warned that urine may leak around the catheters. Incontinence care should be given (see Chapter 4).

Following catheterization of a ureter with a stone in it the patient may have a febrile reaction similar to those that occasionally follow cystoscopic examinations. The care is the same. Since this may be a somewhat traumatic catheterization, the nurse needs to be especially aware of the possibility of pyelonephritis or septicemia. Any decrease in urinary output, pain in the flank or abdomen, fever, or fall in blood pressure should be reported to the doctor at once.

Therapeutic renal irrigations. If the renal stones have recently developed and are phosphatic in makeup, a continuous drip irrigation of the renal pelvis with Renacidin may be ordered in an attempt to dissolve the calculi. Two ureteral catheters are inserted into the renal pelvis via a cystoscopic procedure; the irrigating solution goes into one and returns from the other (or, if only one catheter is used, the fluid drains around it). This may be performed through a nephrostomy tube also. The patient requires constant nursing supervision since any blockage of drainage causes serious distention of the renal pelvis or infiltrates the renal tissue and may thus seriously endanger the patient's life. The procedure may be continued intermittently for several days but should be discontinued if any signs of fever or infection appear. Periodic roentgenograms are taken to determine results. The patient will void since only one ureter is intubated.

Manipulation of a ureteral stone. A stone that has passed to the lower third of the ureter can sometimes be removed by cystoscopic manipulation. Special catheters with corkscrew tips, expanding baskets (see Fig. 3-15), and loops (see Fig. 3-16) are passed through the cystoscope, and an attempt is made to snare the stone. The patient is anesthetized for this procedure. Because the manipulation may not be successful, the doctor usually tells the patient that surgery may be performed while he is still anesthetized. The catheter may become caught and this would necessitate surgical removal of both it and the stone. The aftercare of a patient in whom manipulation has been carried out successfully is the same as that following cystoscopy (see Chapter 6). Usually an indwelling ureteral catheter is left for 24 hours. Any signs suggestive of peritonitis (for example, abdominal pain or fever) or a decreased urinary output should be carefully watched for since the ureter sometimes is perforated during manipulation.

OPERATIVE REMOVAL OF RENAL AND URETERAL CALCULI

A roentgenogram is taken immediately preceding surgery for removal of a ureteral calculus since the stone may have moved and it is desirable to make the incision into the skin directly over the stone. The operation for removal of a stone from the ureter is a ureterolithotomy (Fig. 10-5, *C*). If the stone is in the lower third of the ureter, a lower abdominal incision is made; if it is in the upper two-thirds, a flank approach is used. A nonmuscle-cutting approach is possible if the stone is opposite Petit's triangle (L_3 to L_4). If the patient has a ureteral stricture that causes stones to form, a plastic operation to relieve the stricture may be done as part of the operation·(see Chapter 8).

Removal of a stone through or from the pelvis of the kidney is known as a pyelolithotomy (Fig. 10-5, *A*); removal of a stone through the renal parenchyma is a nephrolithotomy (Fig. 10-5, *B*). Occasionally the kidney may have to be split from end to end (kidney bivalve) to remove the stone; this type of procedure is often necessary to remove a staghorn calculus (one that fills the entire renal pelvis and calyces). Renal roentgenograms are made during surgery to be sure no stone fragments are left behind. Patients in whom an extensive nephrotomy is done may have severe hemorrhage following surgery. Occasionally, if one kidney is severely damaged by the stones and the other kidney has adequate function, a nephrectomy may be performed. Rarely, the ureter is replaced with a segment of ileum to the bladder or skin to allow recurring stones to pass without further surgery.

Nursing care of patient who has a ureteral incision

The patient who has had a ureterolithotomy through a lower abdominal incision needs the routine postoperative care given any patient undergoing abdominal surgery. The incision, however, may drain large amounts of urine for several days to several weeks postoperatively since watertight suturing of the ureter is not performed in order to prevent subsequent constriction as the ureter heals. A tissue drain is placed adjacent to the ureteral incision and may be left in place for several days or a week or more. (For special nursing measures that should be used to care for the draining urinary fistula, see Chapter 4.) Occasionally a ureteral catheter or T tube will be left in place for several days also.

If the ureter has been approached through a flank incision, nursing care includes the general care given any patient after renal surgery (see following discussion) and care of the urinary fistula.

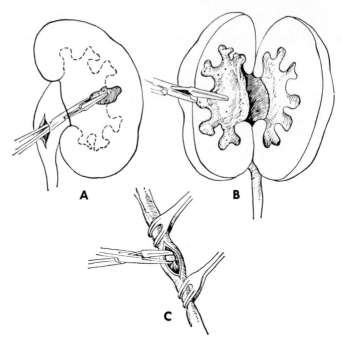

Fig. 10-5. Diagram showing location of calculi in upper urinary tract and surgical approaches used in removing them. **A,** Pyelolithotomy (removal of stone through renal pelvis). **B,** Nephrolithotomy (removal of staghorn calculus by splitting kidney). **C,** Ureterolithotomy (removal of stone from ureter). (From Shafer, K. N., Sawyer, J. R., McCluskey, A. M., Beck, E. L., and Phipps, W. J.: Medical-surgical nursing, ed. 5, St. Louis, 1971, The C. V. Mosby Co.)

Nursing care of patient with flank (kidney) incision

Whenever there has been a flank incision, there are special nursing responsibilities. Because the incision is directly below the diaphragm, deep breathing is painful and the patient is reluctant to take deep breaths or cough or to move about. He tends to splint his chest and therefore is likely to develop atelectasis or hypostatic pneumonia. He needs adequate medication for pain; usually he will require a narcotic every 4 hours for 24 to 48 hours after surgery; after this time the intervals between doses may be gradually increased. After the patient has been given medication to relieve pain and mechanical support (either manual or with a tight many-tailed abdominal binder) has been applied to the incision, he should be encouraged to expand the rib cage fully and to cough. This should be done at least every 1 or 2 hours. Medications may be ordered to loosen the expectorant. Positive-pressure breathing apparatuses with vaporized medicants are most appropriate. Usually an inhalation therapist gives this treatment; however, the nurse should also be familiar with the technique for further support of the patient. While he is in bed, the patient

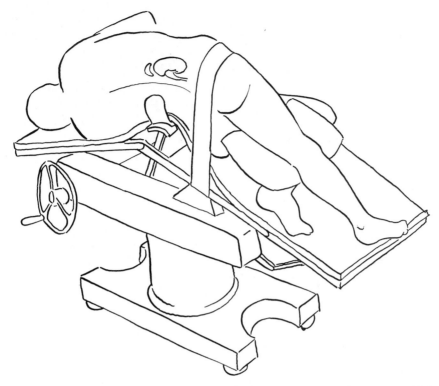

Fig. 10-6. Position of patient for lumbar (flank) approach to kidney. (Unpublished illustration of Dr. B. G. Clarke and Dr. L. Del Guercio.)

should turn or be turned from side to side, and he should be encouraged to get up as soon as ordered. Most patients will be more comfortable turning themselves. After surgery on the kidney the patient can turn to either side unless he has a nephrostomy tube in place. Even then, he can be tilted to the affected side, with pillows placed at his back for support; it must be ascertained that the tube is not kinked and that there is no traction upon it.

The patient often complains of muscular aches and pains after an operation on the kidney. These are caused by the hyperextended side-lying position required for the operation (Fig. 10-6). Support of the part with pillows may give relief. If the discomfort is severe, however, the doctor should be notified, and he may order heat and muscle relaxants.

Following surgery on the kidney, many patients develop abdominal distention. This is usually a result of paralytic ileus of reflex origin. Patients who have had ureteral colic prior to surgery frequently have already developed severe paralytic ileus; this is thought to be related to the reflex gastrointestinal symptoms caused by the pain. Because of the problem of abdominal distention following renal surgery, the patient is often given no food or fluids by mouth for 24 to 48 hours postoperatively. Prophylactically, a gastric tube may be inserted. The passage of flatus as a prevention or treatment of early ileus may be aided by administration of parasympathomimetic or intestinal irritant drugs. Fluids by mouth should be started slowly, and the nurse should watch for signs of distention. It is preferable to give warm fluids. Iced fluids, citrus fruit juices, and milk are usually omitted for several days postoperatively. Most patients tolerate a regular diet by the fourth postoperative day. Fluids of up to 3000 ml. a day are usually ordered if the patient has a sound cardiovascular system.

If distention occurs, rectal and nasogastric tubes may be ordered. Oral intake should be halted. Blood electrolyte imbalance as a cause of ileus should be corrected by the administration of intravenous fluids containing the proper ionic proportions.

Hemorrhage may be a sequel of renal surgery. It occurs more often when the parenchyma of the kidney has been incised since this is a highly vascular structure. (See Chapter 4 for a discussion of hemorrhage in urologic surgery.) The bleeding may occur on the day of surgery, or it may occur 8 to 12 days postoperatively, during the period when tissue sloughing normally occurs in healing. The nurse should closely observe the patient during this period for any signs of hemorrhage. Temperature elevations are cause for equal alarm since they may indicate abscess formation or pyelonephritis. Subsequent septicemia and shock can be catastrophic. Therefore a careful search for the source of infection and institution of vigorous antibacterial therapy are urgent.

A nephrostomy or pyelostomy tube frequently will be inserted following surgery on the kidney. There may be a moderate amount of urinary drainage on the dressing, but if the catheter drains adequately, this problem should be minor. (The care of draining tubes is discussed in Chapter 4.) Saline solution is used as an irrigant to keep the tubes open.

Prophylaxis and home care

Since calculi are likely to recur or develop after surgery on the kidney, patients should understand the importance of following prescribed prophylactic measures. Many patients with a history of renal calculi are advised by their doctors to increase fluid intake for the remainder of their lives. If they have a tendency to form calcium stones, they may also be advised not to consume excess amounts of foods high in calcium content, although adequate nutrition should be maintained. They should be urged to return to their doctor regularly for physical examinations as recommended.

Special medications and diets designed to eliminate conditions conducive to the formation of calculi may be prescribed. If elements found in the stone settle out readily in acid urine, an alkaline-ash diet (Table 4)

Table 4. Food sources of inorganic materials found in urine

Alkaline-ash*	Acid-ash†	Calcium‡	Phosphorus§
Milk	Eggs	Milk	Milk
Fruits, except	Meat, fish,	(1 gm./qt.)	Poultry
cranberries,	poultry	Cheese	Fish
plums, and	Oysters	Green leafy	Cheese
prunes	Breads	vegetables	Nuts
Rhubarb	Cereals		Cereals
Vegetables,	Pastries		Legumes
especially	Puddings		
legumes and			
green vegetables			

*Although meats are acid-ash, small amounts of beef, ham, halibut, veal, trout, and salmon are allowed on an alkaline-ash diet. No other acid-ash foods should be given. Neutral ash foods such as butter, cream, sugar, and tapioca may be used.
†Although fruits and vegetables are basically alkaline-ash, certain ones are allowed on an acid-ash diet. They include watermelons, grapes, fresh pears, grape juice, cherry juice, raspberry juice, fresh peaches, asparagus, fresh peas, pumpkin, squash, turnip, mushrooms, cauliflower, fresh string beans, tomatoes, corn, cranberries, and prunes. Neutral ash foods may be used (see under*).
‡Normal adult allowance is 0.8 to 1 gm.
§Normal adult allowance is 1 to 2 gm.

may be prescribed and an alkalinizing medication such a sodium bicarbonate or potassium citrate given. If the stone forms in alkaline urine, an acid-ash diet (Table 4) may be prescribed and an acidifying drug such as potassium acid phosphate or ascorbic acid may be given.

The Schorr regimen has shown beneficial results in the prevention of phosphatic calculi. A diet containing only 1300 mg. of phosphorus and 700 mg. of calcium daily is prescribed (Table 5), and 40 ml. of aluminum hydroxide gel is taken after meals and at bedtime. The aluminum combines with the excess phosphorus, causing it to be excreted through the bowel instead of through the kidney, thus decreasing the possibility of stone formation. Patients who must have a catheter left in place for long periods of time may be placed on this regimen prophylactically.

Special diets are not easy to continue indefinitely. The nurse who is aware of the patient's diet prescription can often help the patient fit the foods into menus or adjust the ingredients to his cultural diet pattern and his food preferences. If the patient must take a lunch to work or eat in restaurants, he may need guidance in selecting appropriate foods. Many patients on special diets feel they cannot eat at friends' homes; on these occasions the patient usually may eat sparingly of those foods served even though they are not on his diet. He should discuss with his doctor the amount of leeway he may take on such occasions.

Aluminum hydroxide gel tends to constipate some persons. Usually this tendency can be counteracted if they eat more raw fruits and vege-

Table 5. Diet containing 1300 mg. phosphorus and 700 mg. calcium

Foods permitted	Foods prohibited
Milk: 1 cup per day, as beverage or in cooking	Cheeses and cream
Eggs: 1 per day	
Cereals: any dried or cooked refined cereals such as Cream of Wheat, Farina, cornflakes, Rice Krispies, or Puffed Rice; cornmeal, white rice, spaghetti	Whole—grain cereals: Allbran, barley or brown rice, Wheaties, Puffed Wheat, Pep
Bread: white, plain or toasted; rolls or crackers made with refined flour	Breaded foods to excess
Vegetables: at least 2 servings daily besides potato, the servings being taken from the following list: string beans, lima beans, asparagus, beets or beet greens, cabbage, carrots, cauliflower, celery, chard, cucumbers, eggplant, escarole, lettuce, mushrooms, peas, onions, peppers, pumpkin, potatoes, radishes, squash, tomatoes, spinach, turnip	Dried vegetables such as dried peas, beans, or lentils, broccoli, artichokes, Brussels sprouts, or wax beans
Fruits: at least 2 servings daily of any of the following: apples, apricots (fresh or canned), bananas, cantalope, figs, (fresh or canned), grapefruits, oranges, tangerines, grapes, berries in season, peaches, pears, pineapple, plums, rhubarb, fresh juices, tomato juice	Dried fruits such as prunes, apricots, figs, peaches, raisins, dates
Meat: fish, poultry (or cottage cheese as meat substitute), 1 large serving (4 oz.) or 2 small servings (2 oz. each) of the following: beef, veal, chicken, lamb, pork, fish (not breaded)	Brains, sweetbreads, kidney, liver, heart, game (pheasant, rabbit, grouse, deer), fish roe, sardines, herring, smelts, or crab
Desserts: berry or fruit pies, cobblers, gelatin desserts (plain or fruited), fruit ices	Desserts made with milk or cream such as puddings, sherberts; ice cream, cake, or cookies
Fats: butter, oleomargarine or oil, Crisco	Gravies made with milk; mayonnaise
Sweets: sugar, jelly, jam, hard candies	Chocolate to excess; nuts or nut products such as peanut butter
Beverages: coffee, tea, carbonated beverages	Cocoa, Ovaltine, hot chocolate, milk drinks
Soups: broth or consommé	Cream soups or chowder

	Meal plan (sample)*	
Breakfast	**Luncheon**	**Dinner**
Fruit or juice	1 egg (if not for breakfast) or 2 oz. of meat	2-4 oz. of meat, fish, or chicken
Refined cereal or 1 egg	2 vegetables	Potato or substitute
1 cup milk	Salad	Salad
Sugar	White bread or roll	Vegetable
White toast	Butter	Fruit or dessert allowed
Butter	Fruit or dessert	Black coffee
Coffee	Tea with lemon and sugar	Sugar

*Between meals—fruit or fruit juice, if desired.

tables or drink a glass of prune juice each morning. If not, the doctor may order a mild cathartic such as milk of magnesia to be taken at bedtime. Psyllium (Metamucil), a bulk laxative of vegatable origin, may also be ordered. Patients usually are not advised to take mineral oil routinely since it may absorb vitamin A and cause this vitamin to be excreted, thereby lessening the amount available for use by the body. Prolonged use may also lead to bronchial granulomas. Since the patient usually discontinues the regimen because of constipation, the nurse should anticipate this and tell him that bowel regularity can often be maintained by drinking plenty of fluids, eating fresh fruits and vegetables that will add bulk to the diet, and defecating at a regular time each day.

CALCULI OF URINARY BLADDER

Calculi may form in the urinary bladder as a result of infection, obstruction, the presence of foreign bodies such as an indwelling catheter, or failure of the bladder to empty normally, which may occur in neurologic disease.

If bladder diverticula are present, stones are especially likely to form. The patient usually has symptoms of cystitis, but if the stone is large, he may have an intermittent stream and may complain of a heavy feeling in the suprapubic region and decreased bladder capacity. Vesical calculi are usually diagnosed by cystoscopy and cystograms.

Stones may be removed from the bladder through a suprapubic incision (cystolithotomy) or they may be crushed with a lithotrite (stone crusher) (see Fig. 3-10), which is passed transurethrally. The latter procedure is known as a litholapaxy and is applicable to smaller and softer stones.

After removal of vesical calculi the bladder may be irrigated (intermittently or constantly) with an acid solution such as Renacidin to counteract the alkalinity caused by the infection and to help wash out the remaining particles of stone. Renacidin contains 65% organic acids (food acids); it loses its strength in 2 or 3 days and therefore should be freshly mixed. If there has been a suprapubic incision, care of the incision is similar to that following a suprapubic prostatectomy (see Chapter 8).

QUESTIONS

1. What is the significance of urea-splitting organisms in the urinary system?
2. Name several common constituents of urinary tract stones.
3. Which stones are insoluble in acid urine?
4. Which stones tend to be insoluble in alkaline urine?
5. What are some predisposing conditions for stone formation?
6. What endocrine disease can cause stone formation?
7. What metabolic disease can cause stone formation?
8. What diagnostic tests are used to diagnose urinary tract stones?
9. Are most urinary tract stones handled by surgery?
10. Name some noncutting procedures that can be used to remove ureteral stones.

11. Name a solution and the rationale for its use for a bladder irrigation and stone prophylaxis.
12. What is the difference between a pyelolithotomy and a nephrolithotomy?
13. What are the special nursing responsibilities in the care of a patient who has had a stone operation?
14. What is the Shorr regimen in stone management?
15. What instrument is used to remove a bladder stone?

REFERENCES

Abeshouse, G., Abeshouse, B. S., and Doroshow, L. W.: The use of Renacidin as a solvent for vesical calculi, J. Urol. 86:69, 1961.

DeTar, W. T., Fries, J. G., and Crigler, C. M.: Hyperparathyroidism and renal lithiasis, J. Urol. 86:24, 1961.

Marshall, V. F., Lavengood, R. W., Jr., and Kelley D.: Longitudinal nephrolithotomy and the Shorr regimen in the management of staghorn calculi, Ann. Surg. 162:366, 1965.

Mulvaney, W. P., and Henning, D. C.: Solvent treatment of urinary calculi: refinement in technique, J. Urol. 88:145, 1962.

Murphy, F. J., and Zelman, S.: Ascorbic acid as a urinary acidifying agent. 1. Comparison with the ketogenic effect of fasting, J. Urol. 94:297, 1965.

Trinkle, K. J., and Winter, C. C.: Management of ureteral colic due to calculus disease, Ohio Med. J. 58:668, 1962.

Winter, C. C.: Renal calculi: diagnosis and management, Hosp. Med. 2:31, 1966.

Winter, C. C., Roehm, M. M., and Watson, H. G.: Urinary calculi: medical and surgical management, Amer. J. Nurs. 63:72, 1963.

Winter, C. C., Roehm, M. M., and Watson, H. G.: Urinary calculi: nursing care, Amer. J. Nurs. 63:75, 1963.

Yendt, E. R.: Drugs used in management of renal calculi, Canad. Med. Ass. J. 93:315, 1965.

CHAPTER 11

Tumors of urinary tract, including the prostate gland

The cause of hematuria must always be identified. It is probably the most common symptom of neoplasms of the urinary tract. The bleeding is seldom constant, and weeks or months may elapse between episodes of hematuria. Cystitis and fever without associated infection also frequently bring the patient with a tumor of the urologic system to a doctor. A mass may be palpable or sometimes visible in the region of the tumor. Pain, weight loss, and marked pallor are usually late manifestations of tumors anywhere in the urinary tract. As with neoplastic disease elsewhere in the body, early diagnosis offers one of the best prospects of cure.

CYSTS AND TUMORS OF THE KIDNEY

Masses in the kidney may represent fluid-filled cavities or solid tumors. Either may eventually result in obstruction of urinary drainage or destruction of renal tissue.

Solitary cyst of the kidney

A cyst of the kidney is difficult to differentiate from a renal tumor, although a renal mass can usually be revealed by intravenous or retrograde pyelography or by nephrotomography, aortography, or the renal scan. It is usually considered best to explore the mass surgically because solid tumors are not always distinguishable, and even cysts occasionally contain malignant cells. The area of involved cortex is surgically decompressed and unroofed to prevent it from pressing on the renal parenchyma. Multiple cysts are treated in the same way.

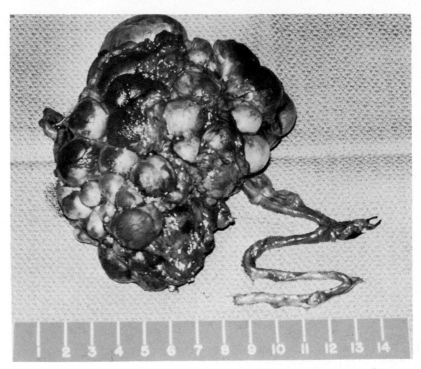

Fig. 11-1. This surgical specimen is a multicystic kidney. In this particular specimen the ureter seen at lower right is of normal caliber. Usually the ureter is atretic. No viable or normal renal parenchyma was found microscopically.

Polycystic disease

Polycystic disease is a familial disease characterized by multiple cysts of both kidneys, which are usually enlarged. The cysts press on the renal parenchyma and ultimately destroy the nephrons. Hematuria, mild hypertension, and flank pain are common.

Unfortunately, there is no specific treatment for this disease. The adult patient may live for many years. He may gradually develop azotemia or uremia and usually dies at a younger than average age, all other circumstances being equal. Babies discovered to have this disease rarely survive.

Unilateral multicystic disease

Some patients are found to have one kidney completely replaced by a multitude of cysts (Fig. 11-1), and nephrectomy is performed since the kidney is useless. The ureter may be normal or atretic. In infants the kidney may be discovered as a mass in the flank, and since no function is discernible, it is to be distinguished from hydronephrosis (in contrast to neoplasm) since some degree of function is usually present in the latter.

Retrograde pyelography should be attempted to clarify the diagnosis pre-operatively.

Neoplasms

Tumors of the kidney are usually malignant. They grow insidiously, producing no symptoms for a long time. Finally, the patient seeks medical care because of hematuria, back pain, weakness, or weight loss. Others have low-grade fever, anemia, or even polycythemia. Unfortunately the hematuria is often intermittent, lessening the patient's concern and causing procrastination in seeking medical care. There are three principal types of renal neoplasms—those arising from embryonic tissues and appearing during infancy and childhood, those arising in the renal parenchyma of adults, and those originating in the renal pelvis or calyces of adults.

Wilms' tumor is an embryonal type of growth and occurs most often in children before the age of 7 years. It is one of the most common neoplasms occurring in children. A mass about the size of a grapefruit or larger in one side of the abdomen may cause the mother to bring the child to a doctor (Fig. 11-2). This may be the only finding, but a low-grade intermittent fever and hematuria are not uncommon. Gastrointestinal symptoms, weight loss, and anemia are late symptoms. Urinary symptoms are rare.

This tumor grows rapidly and metastasizes relatively early, both by direct extension and via the vascular channels. It may invade the renal vein, vena cava, retroperitoneal lymph nodes, spleen, intestine, or liver or go directly to the lungs. Treatment is usually instituted within a day or two of discovery after adequate preoperative evaluation and preparation for surgery have been accomplished. Unfortunately the tumor occurs bilaterally in a small percentage of cases and care must be exercised to study both kidneys by appropriate radiologic tests.

If there is no evidence of metastasis, the usual treatment for Wilms' tumor is nephrectomy followed by a course of irradiation therapy beginning on the operative day. Actinomycin D (Chapter 4) may be used preoperatively and postoperatively and for patients with a recurrence of the tumor.

Tumors of the renal parenchyma are often called hypernephromas or adenocarcinomas. They are the most common tumor seen in the adult kidney and rarely occur before the age of 30 years. They spread through the bloodstream by local invasion and via the lymphatic vessels. Metastases may occur anywhere but are often found in the lungs, liver, long bones, vertebrae, and brain. Therefore chest and bone roentgenograms to detect metastases are always ordered preoperatively. Hematuria is usually a late symptom.

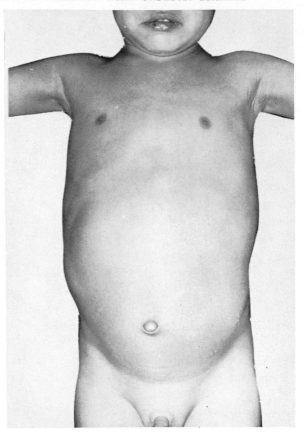

Fig. 11-2. Child with Wilms' tumor. Note protrusion of abdomen and mass visible in right flank. (From Marshall, V. F.: The diagnosis of genito-urinary neoplasms, New York, 1958, American Cancer Society, Inc.)

Small growths in the renal parenchyma may not be apparent in routine pyelograms, but larger masses are frequently detected in this manner. If there is good function of the unaffected kidney, the diseased kidney is removed (nephrectomy) (Fig. 11-3). Removal of a solitary metastasis is often feasible. Preoperative and postoperative irradiation is not used routinely, but this adjunct to surgery is gaining favor. Occasionally, hormonal drugs such as medroxyprogesterone (Provera) and testosterone are used to temporarily halt the growth of inoperable tumors, with a minority of patients responding favorably for variable periods of time. Spontaneous regression of metastases after removal of the primary neoplasm is exceedingly rare. The growth rate of renal adenocarcinoma varies considerably, and some patients have been known to live for many years despite the presence of metastases, the original tumor, or recurrences.

Tumors arising in the renal pelvis or calyces are less common. They are transitional or squamous cell in origin (epitheliomas) and resemble ureteral and bladder tumors. Hematuria is the usual symptom, and pyelo-

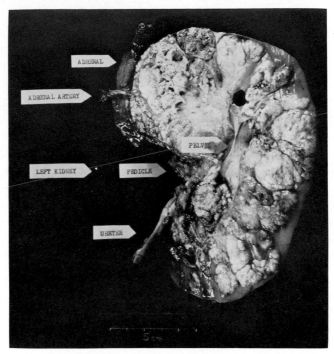

Fig. 11-3. Picture of carcinoma replacing most of the kidney.

grams are the means of diagnosis. Urinary cytologic examinations are often but not invariably positive.

If the tumor is unilateral in nature, not only is a nephrectomy performed but also the entire ureter and a cuff of bladder are resected since the tumor tends to spread along the ureter to the bladder. Most urologists feel that these patients should have periodic cystoscopic and urographic examinations for the remainder of their lives lest such tumors recur in the bladder or remaining kidney or ureter. They are believed to be caused by carcinogens in the urine.

Unfortunately the prognosis for patients of any age with cancer of the kidney may not be good. This is because the patient frequently does not reach the doctor until the disease is far advanced. Only about 35% to 45% of patients with renal parenchymal tumors survive 10 years following nephrectomy. The 10-year survival rate for tumors of the renal pelvis is about 25%. Any person who has or has had hematuria should be urged to see a urologist. Hematuria does not necessarily indicate cancer, nor does the cessation of it mean that there is no malignant disease.

Nursing care after surgery for renal tumors

A nephrectomy is the definitive treatment for renal tumors. This may be performed through a lumbar, transperitoneal, or transthoracic (between the ribs and through the diaphragm) approach. The kidney and surrounding tissue are widely resected in an attempt to remove all adjacent tissues involved in the lesion.

The nursing care following a nephrectomy is similar to that for any patient who has had renal surgery. There should, however, be only a minimal amount of serosanguineous drainage on the dressing. In fact, if the wound is dry and the kidney uninfected, no drain may be left in place. Since the renal vessels, which are normally short, are often involved in the tumor mass, the vessel stumps may be extremely short. Therefore the patient should be observed carefully for signs of internal hemorrhage. If a suture should slip from the stump, death from exsanguination may occur rapidly. Blood is usually kept on call for emergency use. If excessive bleeding occurs, a blood transfusion is started and the patient is returned to the operating room. The incision is then reopened with the patient under anesthesia.

If the thoracic approach is used, the patient may have a catheter placed into the pleural space postoperatively. This should be attached to underwater drainage to prevent air from reentering the pleural cavity and collapsing the lung. The catheter from the chest should always be clamped before any part of the drainage apparatus is disconnected. Deep breathing and coughing are essential.

Any patient who has had a nephrectomy should be observed closely for signs of spontaneous pneumothorax since the pleura is occasionally accidentally perforated. Sudden, sharp chest pain, dyspnea, anxiety, increased diaphoresis, or symptoms of shock such as a rapid pulse rate and falling blood pressure should be reported immediately. Oxygen and a thoracentesis may be required at once as emergency measures, and the patient should be urged to remain very quiet; he will probably be more comfortable in a high Fowler position.

If the renal tumor is inoperable, irradiation over tumor sites or chemotherapy may be ordered as a palliative measure. Surprisingly, an occasional patient with such a hypernephroma may survive for many years.

Occasionally, if the lesion is benign, it is unnecessary to remove the entire kidney. A segmental resection of the kidney is then performed. This is most often done to remove tuberculous and calculous lesions and ischemic (bloodless) areas of the kidney and for the repair of anomalous conditions such as a horseshoe kidney. The nursing care is similar to that required following any operation on the kidney, and careful observation for postoperative hemorrhage is of prime importance.

TUMORS OF THE URETER

Primary tumors of the ureter occur rarely. They are usually transitional or squamous cell carcinoma. Secondary tumors of the ureter are direct extensions from malignancies in the renal pelvis, bladder, bowel, uterus, or ovary. Ordinarily the treatment is removal of the kidney, ureter, and an attached segment of the bladder. The prognosis is poor if the tumor has invaded through the ureter wall. Nursing care during the postoperative period combines that needed by a patient after nephrectomy and that needed by a patient with a segmental resection of the bladder.

TUMORS OF THE URINARY BLADDER

Painless hematuria is the first sign of about 60% of all tumors of the urinary bladder. It is usually intermittent; because of this, patients may fail to seek treatment.

Symptoms of cystitis sometimes are the presenting syndrome of a vesical tumor since the tumor may act as a foreign body irritant in the bladder. Renal failure or pain resulting from obstruction of the ureters may produce the symptoms that cause the patient to seek medical care. A vesicovaginal fistula may be the acute problem. The last two conditions are indicative of a poor prognosis because the tumor has infiltrated deeply to cause these disorders. Certain bladder tumors secrete mucus or slough bits of tumor tissue as ominous signs.

Most bladder tumors start as *papillomas, leukoplakia,* or *chronic cystitis.* Although these conditions may be successfully treated by fulguration, a new tumor may appear as long as 5 years later. Any patient from whom a papilloma has been removed should have a cystoscopic examination every 3 months for 1 year and then every 6 to 12 months since further symptoms may not appear until a new papilloma has become an advanced tumor. This prophylaxis may seem unnecessary and unacceptable to some patients since cystoscopy may be somewhat of an ordeal. The necessity for this procedure should be fully explained by the doctor, and the explanation reinforced by the nurse. Emphasis can be placed on how fortunate it is to discover a bladder tumor in an early stage so that prompt treatment, the only successful management of bladder tumors, can be instituted.

Carcinoma of the bladder is diagnosed by cystoscopy and biopsy. It may be suspected if urinary cytologic findings are positive. Tumor tissue stained from tetracycline therapy may fluoresce under ultraviolet light used in special cystoscopy. The treatment is dependent upon the size of the lesion and the depth of the tissue involvement.

TREATMENT OF VESICAL TUMORS
Transurethral resection and fulguration

Small tumors with minimal involvement of the muscle tissue layer may be adequately treated with transurethral resection and fulguration if they can be reached easily by the resectoscope. The patient may or may not have a Foley catheter in place after this operation. The urine may be pink-tinged, and gross bleeding may be intermittent. Burning on urination may occur and can usually be relieved by adequate fluids, analgesics, and antispasmodics. The patient is usually discharged within a few days after surgery.

Sometimes radon seeds are implanted around the base of a vesical tumor. This is done cystoscopically or through a cystotomy opening after the tumor has been excised and fulgurated. The radioactive radon gas is sealed in gold or platinum encasings that do not have to be removed.

Following surgery the patient may have a cystostomy tube in place, but more often he will have only a urethral catheter. He usually has rather severe cystitis caused by irradiation. Treatment of the cystitis consists of sedatives, antispasmodic drugs, fluids, and analgesics. For the first 2 or 3 days, while the radon is radioactive, the nurse should avoid excessive exposure when caring for the patient (Chapter 4). When a transurethral implant has been performed, the patient can usually be discharged after 3 or 4 days. When a cystostomy has been done, the urethral catheter is removed as soon as the wound has healed and the patient is discharged within a day or two thereafter. This mode of treatment has largely given way to external irradiation.

Segmental resection of bladder

If the tumor involves the dome of the bladder, a segmental resection of the bladder may be done. More than half of the bladder may be resected. Although the bladder may have a capacity of no more than 60 ml. immediately postoperatively, the vesical tissues will regenerate so that within several months the patient is able to retain from 200 to 400 ml. of urine in the bladder if it is normal otherwise. Irradiation tends to reduce bladder capacity.

The decreased size of the bladder, however, is of major importance in the postoperative period. The patient usually returns from surgery with both a cystostomy tube and a urethral catheter in place. Two catheters are used to obviate the possibility of obstruction of drainage since it would take only a very short time for the bladder to become overdistended, and there would be danger of disrupting the vesical suture line. One or both of the catheters may be drained by a suction apparatus. Since the bladder capacity is markedly limited, the catheters frequently cause severe bladder spasm. The cystostomy tube is usually removed 1 to 2 weeks postoperatively. The urethral catheter remains in place until the suprapubic wound is well healed. Sometimes, if the cystostomy wound is not completely healed, the catheter will have to be left in place longer and the patient may be discharged to return later for removal of the tube.

As soon as the urethral catheter is removed, the patient becomes acutely aware of the small capacity of the bladder; he usually will need to void at least every 20 minutes. He needs to be reassured that the bladder capacity will gradually increase. Meantime, he is urged to drink at least 2000 ml. of fluid a day, but he should be given advice on how to time ingestion of the fluids in such a way that he is not a "prisoner in the bathroom." This may be done by taking large quantities of fluids at one time, limiting fluids for several hours before he plans to go out, and taking no fluids after 6 P.M.

Cystectomy

Cystectomy, or complete removal of the bladder, is usually done only when the tumor seems curable. In males the seminal vesicles and prostate are usually removed also. Complete removal of the bladder requires permanent urinary diversion. This may be accomplished by various methods (see discussion on urinary diversion). Rarely is it feasible to replace the bladder in situ with a segment of bowel.

Immediately after the cystectomy the patient is usually acutely ill. Since not only the bladder but also large amounts of surrounding tissue are removed (the male patient also has undergone a radical prostato-seminal vesiculectomy), the patient is subject to circulatory disturbances. These may be surgical shock, thrombosis, or cardiac decompensation. There is a long vertical or transverse abdominal incision, and there may be an additional perineal incision. The abdominal wound is usually reinforced by wire or silk retention sutures. The patient is not allowed anything by mouth for several days and may have a gastric tube connected to suction. Fluids, electrolytes, glucose, vitamins, and perhaps antibiotics are given intravenously. The nursing care is the same as that given any patient after major abdominal surgery plus the routine care for a perineal wound if one is present (see discussion on radical perineal prostatectomy) and care of the diverted urinary drainage. The male patient will be impotent postoperatively if the prostatic capsule has been removed.

Other treatment

Occasionally, if a cancerous lesion of the bladder is small and superficial, *radioisotopes* contained in the balloon of a Foley catheter or *chemotherapeutic agents* (such as thio-tepa) may be inserted into the bladder. The catheter containing radioactive material is attached to drainage, and all urine must be saved and sent to the radioisotope department for monitoring prior to its disposal. (See Chapter 4 for other precautions.) Severe cystitis and proctitis usually result from this treatment, and the patient may be very uncomfortable for several days or weeks. Forcing fluids gives some relief from the symptoms, and urinary antiseptics and antispasmodic drugs are frequently ordered. Care should be taken to keep the stool soft, and a low-residue diet may be ordered.

External irradiation of vesical tumors with x-rays or cobalt is done, especially as a palliative treatment for inoperable cancer. Contraction of the bladder and serious cystitis often occur. If a urinary diversion procedure has been performed, however, irradiation of the bladder may decrease bleeding from the tumor and give relief from pain.

A less than tumoricidal dose of irradiation therapy may be administered 30 days prior to surgical removal of the neoplasm and is known as *combined therapy.*

Chemotherapy such as parenteral 5-fluorouracil may occasionally be used as an adjuvant in treating tumors of the bladder and is most often used for lesions that have already metastasized (Chapter 4).

Urinary diversion

The ureters may be transplanted before the cystectomy or at the same operation. They may be connected to the intact colon (*ureterosigmoidostomy* anastomosis) or a sigmoidal colostomy may be performed to divert the fecal stream and the ureters then transplanted into the rectum (*rectal bladder*). Also, a section of the ileum may be isolated and its blood supply preserved. It is sutured closed at one end and the other end is brought to the skin as an ileostomy. The ureters are transplanted into the proximal end of this segment of ileum (*ileal conduit*). Occasionally one or both ureters are completely removed, necessitating anastomosis of the ileal segment directly to the renal pelvis or pelves. The remaining intestine is reanastomosed. The ureters also may be implanted directly onto the abdomen (*cutaneous ureterostomies* or *loop ureterostomies*). We have a series of patients in whom live omentum has been wrapped around the distal ureter at the skin anastomosis in the expectation that the omentum will prevent stenosis of the ureteral ostia.

The patient whose ureters are transplanted into the bowel is usually happier socially than one with urinary fistulas opening onto the skin, but hydronephrosis and kidney infection frequently occur. The kidney may empty poorly because the rectum normally has a higher pressure than the bladder, or the ureterosigmoidostomy anastomoses may close because of fibrosis. (See discussion on ureteral physiology in Chapter 2.) Conversely, reflux of fecal contents into the ureters and kidneys is not uncommon, although the ureters are placed in a tunnel in the well of the bowel in an attempt to obviate this problem. As the ureters and renal pelves dilate, organisms in the bowel easily start a pyelonephritis. The intestinal tract also has absorptive powers, and waste products in the urine, especially chlorides, may be resorbed, upsetting the electrolytic balance of the body. For these reasons it is better physiologically to transplant the ureters into an ileal conduit or directly onto the skin of the abdomen. When these procedures are done, however, the patient has one or two permanently draining ostomies. These must be cared for by some type of drainage system. This may be annoying and embarrassing, and some patients who are thus encumbered find this an almost impossible adjustment to make. However, if the need for such drainage has been thoroughly explained before the procedure and if the patient is properly instructed in caring for the ostomy and is given continuing psychologic support and encouragement, he can usually adjust. These patients learn to accept the cups, bag, or tubes as the "price they pay for their lives." Some lead relatively happy and productive lives for years. Many are surprised to find they can work, play, dance, swim, have babies, etc. Children adapt very readily.

Ileal conduit (Brinker procedure)

The ileal (or colonic) conduit (see Fig. 8-14) is made in such a way that it will not act as a reservoir but only as a passageway for urine from the ureters to the outside. Because of this, patients with ileal conduits should have less difficulty with electrolytic imbalance than those in whom the bowel serves as a reservoir. Some problems do still occur, however, and signs of renal infection, failure, or electrolytic imbalance such as chills, fever, flank pain, nausea, vomiting, diarrhea, or lethargy should be reported to the doctor.

Care during operative period

The preoperative preparation of a patient who is to have an ileal conduit is quite different from the preparation of a patient prior to a ureterosigmoidostomy. No special diet, antibiotics, cathartics, or enemas are necessary since the ileum is considered sterile. Following an ileal conduit procedure the patient may return from the operating room with catheters inserted through the ileostomy opening to provide for ureteral drainage and anastomotic splinting. The catheters may need to be gently irrigated every day. Sometimes no catheters are used. Mucus will be secreted by the ileal conduit. A permanent or temporary ileostomy bag (usually plastic) is secured over the opening to collect the drainage (see Fig. 4-16).

Regardless of what surgical technique is used, the nurse must carefully watch for any signs indicating distention of the isolated segment of ileum with urine since this may cause the suture line to break or it may cause back pressure on the kidneys. The ureters are anastomosed to the conduit without a tunnel so that reflux occurs readily. Distention of the lower abdomen or decreased urinary output should be reported at once. Failure to empty the collection bag before it is completely full causes back pressure that slows drainage. Swelling about the stoma may also prevent emptying of the conduit. Swelling about the ureteroileal anastomosis or pressure of distended organs against the conduit may prevent drainage from the ureters into the conduit if unintubated. Urinary ileostomy bags that can be attached to a drainage apparatus at night are preferable.

Symptoms of peritonitis (fever, abdominal tenderness, swelling, pain) should be carefully watched for and reported at once. After this type of surgery the intestinal anastomosis may leak fecal material or the ileal conduit may leak urine into the peritoneal cavity. If this happens, an emergency operation to repair the intraperitoneal leak must be performed. Urinary leakage may be retroperitoneal, and if a drain is in place, surgical intervention may be unnecessary.

The patient will usually have a gastric tube in place for several days after an ileal conduit procedure to prevent distention of the bowel with resultant pressure on the intestinal anastomosis. If the tube fails to drain properly or if abdominal distention or cramping occurs, the doctor should be notified. The nurse should note and record the passing of flatus or feces since this indicates patency of the intestinal tract after bowel reanastomosis. After the fourth postoperative day the patient may be given laxatives. The patient progresses from a liquid to a regular diet. (For further details concerning the care of a patient following intestinal anastomosis, see a surgical nursing textbook.)

Care of ileal conduit drainage. The nurse usually changes the temporary plastic ileostomy bags as needed for several days postoperatively. Later the patient is taught to handle this step. A variety of bags are available and instructions for their use will vary (see Chapter 4).

Rectal bladder

The patient with a rectal bladder rarely requires the same care as one with a ureterointestinal anastomosis. There will be no fecal discharge from the anus since isolation of the rectum requires a colostomy. He will need the colostomy cared for postoperatively and will need to be taught to provide this care for himself prior to discharge. The nurse should review colostomy care in a surgical nursing textbook. The anal sphincter must be strong and efficiently controlled to prevent urinary leakage. Therefore small children and elderly patients are not good candidates for this type of diversion.

Cutaneous ureterostomy

When the ureters have been transplanted to the abdominal wall, the patient may have soft rubber catheters in place for about 1 week if the ureters are small. In the pediatric age group the ureters are often dilated and do not need to be splinted. It is important that the catheters drain adequately so that hydronephrosis does not develop. (See discussion on maintenance of drainage and catheter care in Chapter 4.)

Use of ureterostomy cups. If cutaneous ureterostomies heal properly,

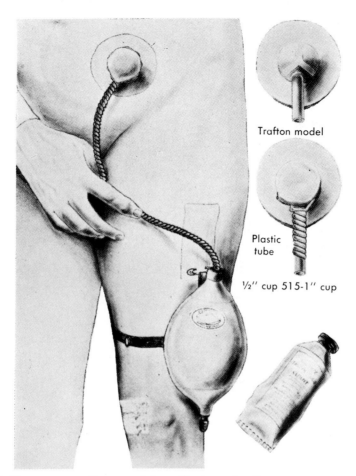

Fig. 11-4. Singer cup appliance used for collecting urine from cutaneous ureterostomy.

the patient can use ureterostomy cups or ostomy bags instead of catheters for drainage. Singer or Whitmore cups are the type commonly used (Figs. 11-4 and 11-5). The cups are applied to the skin with adhesive disks and may require changing only every 2 or 3 days. The technique for applying the cup is not difficult, but it does take practice. With guidance, the patient can often apply it himself after the first time. When the cup is first applied, the nurse must make sure that there is adequate drainage from the kidney. If the patient complains of any back pain, the cup should be removed at once and reapplied. Sometimes obstruction to drainage is caused by angulation of the ureter or by temporary ureteral edema. If the ureter is angulated or if there is stomal stenosis, the kidney will have to be drained permanently with a catheter.

A written procedure such as the following on home care of ureterostomies with cups is helpful to the patient.

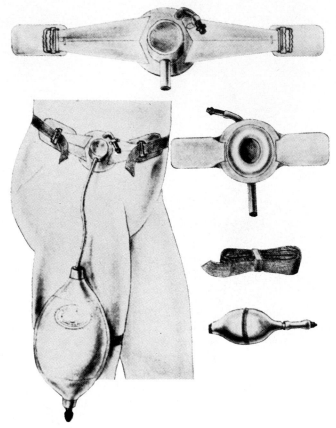

Fig. 11-5. Whitmore cup appliance used for collecting urine from cutaneous ureterostomy.

Home care of ureterostomies with Singer cups

You are being sent home with cups because your doctor believes they will be more convenient for you than catheters. It is extremely important that you follow this plan of care to keep the skin in good condition.

Equipment needed for changing cup

1. Ureterostomy cup with tubing coil
2. Skin cement or adhesive disks
3. Leg bag or urinal with 2 straps
4. Cotton-tipped applicators
5. Tincture of benzoin
6. Can of cement solvent
7. Absorbent cotton and mesh gauze
8. Small tube brush
9. Clean soft rags or cheesecloth
10. Paper bag for waste
11. Vinegar
12. Deodorant powder or tablets

Other equipment needed

1. 6 glass or plastic Y connectors (8 mm. diameter)
2. 8 straight glass or plastic connectors (8 mm. diameter) if 2 urinals or 2 night bottles used
3. Latex rubber tubing (8 mm. bore), 4 feet (if 2 night bottles are used, 8 feet)
4. Large glass bottle or floor bag

Procedure for changing cup

1. Collect all equipment on a tray and go to bathroom.
2. While running bath water, sit near tub and, with small cloth saturated with cement solvent, rub along upper edge of cuff until it begins to separate from skin.

Note: Solvent is inflammable! Do not smoke or be near an open flame such as pilot light on stove while using solvent!

3. Grasp loosened edge of cuff and gently pull away from skin, continuing to apply solvent-saturated cloth until cup is completely separated from skin.
4. Clean remaining cement from skin.

Note: If you have two sets of cups, you may prefer to do steps 5 and 6 after you have replaced clean cups.

5. Wash cup thoroughly with soap and warm water. Soak it in vinegar solution (4 tablespoons of distilled vinegar to 1 pint of water) for 15 minutes. Run tube brush through connectors. Rinse with cold water containing deodorant powder. Dry cups thoroughly.
6. Cement does not need to be cleaned from cup each time cup is changed but only when cement is about ⅛ inch thick. Then most of it can be easily peeled off with your fingers. Remove remainder with cement solvent.
7. Get into bathtub with water at waist level or shower and bathe thoroughly. Do not rush this bath, which is not only for cleansing but also for soothing ureteral openings.
8. After drying yourself completely, you are ready to reapply cups. If skin or ureteral bud is irritated, however, you should first lie under a heat lamp for 20 minutes. Use a bridge or a gooseneck lamp with a 60-watt bulb. Place it 2 feet above your abdomen. **Do not use a sun lamp.** Karaya powder may be applied first.
9. Secure urinal to your leg with leg straps. It is necessary to wear only one urinal, but some people are more comfortable with two. To give better support to bag, take a double piece of tape (1½ by 4 inches) and, after fastening a large safety pin through it, put it on your leg about 1 inch above the bag. If you prefer, the bag can be suspended from a belt placed around your waist.
10. Place cup over ureterostomy with ureteral opening in center of opening of cup.
11. Holding cup in position, dip a cotton-tipped applicator in tincture of benzoin and trace outline of cup on skin.
12. Removing cup, place a tightly rolled piece of gauze over ureteral openings or cotton applicators in openings. You will need to have several of these ready for use.

Note: If at any time during the following steps the gauze or cotton becomes wet, change quickly to a dry piece. Any urine running over skin will cause cup to leak.

13. Holding gauze in place, once again thoroughly wash and dry skin around bud in order to remove any urine.
14. With tincture of benzoin, paint area within circle that you traced on skin.
15. Be sure cup is dry, and then apply a continuous stream of cement to cup and smooth it with your finger or a small brush. Set cup aside. Or use adhesive disk.

16. Apply a continuous stream of cement to painted area of skin, and, getting into a position so that the abdomen is as free from wrinkled skin as possible, smooth this paste with your finger or a brush. Or use adhesive disk.

Note: When applying cement, use long strokes rather than dabbing. Try not to go back over areas already covered, because this tends to pull the cement off.

17. Keeping in position as above, take a deep breath and hold it to make your abdomen firm. Immediately place lower cuff of cup, with outlet in position to attach to urinal, on benzoin line and press firmly. Remove gauze and bring upper part of cup into position. Hold it securely for about 2 minutes.
18. Attach outlet of cup to leg bag.

Note: If cup starts to leak at any time, dry loosened area under cuff with a cotton-tipped applicator and try to patch it by putting cement on with an applicator. If unsuccessful, remove cup and reapply. Edges may be sealed with paper tape.

Emptying leg bag

1. Standing over toilet, turn screw on bottom of bag one-half turn.
2. Allow to drain and retighten.

Preparation for sleep

1. Remove urinal and day tubing and wash thoroughly with soap and water.
2. Soak urinal and tubing in vinegar solution for 15 minutes.
3. Run tube brush through connectors and into top of urinal.
4. Rinse with cold water containing deodorant.
5. Hang up to dry and air overnight.
6. Attach your drainage appliance to tubing. Allow it to drain into a large bottle at side of bed. Cut 4 feet of tubing (2 feet go to bottle and 2 feet should be on bed to allow you to turn over without pulling cup off).

ALTERNATE METHOD FOR STEP 6. Take a clean plastic urinal and pin it, by loop at top, to side of mattress. Attach about 2 feet of tubing between it and cup.

Note: When you lie down, your drainage apparatus must be at a level lower than the body or you will have pain because your kidney cannot drain properly. You will also have leakage around cup.

Care of night equipment

Daily. Wash bottle or urinal and all tubing thoroughly with soap and water. Soak for 15 minutes in vinegar solution (4 tablespoons to 1 pint of water). Rinse with cold water containing deodorant.

Twice a week. Boil tubing and bottle for 10 minutes. (This controls odor and ensures cleanliness.)

Suggestions on general care

1. It is easier to change cup if you have not had any fluids for 3 or 4 hours since there will be less urine flowing. However, you must still plan to drink at least 2 quarts of fluid a day.
2. If cup leaks:
   a. Review your method of changing it carefully. You may not be getting skin cleaned and dried properly.
   b. Check to see that all tubing and connections are clean. Crystals should not form in it if you care for it each day as outlined.
   c. Check to see that no part of tubing or bag is kinked.
   d. Be sure that you always have your drainage container at a level lower than opening of ureters.

    e. Be sure leg bag is closed tightly. You may need a new washer in bottom of bag.

    f. If all of the preceding steps have been checked and you still have trouble, return to clinic or to your personal physician.

3. If skin becomes reddened and sore:

    a. Increase length of time you are spending in your daily tub bath and apply karaya powder.

    b. Use heat lamp 20 minutes each time cup is taken off. (See step 3 of routine procedure.)

    c. Do not be afraid to reapply cup; the oxide in cement has healing properties, as does pressure of cup.

    d. Some people find it helps to remove the cup applied with cement for several nights and to apply a Whitmore cup, which is held in place with an inflated cuff and a belt, not by cement.

    e. If these methods are not satisfactory or if the skin is oozing, return to clinic or to your private doctor. A catheter will probably be inserted for several days until the skin heals.

4. If ostium swells or becomes irritated:

    a. Be sure that you are changing cup every day and soaking in a tub of warm water 15 minutes.

    b. Use heat lamp.

    c. Be sure you are using drainage with an air outlet at night.

    d. You might try placing a No. 20 hypodermic needle into tubing (place with hub uppermost) to provide an air outlet during day.

    e. If stoma is so swollen that cup irritates it, plastic postoperative ileostomy appliances or pads may be used. Close bottom of bag with a rubber band. You must empty it about every 2 hours; otherwise the weight will pull the bag off. Wear this for several days or until swelling subsides.

    f. If there is no improvement, return to clinic or see your personal physician.

5. Sports, including swimming:

    a. If your doctor does not limit your activity for some other reason, your ureterostomies should not keep you from participating in any activity.

    b. If you wish to go swimming, you may wear plastic ileostomy appliances. If you do not wear a tight bathing suit, no one will notice these appliances.

6. Most persons carry a tube of cement and several applicators in their pocket or handbag at all times. They seldom need to use these, but it is reassuring to have them. Wearing a girdle or a surgical belt over cups may also make you feel more secure.

7. If you are going away on a trip, you will need to remember to pack your night drainage equipment and a supply of equipment to change cups.

8. If you follow directions for caring for equipment, there should be no problem of odor.

9. If you have back pain or any other unusual symptoms, return to clinic, call your personal physician, or go to a hospital emergency room.

10. Protect your bed with a full-length piece of plastic, for you may accidently kink the tubing while you are asleep. This may cause a leak in the system.

Use of ureteral catheters. If the kidneys do not drain properly when ureterostomy cups are used, the patient must wear ureteral catheters (Figs. 11-6 to 11-8). Patients are taught to irrigate these each day. (See discussion of home care of catheters in Chapter 4.) Most patients return to the doctor every 2 to 4 weeks to have the catheters changed; some are taught to change their own catheters. Latex rubber many-eyed Robinson or whistle-tip catheters (Chapter 3) usually give the best drainage and

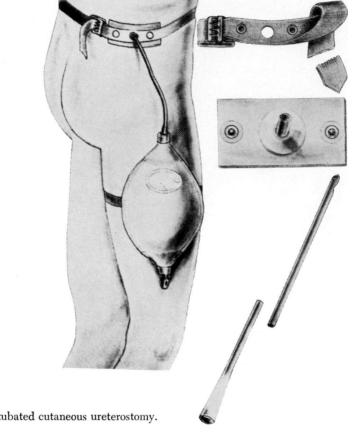

Fig. 11-6. Intubated cutaneous ureterostomy.

cause the least trauma to the ureteral tissues. The catheters are anchored to the skin with adhesive tape or a catheter disk with a belt, and they are attached by tubing to a drainage receptacle (Chapter 4).

If the patient is to change his own catheters, he should change one catheter each day while he is in the hospital to get the needed practice. This procedure should not be taught until he has mastered the procedure for irrigation. It is helpful to review the anatomic placement of the catheters with the patient, using diagrams. The doctor or nurse specialist should give the first instruction. The nurse who is to do the follow-up teaching should be present. The patient should be referred to a public health nurse for additional assistance.

A written procedure such as the following for changing ureterostomy catheters is helpful to the patient.

Changing ureterostomy catheters

For your convenience the doctor is going to have you learn how to change your own catheters. This should be done only once a week unless a catheter is not draining properly.

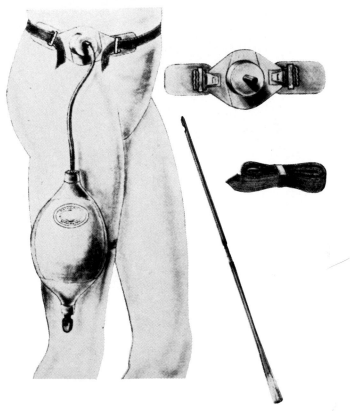

Fig. 11-7. Another example of intubated cutaneous ureterostomy or nephrostomy.

Equipment needed to change two catheters

1. All equipment used for irrigation of catheters
2. Clean, marked catheters (same size as catheters to be removed)
3. Two pairs of forceps with a 15-inch string tied to each handle
4. Lubrication jelly

Procedure

1. Prepare and assemble equipment exactly as for irrigation.
2. Place all equipment in pot, winding strings around handle of pot. Catheters do not need a string attached since you can pick them out with forceps.
3. Boil and cool equipment in same manner as for irrigation.
4. Cut 4 pieces of plastic adhesive tape (1 by 4 inches).
5. Prepare irrigation materials so as to be ready to irrigate. Leave forceps and catheters in pan. All equipment should be within convenient reach.
6. Loosen old tape from skin around one catheter. Do not remove catheter.
7. Cleanse skin with solvent, wash with soap and water, and dry. Apply tincture of benzoin to skin and allow this to dry. Apply first piece of adhesive tape.

Note: Solvent is inflammable! Do not smoke or be near an open flame such as pilot light of stove while using it!

8. Remove old catheter, putting it in basin for drainage returns. Pick up one

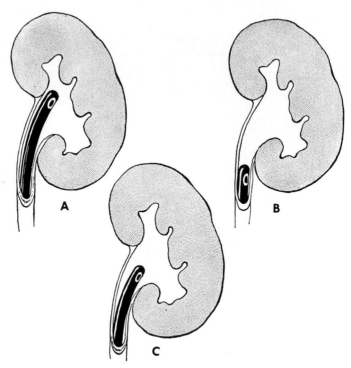

Fig. 11-8. Schematic drawing to show correct position of ureteral catheter in renal pelvis. **A,** Catheter inserted only far enough to obtain urine. **B,** Catheter pulled back to point at which drainage of urine ceases. **C,** Catheter then reinserted 2.54 cm. (1 inch). In final position, urine should drain freely, leaving none in any portion of renal pelvis. (From Shafer, K. N., Sawyer, J. R., McCluskey, A. M., and Beck, E. L.: Medical-surgical nursing, ed. 2, St. Louis, 1961, The C. V. Mosby Co.)

pair of forceps by string. Gather string into palm of hand. Grasping catheter with forceps about ½ inch from end that will go into ureter, pull it out of of pot. Grasp irrigating end of catheter, about 2 inches from end, in your left hand.

Note: Do not lock forceps. Hold them gently closed around catheter.

9. Hold your left hand high so that catheter will not touch skin. Get into a sitting or semireclining position, whichever seems easier for you. Insert lubricated tip of catheter into opening of ureter. As you take deep breaths and blow them out, push catheter in with forceps. If you feel an obstruction, take another breath and catheter will probably slide in. If you cannot get catheter in easily, stop and notify hospital doctor or your personal physician.

Note: Be sure to gradually lower your left hand as you insert catheter so as to allow a slack section of catheter to push into ureter.

10. Insert catheter up to mark. (This will originally be determined in the hospital, and you should mark this point on each new catheter with colored fingernail polish.) Most patients will find that the catheter drains and irrigates best when it is inserted about 7 or 8 inches, but this will be individually determined by your doctor and may be different on each side.

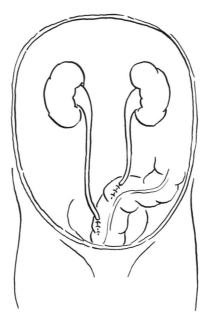

Fig. 11-9. Ureterosigmoidal anastomosis. (Unpublished illustration of Dr. B. G. Clarke and Dr. L. Del Guercio.)

Ureterointestinal anastomosis (ureterosigmoidostomy)

When the ureters are transplanted into the bowel (Fig. 11-9), special preparation and care are necessary.

Preoperative care. If the ureters are transplanted into the colon, the patient is given a bowel preparation (a nonresidue diet for 3 days and neomycin enemas 12 hours before surgery). The nurse should give 200 to 300 ml. of the enema and ask the patient to retain it as long as possible. This gives evidence of anal sphincter control and helps the patient to begin, preoperatively, to adjust to fluid in the bowel. It must be remembered that bowel preparations vary considerably among surgeons.

Postoperative care. Postoperatively, a large tube (30 Fr.) is left in the rectum to drain the urine. It is secured in the gluteal fold with a double-flap adhesive tape anchorage or by sutures. (See the procedure for rectal tube drainage of urine on p. 308.) If the tube becomes obstructed despite irrigations during the first 4 or 5 days, the doctor should change it since there is danger of perforating the newly operated tissues. A sterile tube is used, and it is inserted only 4 inches since the anastomosis is about 6 to 8 inches above the anus. Because of its local anesthetic effect, tetracaine ointment may be used to lubricate the tube for insertion. The urinary output should be carefully measured and recorded. Usually the ureters are intubated with catheters that are brought out the anus and attached to the buttocks by sutures. They may require irrigations to keep them patent. They are marked right and left.

The rectal tube usually is not discontinued until the eighth postoperative day, and the ureteral tubes slip out by the tenth day or are removed. The rectal tube may be removed for the patient to defecate and then reinserted. A low-residue diet is usually ordered until the tubes are removed. When drainage is first discontinued, the patient has diarrhea-like bowel movements; therefore the tube is replaced for several nights to prevent loss of sleep. Until the bowel adjusts to being a reservoir for urine, the stool will be soft, but the patient will be able to tell when he needs to void and when he needs to defecate. He should be able to retain about 200 ml. of urine.

Preparation for discharge. The patient needs specific instructions prior to discharge. He should void (rectally) every 2 to 4 hours in the daytime and once or twice at night to minimize the resorption of waste products and to improve the emptying of the kidneys. Some doctors prefer that the patient insert a rectal tube and connect it to drainage each night. The patient should report any nausea, vomiting, fever, or lethargy to the doctor; these symptoms are suggestive of electrolytic imbalance and/or pyelonephritis, and alkalinizing drugs or antibiotics may be prescribed. The patient with a ureterointestinal anastomosis should never again need a laxative or enema. If the patient is ever readmitted to a hospital, he should tell the hospital personnel that he voids through the rectum. He ordinarily may eat a regular diet, and his physician will usually want him to drink at least 1000 ml. of fluid daily. A written procedure for rectal tube drainage is helpful; the following is an example.

Rectal tube drainage of urine

You will need the following equipment:
1. Plastic tubing (8 mm. diameter), 4 feet, with connector
2. Tetracaine ointment
3. Tincture of benzoin
4. No. 28 rectal tube
5. Plastic tape (1-inch width)
6. Plastic collecting bag or bottle

Procedure

1. Attach rectal tube to the drainage tubing that empties into the plastic bag at side of bed.
2. Lubricate rectal tube with tetracaine.
3. Cut four 6-inch strips of 1-inch plastic tape.
4. Paint the skin under buttock on the side that will be toward the bottle with tincture of benzoin. (Use a cotton-tipped applicator stick, and allow it to dry thoroughly.)
5. Apply two pieces of tape to the skin.
6. When you are in bed, insert the rectal tube 4 inches. Place the other pieces of tape over the rectal tube and the first tapes. Run your fingers along the rectal tube to secure the tape.

Note: It is wise to have toilet tissue at the bedside to wrap the tube in when you remove it in the morning. You may wish to protect the bed from any leakage by using a piece of plastic (a plastic tablecloth, for example) under the sheets and large pads over the sheet, or a diaper may be worn.

Care of night equipment (do daily)

1. Wash bottle, rectal tube, and all tubing thoroughly with soap and water.
2. Soak rectal tube and drainage tubing for 15 minutes in benzalkonium solution (1:750).
3. Rinse rectal tube and tubing with cold water containing deodorant powder.
4. Boil the rectal tube for 10 minutes. (This will control odors and ensure cleanliness.)

Nephrostomy

If the ureters become strictured and the kidneys drain inadequately, permanent nephrostomy tubes may need to be inserted into the renal pelves to divert the urine. This is usually done as a last resort (see Fig. 8-13). Temporary nephrostomy drainage is frequently necessary when plastic repair of the ureters or lower urinary tract requires urinary diversion. (See Chapter 4 for care of nephrostomy tubes.)

CANCER OF PROSTATE GLAND

Autopsy examinations have shown that from 15% to 20% of all men past 50 years of age have microscopic carcinoma of the prostate. Although many of these men do not have clinical symptoms, it is known that the incidence of clinical cancer of the prostate increases with advancing age. With an increase in life expectancy, the incidence of cancer of the prostate probably will rise.

Diagnosis

Cancer of the prostate is most often diagnosed when the patient seeks medical advice because of symptoms of prostatic obstruction caused by a local growth in the prostate gland or because of sciatica (pains in the lower back, hip, and leg) caused by metastases of the cancer to the bones. In the late stages the patient will exhibit the symptoms and signs of any terminal disease (anorexia, pallor, weakness, weight loss, etc.). Cancer of the prostate gland frequently occurs concurrently with benign prostatic hypertrophy, which may cause the obstruction, or the cancer itself may be so far advanced as to cause obstruction.

Since cancer of the prostate that causes obstruction of the urethra or results in back and leg pains may be too far advanced for curative treatment, one can readily understand the need for men past 45 years of age to have rectal examinations as a part of the yearly physical examination. Most carcinomas of the prostate gland are adjacent to the rectal wall and thus can often be detected prior to symptomatic disease by rectal examination. Most curable lesions are asymptomatic and therefore can be

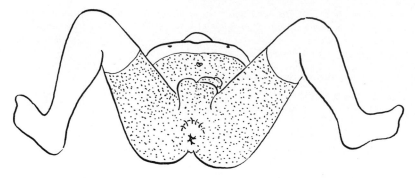

Fig. 11-10. Area prepared and incision used for perineal surgery. (Unpublished illustration of Dr. B. G. Clarke and Dr. L. Del Guercio.)

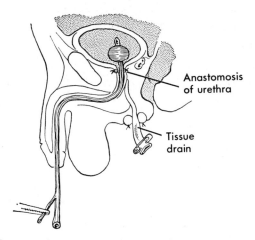

Anastomosis
of urethra

Tissue
drain

Fig. 11-11. Radical perineal prostatectomy. Note that prostatic fossa is not present; prostate gland and prostatic urethra have been resected and urethra anastomosed to bladder. Note placement of tissue drain between scrotum and rectum. In simple prostatectomy there is no urethral shortening; posterior part of prostatic capsule is incised. Incision and drain are similar. (From Shafer, K. N., Sawyer, J. R., McCluskey, A. M., Beck, E. L., and Phipps, W. J.: Medical-surgical nursing, ed. 5, St. Louis, 1971, The C. V. Mosby Co.)

diagnosed only in the course of routine physical examinations that include rectal palpation of the prostate gland. The doctor usually takes a biopsy of suggestive masses.

Prostatic biopsies may be obtained either by excision of a core of tissue through a specially designed needle or by obtaining a specimen of tissue through a surgical incision. Both of these procedures are carried out under sterile conditions using local or general anesthesia.

Surgical biopsy. A prostatic biopsy specimen can be obtained by making a small incision in the perineum between the anus and the scrotum (Fig. 11-10). The dressing is usually held in place by a two-tailed binder.

The patient must be instructed to be careful not to contaminate the incision while cleansing himself following defecation. If the incision is accidentally contaminated, the area should be carefully cleansed. Irrigation of the perineum using sterile benzalkonium chloride sponges is sometimes ordered routinely following defecation. A heat lamp with a 60-watt bulb placed 12 inches from the perineum is often used two or three times a day to encourage healing. The patient must be in a position in which the scrotum is elevated so that the heat strikes the incision. This is best accomplished by allowing the scrotum to rest on a wide piece of adhesive tape extending from thigh to thigh (see Fig. 9-2). Occasionally an exaggerated Sims position gives satisfactory wound exposure. When the sutures have been removed, sitz baths are often ordered instead of the lamp treatment, and these add a great deal to the general comfort of the patient. The patient usually remains in the hospital until the laboratory findings are reported.

Needle aspiration biopsy. A patient who has a needle aspiration biopsy usually does not need to be hospitalized. He has no dressings and will rarely require any special care. He should bathe as usual and inspect the aspiration site for redness. If redness appears or if he has other symptoms suggestive of infection (for example, fever), he should call his doctor.

Transrectal needle or surgical biopsies may also be used. Some surgeons prepare the rectum with neomycin enemas and prescribe neomycin orally preoperatively and postoperatively.

An elevated level of acid phosphatase in the blood is usually indicative of cancer of the prostate, but since the acid phosphatase produced by prostatic cancer is not absorbed by the blood until the lesion has extended beyond the prostatic capsule, it is not a useful technique for early diagnosis.

Surgical treatment

In patients in whom a diagnosis is made prior to local extension of the cancer or metastasis, a radical resection of the prostate gland is usually curative. The entire prostate gland, including the capsule, seminal vesicles, and the adjacent tissue, is removed. The remaining urethra is then anastomosed to the bladder neck. Since the internal and external sphincters of the bladder lie in close approximation to the prostate, it is not unusual for the patient to have some degree of urinary incontinence following this type of surgery. He also will be both impotent and sterile. The perineal approach is often used (radical perineal prostatectomy), but the procedure may be accomplished by the retropubic route (radical retropubic prostatectomy) (Fig. 11-11).

The patient is usually given a bowel preparation before perineal surgery to prevent fecal contamination of the operative site. This may include enemas containing neomycin. Postoperatively, the patient with a perineal incision may be kept on a low-residue diet until wound healing is well advanced. Codeine may also be prescribed to inhibit bowel action. Later, stool softeners are ordered.

If the retropubic approach is to be used, the patient usually is given routine preoperative care. Usually no special diet is needed before or after surgery.

Regardless of the surgical approach, the patient returns from surgery with a urethral catheter to drain the bladder. Inadvertent removal of the catheter would produce an awkward situation since it might be impossible to reinsert. Its retention in the bladder is so vital to the success of the operation that, in addition to catheter balloon inflation, it is fixed in place either by suture or tape. A large amount of urinary drainage on the dressing for a number of hours is not unusual. This should rapidly decrease. There should not be the amount of bleeding that follows other prostatic surgery and, since the catheter is not being used for hemostasis, the patient usually has fewer bladder spasms. The catheter is used both for urinary drainage and as a splint for the urethral anastomosis; therefore care should be taken that it does not become dislodged or blocked. The catheter is usually left in place for 2 weeks. A tissue drain is removed 24 to 48 hours after perineal surgery unless otherwise ordered by the surgeon. A suprapubic drain remains longer.

The care of the perineal wound is the same as that following a perineal biopsy, although healing is usually slower. If there has been a retropubic surgical approach, the care of the incision and possible wound complications is the same as that for a simple retropubic prostatectomy (Chapter 8).

Since perineal surgery causes relaxation of the perineal musculature, the patient who has had a perineal prostatectomy may suddenly have fecal incontinence. This is upsetting for the patient and sometimes can be avoided by starting perineal exercises within a day or two after surgery. Control of the anal spincter usually returns readily. Perineal exercises should be continued even after anal sphincter control returns since they also strengthen the urethral sphincter. Unless the urethral sphincter has been permanently damaged, the patient who has practiced perineal exercises will usually regain urinary control more readily after removal of the catheter. (See Chapter 4 for a discussion of perineal exercises.)

The patient with carcinoma of the prostate gland is often depressed after surgery because he suddenly realizes the implications of the disease and of being impotent and perhaps incontinent. He usually has been told by the doctor before the operation of these possible consequences, but he may not have fully comprehended their meaning. He needs to be encouraged, and provision should be made to keep him dry (see discussion on care of incontinent patients in Chapter 4) so that he will feel able to be up and to socialize with others without fear of wetting himself after the catheter is removed. Until the doctor has ascertained that return of urinary sphincter control is unlikely, the use of a shower cap (described in Chapter 4) or training pants is preferable since this gives some protection but not enough to discourage the patient from attempting to regain control of micturition.

Conservative treatment

When cancer of the prostate gland is inoperable, the *Huggins treatment* may be used. This is based on elimination of androgens by removal of the testicles and/or giving estrogenic hormones. Occasionally it is necessary to resect the prostate gland to relieve obstruction. This is most often done transurethrally (Chapter 8).

In the Huggins treatment the estrogen given is usually stilbestrol, 1 to 3 mg. a day. This frequently will relieve the pain and sometimes will decrease obstruction sufficiently to obviate the need for a prostatectomy. Stilbestrol may produce nausea and causes engorgement and tenderness of the breasts of the male patient (gynecomastia). The latter can be prevented by delivering a single dose of x-ray therapy to the breasts before commencing the hormone therapy. Severe side effects should be reported to the doctor so that the dosage or type of estrogenic preparation may be adjusted. High doses of female hormone predispose to sodium retention and congestive heart failure.

When symptoms begin to recur or if the patient is extremely uncomfortable and needs immediate relief when the diagnosis is first made, a bilateral orchiectomy (castration) is done. This is not a severe operative ordeal and is often done under local anesthesia. The patient's permission for sterilization must be obtained (Chapter 4); if he is married, he is usually urged to discuss the operation with his wife. This surgery eliminates the testicular source of male hormones and seems to cause regression or at least slows the growth of the cancer. The great advantage of castration is that the treatment is always working whether or not the patient is reliable about taking his medicine. Relief, as the result of palliative treatment via castration and estrogens, is quite dramatic in many patients. This result is of variable duration, however, ranging from only a few months to many years or even the remainder of the patient's normal life expectancy.

Remission may also sometimes be obtained for patients who have further symptoms of prostatic carcinoma after castration and estrogen therapy by judicious manipulation of the function of the adrenal glands.

These organs, like the testes, produce androgens, although to a lesser degree (Chapter 2). The function of the adrenal glands may be suppressed indirectly by administration of cortisone or cortisone-like substances. The drug supplies the adrenal hormone essential for life processes (Chapter 2), and its presence in the bloodstream suppresses secretion of adrenocorticotropic hormone (ACTH) from the pituitary gland. ACTH is essential for the stimulation of secretion of androgens (and cortisone as well) from the adrenal glands. (See Chapter 14 for a discussion of the patient receiving cortisone therapy.) A hypophysectomy (neurosurgical removal of the pituitary gland) or ablation with injected radioisotopes may also be done to produce the same results. After this operation the patient will always need substitution of essential hormones, the secretion of which is stimulated by pituitary hormones. The adrenal glands themselves may also be removed. (See Chapter 14 for a discussion of this procedure and the care of the patient.) The selection of patients for these added palliative treatments remains a matter of medical judgment based on many clinical and endocrinologic considerations.

HEMATOSPERMIA

Hematospermia is blood in the ejaculate. This is almost always alarming to the patient and can occur at any age. It is usually harmless and is not associated with infection or tumor. Malignancy of the seminal vesicles is rare.

CARUNCLE OF FEMALE URETHRA

Caruncles or nonmalignant tumor growths resulting from chronic urethral irritation are fairly common in women of 40 to 65 years of age. They occur at the meatus as a small red tumor, and if they are large enough, they can obstruct the urethra, but more often they become excoriated and bleed. The most common symptom is painful urination. They are removed by cauterization (see discussion on treatment of vesical tumors) or surgical excision or regression is produced by applications of estrogen cream and/or podophyllin. Following healing, periodic dilatation of the urethra is usually necessary for a time. Caruncles frequently recur. Biopsy may be necessary to rule out carcinoma. Prolapse of the posterior urethral lip is often confused with a caruncle.

CARCINOMA OF URETHRA

Carcinoma of the urethra is rare and usually of the adenocarcinoma variety, although squamous and transitional cell tumors occur also. The patient notes dysuria, hematuria, and difficult micturition. It may be mistaken for a stricture. The tumor is visualized by urethroscopy. Treatment varies from local extirpation to radical surgical excision or irradiation. The prognosis is grave for patients with advanced infiltrative lesions. Tumors near the meatus may metastasize to the inguinal nodes, but most spread to the pelvic lymph channels.

CANCER OF PENIS

Carcinoma of the glans penis is uncommon. It is practically never seen in men who have been circumcised in infancy; this is a good reason for circumcising male babies. The lesion may originate as a local irritation that itches and has a slight purulent discharge resulting from secondary infection. It may be only a scaly, patchlike area, or it may be an ulcerating sore that will not heal. Metastasis is usually to the inguinal and femoral nodes and later to the iliac and abdominal nodes.

The treatment is local excision for small, early lesions, but for extensive growths the therapy is partial or complete amputation of the penis. If the amputation must be complete, a permanent perineal urethrostomy must be done to provide urinary drainage (Chapter 8). If there is early lymph node involvement, bilateral inguinal lymph node dissections are done. Large amounts of tissue are removed from the groin during a radical inguinal node dissection, and the skin may be left avascular. Muscle and skin grafts aid in the healing of radical node dissection wounds. Pressure dressings are applied and drainage tubes may be connected to suction. Lymph and serum may collect under the skin for days after healing, and repeated aspirations may be necessary. The tissue over the inguinal incisions frequently sloughs, and after the sutures are removed, use of a heat lamp is frequently ordered. No more than a 60-watt bulb should be used, and the lamp should be placed 2 feet above the area to prevent burning the tissue. The wounds heal slowly at best, and the patient may become quite discouraged. Diversional occupations and socializing with other patients may help to pass the time and keep the patient from thinking too much about himself.

X-ray therapy to local and metastatic lesions may be used alone or in conjunction with surgery. Total penile amputation is psychologically traumatizing to the man; he is impotent, his body form is mutilated, he may have to sit to void, and he may know or suspect that he has cancer. He is usually quite depressed and is reticent to express his feelings. If he has to use a bedpan or sit to void, he should be assured of privacy. The change in the voiding position itself is a tremendous adjustment for most men. Psychiatric assistance may be needed by the patient. A psychiatric consultant may be able to help the nurse plan for his care more effectively. Partial amputation is usually handled with less psychogenic stress.

If the course of cancer of the glans penis is not checked, severe lymphedema of the legs occurs and there is extensive local spread of the ulcerat-

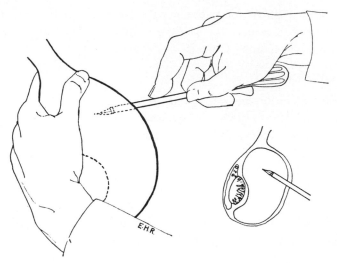

Fig. 11-12. Aspiration of hydrocele. (From Pelouze, P. S.: Office urology, Philadelphia, 1940, W. B. Saunders Co.)

ing lesion. Death may be caused by hemorrhage following erosion of the femoral vessels.

SCROTAL AND TESTICULAR MASSES

Immediate medical attention should be sought for any swelling of the scrotum or of the testicles within it. Scrotal enlargements must be diagnosed accurately. They should never be treated symptomatically by the patient with suspensories, which may give temporary relief and encourage procrastination in seeking medical attention.

Hydrocele

A painless swelling of the scrotum may be caused by a condition known as hydrocele. This is a benign collection of fluid within the tunica vaginalis. The cause is usually unknown, although it may follow trauma to the scrotum or inflammation of the epididymis or testis. It will transilluminate in a darkened room when a flashlight is used. This helps to differentiate it from a hernia or solid tumor. It may be unilateral or bilateral, and it frequently occurs in newborn male babies. Occasionally a hydrocele is treated by aspirating the fluid (Fig. 11-12) and injecting a sclerosing drug such as urea or quinine hydrochloride into the scrotal sac. This may require repetition. Excision of the tunica vaginalis (hydrocelectomy) is the preferred treatment. Unless associated with a hernia, hydroceles in newborn infants are usually not treated since they tend to regress spontaneously. Following a hydrocelectomy, a drain is left in place, the scrotum is elevated, and a pressure dressing applied. The patient should be observed carefully for any symptoms of hemorrhage; bleeding may not be external. The patient needs a scrotal support when he is up and about and may still require one after he is discharged from the hospital. He should have two scrotal suspensories since one should be washed each day. Immediately after operation or following an infection, most patients require an extra large suspensory, and sometimes an athletic support (jockstrap) or Jockey shorts are used.

Spermatocele

A spermatocele is a nontender cystic mass containing milky fluid and sperm; it is attached to the epididymis. Excision is usually unnecessary because the lesion is benign, usually small, and asymptomatic. It should be diagnosed by a doctor, however. The larger cysts transilluminate. If the spermatocele causes symptoms and the patient does not want it surgically removed, a scrotal suspensory may be ordered to give relief from discomfort.

Varicocele

A varicocele is a dilatation of the pampiniform plexus of veins superior to or around the testis. It is commonly seen on the left side only, probably because the left spermatic vein is much longer than the right and has fewer competent valves. It usually appears at puberty and feels to the examiner like a "bag of worms"; it empties when the patient is recumbent. A varicocele that appears suddenly later in life on either side is suggestive of an abdominal tumor. The use of a scrotal support is usually all that is necessary to relieve any dragging sensation, but surgical ligation of the veins may be required. If there is an associated infertility problem, the varicocele may be blamed for increased intrascrotal heat and it is often removed because of this reasoning. The testis may be atrophic preoperatively or this may occur as a sequela of the operation.

Torsion of spermatic cord

Torsion of the spermatic cord causes sudden, severe scrotal pain that is unrelieved by rest or support. If often follows activity that puts a sudden pull on the cremasteric muscle, such as may occur from jumping into cold water; occasionally it may be spontaneous or occur during sleep. It occurs most often in adolescent boys and young men, and it is possibly due to congenital absence of the lateral attachments of the testis and epididymis in the scrotum. An operation to reduce and fix the twisted organs may be necessary, and this must be done within a few hours in order to reestablish the blood supply and preserve fertility and viability of the testis. Interruption of the testicular blood supply for longer periods is likely to result in necrosis of the organ. Bilateral exploration of the scrotum and surgical fixation of both testes must be done since the malformation is often bilateral.

Testicular neoplasm

Nearly all testicular tumors are derived from germinal cells and are malignant. Of these cancers, 40% are seminomas; these are radiosensitive. The others are usually relatively radioresistant teratocarcinomas, embryonal carcinomas, and choriocarcinomas.

Cancer of the testicle is usually painless, but it may be accompanied by an aching or dragging sensation in the groin and by swelling of the testicle. The swelling is often first discovered by the patient while bathing or following injury (but usually is not caused by the trauma). Testicular swelling should always cause suspicion of neoplasm of the testicle and immediate medical attention should be encouraged. This condition usually is seen in men between 20 and 35 years of age. Only about 1% of the deaths due to malignant growths in men are caused by testicular neoplasms. If treated relatively early, the prognosis is quite good.

An undescended testicle is about twenty times more likely to become malignant than one that is in the scrotum at birth or descends shortly thereafter. This is an important reason for encouraging parents to consent to surgical intervention to bring the undescended testicle of a young boy into normal position. This does not exclude the possibility of the subsequent occurrence of a neoplasm, but the testicle is located in a position where it may be examined carefully and regularly.

Men with a testicular swelling that the doctor suspects is malignant may be asked to collect a first-voided morning urine specimen. This is sent for an Aschheim-Zondek test or another standard test for detection of pregnancy in women. In one type of testicular tumor, choriocarcinoma (the type with the poorest prognosis), there are chorionic gonadotropins circulating in the bloodstream. These are hormones ordinarily secreted only by the ovaries during pregnancy. They are excreted in the urine and give a positive Aschheim-Zondek reaction. With all types of testicular tumors, the testicle and spermatic cord are surgically removed (high orchiectomy). Unless testicular cancers are diagnosed and treated early, the prognosis is likely to be poor since there may be widespread metastasis. Early diagnosis, radical surgery, and supervoltage radiation, however, give a high percentage of 5-year cures, especially with seminomas.

The patient with cancer of the testicle is usually given a course of radiation therapy (abdominal and mediastinal lymph nodes), and a radical node dissection as high upward as the diaphragm may be done. This dissection should be bilateral. A thoracoabdominal or extensive transabdominal incision may be used. There are few complications following a radical node dissection. Active turning and leg and arm movement are essential to prevent postoperative pneumonia and thrombosis. Deep breathing should be encouraged at hourly intervals. A turning sheet for rotating the patient and a chest binder for thoracic support are usually helpful.

The patient is extremely uncomfortable and needs frequent and large doses of narcotics and sedative drugs.

If the patient practices voiding in the recumbent position preoperatively, postoperative catheterization may not be necessary.

Since irradiation therapy may be begun as early as the day after orchiectomy, the patient may begin to experience the effects during his hospital stay (Chapter 4). Some patients are not given this treatment until after discharge from the hospital, or if it is started in the hospital, they may complete it as an outpatient. (See Chapter 4 for the instruction the patient needs in these instances.)

Patients and their families may be extremely upset by the diagnosis of neoplasm of the testicle. When an early diagnosis has not been made, the doctor frequently is quite frank with the family and with the patient because he believes the man needs to be able to make the necessary arrangements to provide for his family. The patient's prognosis in some instances of late treatment may be measured in only months. Chemotherapy may produce occasional good palliative results. Some patients are openly depressed; others seem to be "taking it too well." The nurse should listen carefully to both the patient and his family and, if it is indicated, should suggest that help be obtained from others such as a social worker, clergyman, or physician. A psychiatric consultant may be able to help the nurse give realistic support to the patient and his family.

QUESTIONS

1. Hematuria almost always requires what types of urologic examinations?
2. What is the most common cause of hematuria in a child?
3. Hematuria in an adult is a warning signal for what serious disease?
4. What is the differential diagnosis of a mass lesion of the kidney?
5. Can a neoplasm ever grow in the wall of a cyst?
6. What is the difference between multicystic disease and polycystic disease?
7. Name three types of neoplasm of the kidney.
8. What is the usual treatment of Wilms' tumor?
9. Wilms' tumor must be differentiated from what other masses in the kidney region?
10. What is the usual treatment for a hypernephroma?
11. What is the usual treatment for transitional cell carcinoma of the renal pelvis?
12. Name three approaches for removal of a neoplasm of the kidney.
13. Why must the dressing be watched carefully after a nephrectomy?
14. What complication can occur immediately after transthoracic nephrectomy?
15. What is the most common neoplasm encountered in urologic practice?
16. Name four methods of treating bladder neoplasm.
17. In a male, what other organs are usually removed along with the bladder for carcinoma?
18. What other modalities are used for treating bladder cancer besides surgery?
19. Name five types of urinary diversion above the bladder level. Explain the advantages and disadvantages of each.
20. When are catheters used for cutaneous ureterostomies?
21. Outline the procedure for a bowel preparation for a patient who is to have a ureterosigmoidostomy.

22. What are the presenting symptoms or signs of cancer of the prostate in most patients?
23. Describe two methods of prostatic biopsy.
24. What is the curative surgical procedure for carcinoma of the prostate?
25. What is the medical management of incurable carcinoma of the prostate?
26. What is the advantage of orchiectomy over stilbestrol for carcinoma of the prostate?
27. What is the significance of blood in the semen?
28. What is a carnucle?
29. What is the prophylaxis for carcinoma of the penis?
30. Name three types of surgical management for carcinoma of the penis.
31. Which scrotal tumor will transilluminate?
32. What is the significance of a varicocele?
33. Why is torsion of the spermatic cord an emergency situation?
34. Outline the management of neoplasms of the testis.
35. What is the relationship between undescended testis and neoplasm of the testis?
36. In addition to surgery, what other therapy is available for neoplasms of the testis and their metastases?

REFERENCES

Amador, E., Dorfman, L. E., and Wacher, W. E. C.: Urinary alkaline phosphatase and LDH activity in the differential diagnosis of renal disease, Ann. Intern. Med. **62:** 30, 1965.

Arey, J. B.: Abdominal masses in infants and children, Pediat. Clin. N. Amer. **10:**665, 1963.

Bakker, N. J., Tjabbes, D., and DeVoogt, J. H.: Experiences with ureterocolonic anastomosis after Mathisen, J. Urol. **104:**824, 1970.

Barnes, R. W., Bergman, R. T., Hadley, H. L., and Dick, A. L.: Early prostatic cancer: long-term results with conservative treatment, J. Urol. **102:**88, 1969.

Beggs, J. H., and Spratt, J. S., Jr.: Epidermoid carcinoma of the penis, J. Urol. **91:** 166, 1964.

Bennett, A. H., and Harrison, J. H.: A comparison of operative approach for prostatectomy, 1948 and 1968, Surg. Gynec. Obstet. **128:**969, 1969.

Brady, T. W., Mebust, W. K., Valk, W. L., Foret, J. D., and Sloss, T. B.: Cutaneous vesicostomy reappraised, J. Urol. **105:**81, 1971.

Cass, A. S.: Transurethral prostatic resection without catheter drainage, J. Urol. **101:** 750, 1969.

Cooke, J. M.: Nephroureterectomy performed for a tumor of the renal pelvis of the kidney, Nurs. Mirror **121:**311, 1965.

Cox, C. E., Lacy, S. S., Montgomery, W. G., and Boyce, W. H.: Renal adenocarcinoma: 28-year review, with emphasis on rationale and feasibility of preoperative radiotherapy, J. Urol. **104:**53, 1970.

Creevy, D. D., and Tollefson, D. M.: Ileac diversion of the urine and nursing care of the patient with ileac diversion of the urine, Amer. J. Nurs. **59:**530, 1959.

Doolittle, K. H., Klotz, D., Bennett, J. E., and Winter, C. C.: The management of extensive lesions of the male genitalia, Amer. Pract. **13:**655, 1962.

Dow, J. A.: Technique of cryosurgery of prostate, J. Urol. **105:**286, 1971.

Ellis, L. R., Udall, D. A., and Hodges, C. V.: Further clinical experience with intestinal segments for urinary diversion, J. Urol. **105:**354, 1971.

Flinn, R. A., King, L. R., McDonald, J. H., and Clark, S. S.: Cutaneous ureterostomy: alternative urinary diversion, J. Urol. **105:**358, 1971.

Flocks, R. H., and Culp, D. A.: Surgical urology, Chicago, 1967, Year Book Medical Publishers, Inc.

Fox, J. E.: Reflections on cancer nursing, Amer. J. Nurs. **66:**1317, 1966.

Franks, L. M.: Carcinoma of the prostate, Nurs. Mirror **123:**VIII-X, 1967.

Freney, M. A. C.: A dynamic approach to the ileal conduit patient, Amer. J. Nurs. **64:**80, 1964.

Glenn, J. F., and Boyce, W. H.: Urologic surgery, New York, 1969, Harper & Row, Publishers.

Grout, D. C., Grayhack, J. T., Moss, W., and Holland, J. M.: Radiation therapy in treatment of carcinoma of prostate, J. Urol. **105**:411, 1971.

Guinn, G. A., and Ayala, A. G.: Male urethral cancer: report of 15 cases including primary melanoma, J. Urol. **103**:176, 1970.

Hanash, K. A., Taylor, W. F., Greene, L. F., Kottke, B. A., and Titus, J. L.: Relationship of estrogen therapy for carcinoma of prostate to atherosclerotic cardiovascular disease: clinicopathologic study, J. Urol. **103**:467, 1970.

Hawtry, C. E.: Fifty-two cases of primary ureteral carcinoma: clinical-pathologic study, J. Urol. **105**:188, 1971.

Howard, R.: Actinomycin D in Wilms' tumor: treatment of lung metastasis, Arch. Dis. Child. **40**:200, 1965.

Ichikawa, T., Nakano, I., and Hirokawa, I.: Bleomycin treatment of tumors of penis and scrotum, J. Urol. **102**:699, 1969.

Jewett, H. J.: Case for radical perineal prostatectomy, J. Urol. **103**:195, 1970.

Jewett, H. J., King, L. R., and Shelly, W. M.: A study of 365 cases of infiltrating bladder cancer: relation of certain pathological characteristics to prognosis after extirpation, J. Urol. **93**:668, 1964.

Kerr, W. K., Barkin, M., and Severs, P. E.: The effect of cigarette smoking on bladder carcinogens in man, Canad. Med. Ass. J. **93**:1, 1965.

Kiesewetter, W. B., and Mason, E. J.: Malignant tumors in childhood, J.A.M.A. **172**:1117, 1960.

King, L. R., and Scott, W. W.: Ileal urinary diversion, J.A.M.A. **181**:831, 1962.

Kopecky, A. A., Laskowski, T. Z., and Scott, R. Jr.: Radical retropubic prostatectomy in treatment of prostatic carcinoma, J. Urol. **103**:641, 1970.

Lapides, J., Koyanagi, T., and Diokno, A.: Cutaneous vesicostomy: 10-year survey, J. Urol. **105**:76, 1971.

Malis, I., Cooper, J. F., and Wolever, T. H. S.: Breast radiation in patients with carcinoma of prostate, J. Urol. **102**:336, 1969.

Marshall, F. C., Uson, A. C., and Melicon, M. M.: Neoplasms and caruncles of the female urethra, Surg. Gynec. Obstet. **110**:723, 1960.

McCoy, R. M., Klatte, E. C., and Rhamy, R. K.: Use of inferior venacavography in evaluation of renal neoplasms, J. Urol. **102**:556, 1969.

Mossholder, I. B.: When the patient has a radical retropubic prostatectomy, Amer. J. Nurs. **62**:101, 1962.

Prout, G. R., Jr., et al.: Irradiation and 5-fluorouracil as adjuvants in management of invasive bladder carcinoma. Cooperative group report after 4 years, J. Urol. **104**:116, 1970.

Prout, G. R., Jr., et al.: Preoperative irradiation as adjuvant in surgical management of invasive bladder carcinoma, J. Urol. **105**:223, 1971.

Roen, P. R.: Atlas of urologic surgery, New York, 1967, Appleton-Century-Crofts.

Silber, I., and McGavran, M. H.: Adenocarcinoma of prostate in men less than 56 years old: study of 65 cases, J. Urol. **105**:283, 1971.

Straffon, R. A., Kyle, K., and Corvalan, J.: Techniques of cutaneous ureterostomy and results in 51 patients, J. Urol. **103**:138, 1970.

Strahan, R. W.: Carcinoma of the prostate: incidence, origin, pathology, J. Urol. **89**:875, 1963.

Uson, A. C., Wolff, J. A., and Tretter, P.: Current treatment of Wilms' tumor, J. Urol. **103**:217, 1970.

Walsh, M. A., Ebner, M., and Casey, J. W.: Neo-bladder, Amer. J. Nurs. **63**:107, 1963.

Whitmore, W. F.: Wilms' tumor and neuroblastoma, Amer. J. Nurs. **68**:527, 1968.

Williams, C. M., and Greer, M.: Homovanillic acid and vanilmandelic acid in diagnosis of neuroblastoma, J.A.M.A. **183**:836, 1963.

Young, J. D., and Aledia, F. T.: Further observations on flank ureterostomy and cutaneous transureteroureterostomy, J. Urol. **95**:327, 1966.

CHAPTER 12

Neurogenic disorders of urinary bladder

Neurogenic vesical dysfunction is still an incompletely understood and a highly controversial subject since the physiology of micturition (Chapter 2) is not yet satisfactorily explained. Neurogenic vesical disorders include all types of dysfunction of the bladder resulting from lesions of the central and peripheral nervous systems. There are three predominant symptom complexes:

1. Bladders with inadequate proprioceptive innervation or weak detrusor response become overfilled and are incapable of complete emptying. "Overflow" voiding occurs; micturition is infrequent, with little force, in small quantities, and often uncontrolled.

2. Bladders with intact reflex arcs but inadequate central nervous system controls have hyperactive detrusor action. "Precipitate" voiding occurs.

3. Bladders with neurogenic damage to the sphincters tend to leak urine persistently.

Nerve damage in the sacral segments of the spinal cord or the cauda equina may interrupt afferent, efferent, or central components of the reflex arc or a combination of these (lower motor neuron bladder). The bladder tends to be of the hypotonic, the "overflow," or the flaccid type.

When damage is higher in the spinal cord, the reflex arc for voiding persists but its action is deranged (upper motor neuron bladder). A hypertonic type of bladder usually appears with precipitate, often incontinent, voiding.

A variety of terms are applied to these two basic types of disorders, respectively: lower motor neuron bladder and upper motor neuron bladder; autonomous bladder and automatic bladder; and tabetic bladder and reflex bladder. In the hypotonic bladder, residual urine is the principal problem and causes overflow incontinence and urinary infection. In the hypertonic bladder, precipitate voiding, often with incontinence, ureteral reflux, and hydronephrosis are likely to occur.

Urinary infection is the main cause of death in these patients, and urinary incontinence is the main cause of disability. Incontinence, moreover, produces further disability by contributing to dermatitis and decubitis ulcers.

The sexual function in patients with paraplegia is almost always impaired. Most male patients with upper motor neuron disease are capable of penile erection, but fewer are capable of ejaculation and fewer still of paternity. Patients with complete lower motor lesions are impotent.

NEUROGENIC BLADDER

Causes. The most frequent cause of severe neurogenic bladder disorder is injury of the spinal cord. After most spinal injuries, spinal shock (complete loss of reflex activity below the lesion) appears and persists for many days or weeks. The bladder is flaccid, and urinary retention occurs. Later, the bladder tends to become spastic, with loss of its ability to accommodate readily and quickly to an increase in urinary volume. The severity of the bladder symptoms is dependent on the site and extent of the cord lesion. Degenerative spinal cord diseases such as multiple sclerosis, syringomyelia, and others may cause bladder difficulties. Acute poliomyelitis is sometimes accompanied by motor paralysis of the bladder; this is usually not permanent. Tabes dorsalis frequently causes a hypotonic bladder disorder because of faulty proprioception and overfilling.

Diabetes mellitus, arteriosclerosis, and pernicious anemia may cause peripheral neuropathy, which results in bladder paralysis. Chronic overfilling of the bladder caused by prostatic obstruction sometimes causes decompensation of detrusor reflexes and a form of myogenic bladder. This is usually reversible. Myelomeningocele (spina bifida) in infants and children is a frequent cause of vesical dysfunction. Acute postoperative urinary retention is a form of neurogenic bladder dysfunction resulting in overfilling of the bladder. Soon after surgery it may be caused by the aftereffects of anesthesia; later it may be caused by local pain. It can usually be relieved by allowing the patient to stand or sit to void, by administration of parasympathomimetic drugs, or by one or two aseptic catheterizations.

Symptoms. The effects of lesions of the spinal cord or peripheral nerves on micturition depend on the part of the physiologic process interrupted. To have voluntary control of micturition, one must have perception of the desire to void, the ability to inhibit or postpone urination until a suitable place to void is reached, and the ability to initiate urination at will.

A hypogastric (presacral) nerve section causes only slight interference with micturition because these nerves apparently contain few efferent or afferent fibers essential to the process. Section of the pudendal nerves, however, seems to have a marked effect on micturition since it paralyzes the external sphincter. Bilateral section of the posterior sacral nerves, which carry the afferent fibers of the pelvic and pudendal nerves to the spinal cord, causes severe dysfunction of micturition. There is immediate loss of the urethrobladder reflex, but after a period of overdistention and overflow the bladder may become "automatic" or "reflex," that is, may automatically empty at regular intervals. Sensations of distention via the pelvic nerves are lost, but the intact hypogastric nerves (carrying sympathetic fibers from the bladder) apparently provide afferent impulses necessary for a urethrobladder reflex. Micturition in the presence of a "reflex" bladder can sometimes be initiated by pinching or stroking trigger areas along the thigh or abdomen.

Destruction of the sacral segment of the spinal cord such as occurs in patients with lesions of the cauda equina or bilateral section of the pelvic nerves, which carry both motor and sensory fibers controlling micturition, interrupts all motor impulses to the bladder as well as the afferent impulses traveling from it via the pelvic and pudendal nerves. The reflex arc for micturition is interrupted, and the bladder is completely isolated from central control. The desire to urinate is abolished, although there may be some vague sensations of fullness in the suprapubic or perineal areas, which may be transmitted via the sympathetic fibers carried by the hypogastric (presacral) nerves. The patient cannot inhibit or initiate micturition, and the bladder becomes distended and overflow incontinence ensues. A large quantity of residual urine remains. This type of bladder is described as nonreflex, autonomous, or flaccid. Varying degrees of apparent reflex activity may return either because destruction of the reflex was incomplete or as a possible function of ganglion cells in the bladder wall. Children with myelomeningocele (spina bifida) present a similar situation. The perineal muscles, including the external sphincter, however, may under these conditions be paralyzed, allowing constant dribbling of urine.

Destruction of the afferent and central elements of the reflex arc, such as occurs in tabetic lesions, produces a hypotonic bladder with a large capacity. Progressive sensory loss causes the patient to have decreasingly less recognition of a need to void; distention of the bladder results. If the bladder neck is unobstructed, the patient can usually empty his bladder completely by applying manual pressure over the suprapubic region (Credé maneuver) combined with abdominal straining (Chapter 4). The detrusor action of the bladder muscles is not absent but cannot in these patients be called into action by adequate sensory impulses. Complete loss of bladder sensation also may occur when both the hypogastric and pelvic nerves are severed or when the spinal cord is transected above the point of entry of fibers from the hypogastric nerves.

When the spinal cord is transected above the sacral region, normal micturition is impossible. All central (voluntary) control of voiding is eliminated. However, the reflex arc is intact, and after recovery from spinal shock the bladder may automatically empty at regular intervals. These intervals are determined by the degree of filling of the bladder that will cause enough sensory impulses to be sent into the spinal cord to initiate the reflex action. The patient has no direct sensation of bladder distention but may experience chills, tremulousness, perspiration, or headaches because of hypertension. The bladder muscle is usually hyperactive, but the bladder frequently empties incompletely.

Lesions of the cerebral cortex may prevent adequate voluntary control of the bladder. The patient usually has difficulty starting or stopping the urinary stream at will, and urgency incontinence is common, probably as a result of inadequate inhibitory control of the urethrobladder reflex by higher centers. It is thought that incontinence in elderly persons that is unexplained by other causes may be cerebrocortical in origin.

Diagnostic procedures. Every patient with a neurogenic bladder has to be assessed individually in terms of his underlying neurologic disease and difficulties in micturition. He frequently requires the combined care of the neurologist, internist, psychiatrist or psychologist, orthopedist, physical therapist, vocational guidance counselor, and urologist. Since it is impossible within the limits of this chapter to consider the varied aspects of care necessary for patients with various underlying causes of neurogenic bladders, only the problems directly related to the difficulties in voiding will be discussed. Medical and neurologic textbooks and nursing books dealing with the general care of patients with neurologic disorders should be consulted when the nurse is called upon to care for patients with such disorders.

In determining the type, level, and severity of neurologic disorders involving the bladder, the nurse can be most helpful to the physician by making and recording detailed accurate observations of the patient's voiding pattern (Chapter 5) as well as of motor and sensory function of all other parts of his body. It is important to observe all function, gait, and abnormal responses to cutaneous heat, cold, and pain as well as to know what maneuvers the patient uses to initiate micturition.

The physician takes a careful history of the patient's difficulty in voiding, and a complete urologic examination (Chapter 5) is performed to ascertain the status of the entire urinary system. The motor and sensory power of the bladder is tested by cystometry, the equivalent of a neurologic examination of the bladder.

Cystometry. When a cystometric examination is made, the patient is

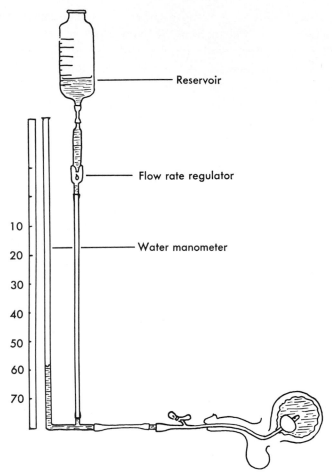

Fig. 12-1. Diagram of apparatus used for cystometric examination. (From Clarke, B. G., and Del Guercio, L.: Urology, New York, 1956, McGraw-Hill Book Co.)

first asked to empty the bladder as completely as possible. A size 18 Fr. two-holed (Robinson) catheter is then inserted into the bladder through the urethra and is taped in place; a Foley catheter may also be used. After the residual urine is collected and measured, the catheter is connected to an irrigating and manometric system from which the air has been expelled.

The simple water manometer (Fig. 12-1) is usually used, although mercury or aneroid (Lewis) manometers are sometimes employed. An irrigating bottle, calibrated in not more than 50 ml. divisions and equipped with a drip-o-meter, is needed. The rubber tubing from this is attached to one arm of a glass Y tube. The other arm of the Y tube is attached to rubber tubing running to a glass tube 120 cm. in length and with a bore 4 to 5 mm. in diameter. The glass tube is attached vertically to a board

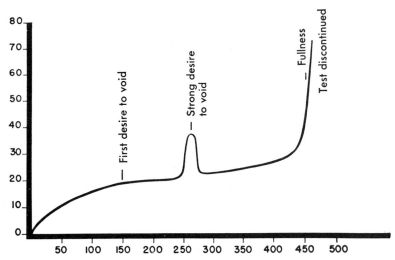

Fig. 12-2. Normal cystogram. (From Clarke, B. G., and Del Guercio, L.: Urology, New York, 1956, McGraw-Hill Book Co.)

calibrated in centimeters, and it is placed so that the zero mark is level with the symphysis pubis of the patient. After the Y tube is attached to the catheter and 50 ml. of irrigating fluid allowed to enter the bladder, the glass tube should be adjusted so that the meniscus of the column of water is approximately at the zero level on the calibrated board.

One of two methods may be used to perform the test. The irrigating fluid (sterile physiologic sodium chloride) may be allowed to drip continuously into the bladder at the rate of about 120 drops per minute or 50 ml. may be instilled into the bladder at intervals. Regardless of the method used to instill the fluid, manometric readings are taken and recorded on a graph after regular increments (usually 50 ml.). The bladder usually is allowed to fill, and measurements are recorded at regular intervals until the patient feels the urge to void or until the doctor believes no more fluid should be instilled. If the fluid is being intermittently instilled, the manometric reading should not be recorded until the pressure stabilizes since rapid instillation causes a momentary abnormal increase in intravesical pressure as the bladder muscle accommodates to the stretch. The patient is asked to indicate the first feeling of fullness, the first desire to void, and feelings of discomfort and urgency. Urgency is always associated with bladder contraction. Each of these sensations is noted on the graph (Fig. 12-2).

Upon conclusion of the cystometry test, the anal sphincter test is performed. With his gloved finger in the rectum, the examiner gives the Foley catheter a sudden tug. Contraction of the anal sphincter indicates that the neural arc S_2 to S_4 is intact and most likely the neurogenic bladder is

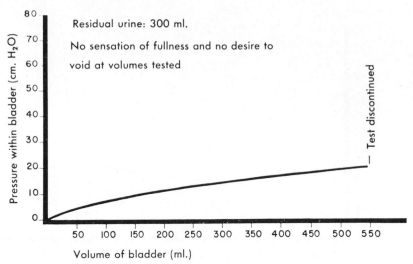

Fig. 12-3. Cystogram typical of stage of "spinal shock." (From Clarke, B. G., and Del Guercio, L.: Urology, New York, 1956, McGraw-Hill Book Co.)

upper motor neuron in type. Pure lower motor neuron bladder dysfunction will be accompanied by an absent bulbocavernosus reflex. The bladder sensory arc may next be tested by instilling ice water into the bladder. (Catheter bag is now deflated.) In the upper motor neuron bladder the catheter and water will be expelled quickly.

The external urinary sphincter resistance can also be measured by inserting a catheter in the anterior urethra and noting the pressure necessary to open the closed sphincter.

"Cord" bladder

"Cord" bladder is a term used for vesical dysfunction resulting from lesions of the spinal cord.

Acute stage. Following acute spinal cord injury or disease, the bladder is atonic, and adequate drainage must be maintained. There may be no reflex activity below the level of the lesion for many days or weeks. This is known as the stage of spinal shock (Fig. 12-3). The treatment for urinary retention is usually aseptic intubation of the urethra and bladder with a small (16 or 18 Fr.) Foley balloon catheter with a 5 ml. balloon; the catheter is attached to continuous drainage apparatus. Occasionally a suprapubic cystostomy will be performed. Catheter drainage is required in either situation until neurologic evaluation shows stabilization and beginning recovery of spinal cord function. This may be several days or several months after onset of the acute stage.

During the acute stage of dysfunction the nurse plays an exceedingly important role in maintaining the patient in good physical condition. Some patients die from infections secondary to decubitus ulcers, hypostatic pneumonia, or urinary tract infection during this stage. The patient's position should be changed frequently. By this means, pressure areas may be prevented or, if they develop, they can be detected and treated immediately. If the patient cannot be moved, a Stryker frame or Foster bed may be used so that he can be shifted at intervals from his back to his abdomen. Adequate dietary intake should be encouraged and fluids forced. Every means to prevent infection should be employed; these include scrupulous maintenance of aseptic techniques and isolation of the patient from anyone with upper respiratory, staphylococcal, or other known infections.

Movement of all joints through the full range of motion should be carried out at least twice a day. The patient should be encouraged to actively move unparalyzed parts. The nurse should passively exercise all paralyzed parts unless there are contraindications. Proper alignment of all paralyzed parts should also be maintained. Paralysis involving the perineal area often causes the penis to lie in such a way that the urethra is sharply angulated; taping the penis back onto the abdomen prevents angulation and the development of urethral fistulas as the result of pressure from the catheter against the sharply bent penoscrotal angle.

During the catheter drainage phase, immobilization causes demineralization of bones, which results in hypercalciuria with serious danger of stone formation in the kidneys and bladder. Generous dietary intake of fluids and active movement by the patient help prevent stone formation in the kidney or bladder. Drugs such as ascorbic acid taken orally every 4 to 6 hours tend to acidify the urine and minimize precipitation of calcium in the urine. Nevertheless, 25% of patients with neurogenic bladder disease sooner or later develop urinary stones (Chapter 10). Urinary tract infection may be lessened by periodic irrigations of the bladder. These can be provided by manually or electronically operated aseptic closed systems or by automatic siphonage ("tidal") devices. (See discussion on catheter care and irrigation in Chapter 4.) In all such systems, care must be taken not to overfill the bladder and allow reflux of infected urine into the kidneys. Ascending pyelonephritis is manifested by fever and chills and requires prompt and vigorous treatment.

Recovery stage. The recovery motor and sensory power of the bladder is tested by cystometry at intervals of 4 to 5 weeks until the patient becomes catheter free (Fig. 12-4). After there is some evidence of return of detrusor activity and, preferably, when the patient has begun to show some degree of ambulation and self-sufficiency, trials are made of voiding. This may be 3 to 6 months after the acute stage.

When bladder rehabilitation is started, the nurse plays an important role. She, the doctor, and the physical therapist usually combine their efforts. Before the program is started, the problems to be overcome, the

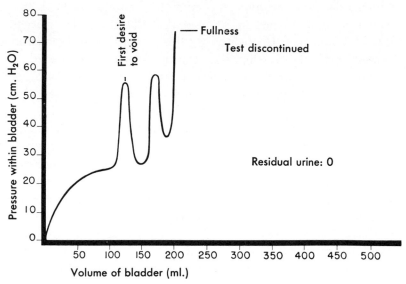

Fig. 12-4. Cystogram typical of recovery from "spinal shock" with development of an automatic bladder. (From Clarke, B. G., and Del Guercio, L.: Urology, New York, 1956, McGraw-Hill Book Co.)

physiologic status, and the probable degree of bladder rehabilitation that can be expected must be carefully evaluated as well as the patient's attitude toward his condition since this affects his progress in rehabilitation. Based on this evaluation, a program individually designed for the needs of each patient is undertaken. Unless the bulbocavernosus reflex is intact, there is little hope that the patient may become catheter free. Patients who are unlikely to become catheter free should not be led to expect they will be; their rehabilitation program should be directed toward life with a catheter (Chapter 4).

It is important for both the patient and the nurse to know that bladder rehabilitation usually takes weeks and even months to accomplish. The patient often becomes discouraged by continued incontinence and needs much encouragement to continue the program. It is helpful if the patient is taught something about the physiology of voiding so that he can better understand his own problems and help in overcoming them.

Depending on the degree of nerve damage, the patient may be able to void voluntarily; he may not need a catheter but yet need to rely on an external collecting device because of imperfect control; or he may require continued use of catheter drainage because a large quantity of residual urine remains in his bladder after voiding or because he has a persistent vesicourethral reflex. If a carefully planned program for rehabilitation is conscientiously carried out, a large percentage of paraplegic patients, however, are able to become catheter free.

Bladder training. Often before a catheter is removed, a period of bladder training designed to increase the volume of urine tolerated by the bladder is undertaken. Not all specialists are in agreement as to the need for this tedious and time-consuming procedure. It is done for the patient with an automatic or reflex bladder since the bladder muscle tends to be quite spastic; it is also used for any patient who has had the bladder constantly drained over a long period. Bladder training is designed to make involuntary or reflex emptying of the bladder more efficient.

Bladder training is carried out by clamping the catheter during the daytime for prescribed periods of time (often 1 to 3 hours). Then it is opened and, instead of letting it drain passively, the patient tries to void through it by abdominal straining. The interval during which the catheter is clamped is gradually increased as the bladder tolerates each increase without incontinent automatic voiding around the catheter. The maximum interval is usually 3 hours. Until a maximum interval has been reached, the regimen is usually carried out only during the day; straight drainage or tidal drainage is resumed at night. Later, the regimen is continued day and night for a period of time. Bladder training programs for patients with complete reflex bladders may need to extend over a period of 2 months or more.

Reeducation for control of micturition. Voluntary control of micturition is a learned process. Depending on the extent of nerve damage, the patient with a "cord" bladder must learn to control micturition by other means than the usual since normal pathways for voluntary control of micturition are interrupted.

The program of reeducation can and should be started during the period of bladder training, but it is only after the catheter is finally removed that active participation by the patient becomes mandatory to the success of the program. One of the first things a patient should aim for is to try to recognize some sensory manifestation that indicates impending micturition. Common manifestations (much different from those felt by normal persons with full bladders) are restlessness, sweaty or chilly sensations, or vague feelings of fullness in the upper abdomen. By learning to recognize and respond at once to the cue of a full bladder, the patient often is able to get ready to void before the bladder empties.

The patient with a reflex or automatic-type bladder may be able to initiate micturition prior to the period of automatic urination by stimulating so-called trigger areas. These areas are often found along the inner aspects of the thigh or along the lower abdomen and can be triggered manually by brushing motions or pinching. Tugging pubic hair or anal stimulation will often cause the bladder to contract.

The patient with a nonreflex or autonomous bladder can often initiate micturition by exerting pressure over the bladder. This may be done by contracting the abdominal muscles and straining down, by leaning acutely forward (this is more useful for women), or by exerting manual pressure over the lower abdomen. The latter is known as the Credé method and is discussed in detail in Chapter 4. A patient with a normal or reflex bladder cannot initiate voiding in this way, but it is a helpful method for use during voiding to ensure complete emptying of the bladder. Residual urine is a problem with most types of neurogenic bladders since the detrusor action apparently is either too weak or is sustained for too short a time to ensure emptying or the urinary sphincter offers too much resistance.

Automatic and autonomous bladders empty at intervals regulated by the intravesical pressure. The level of intravesical pressure is usually determined by the amount of urine in the bladder. It is therefore important for the patient to become aware of the amount of fluid that his bladder will hold without emptying and to determine a schedule of fluid intake that will provide for his needs yet allow his bladder to empty at intervals acceptable to his life pattern. The nurse should work very closely with the patient to determine this (Chapter 4). It is often a time-consuming process that may require days or weeks of trial and error. Detailed records of the amount of liquid intake and the volume of urine voided during each interval should be kept and carefully examined in relation to the time as well as the amount of urinary output. In the years ahead of him, however, this type of regulation can make the patient's life much happier. By following a careful intake schedule, he may plan for voiding by the clock and can be prepared for it or, if possible, he may plan to initiate voiding prior to the period of automatic emptying of the bladder.

Most patients who are planning to go somewhere that voiding will be inconvenient for several hours sharply limit their fluid intake for 2 or 3 hours beforehand. Many patients find it more convenient to limit fluids in the evening so that they are not accidentally incontinent during the night. Great care must be taken that a patient does not sharply curtail his total daily fluid intake, however, since urinary tract infection is an ever-present problem with "cord" bladders. He should plan to take 2000 to 2500 ml. of fluid in each 24-hour period unless this amount of fluid is contraindicated for some reason. Since alcohol, caffeine (coffee), and theobromine (tea) tend to stimulate urinary flow and upset the voiding pattern, it is wise to avoid them.

Usually the patient feels more secure if he wears some type of external protection in case of accidental dribbling. Men often use a rubber urinal (Chapter 4). A penile clamp should not be used since the lack of sensation of a full bladder increases the danger of ureteral reflux of bladder urine. Because the skin of the penis lacks sensory innervation, pressure from clamps may also easily cause skin ulcers. Women most often use protective panties.

Surgical treatment. The patient is followed carefully on the basis of symptoms, urinalysis, residual urine determinations, and cystometric findings. If during recovery a patient does not void successfully, secondary causes of failure to void are sought and, if present, are corrected. Secondary causes are common because of the very nature of the paraplegic process; they include strictures and diverticula of the urethra, contractures of the bladder neck, calculi of the bladder as well as of the kidneys, and prostatic obstruction.

If, after a year or so of bladder training and after correction of such structural hindrances to voiding as may be present, a patient with a hypertonic bladder fails to show good progress, he can sometimes be helped by an injection of alcohol into the subarachnoid space or by neurotomy designed to counteract spasticity of the bladder muscles by converting an upper motor to a lower motor neuron neurogenic bladder. In patients with hypotonic vesical dysfunction, emptying is sometimes improved by transurethral resection of the internal vesical sphincter. The operative reduction of sphincter resistance combined with manual pressure over the suprapubic area (Credé maneuver) to stimulate or reenforce voiding seems to help.

For a small group of patients, when all other methods fail, urinary diversion by cutaneous ureterostomy or by ileal conduit (Chapter 11) may be employed to convert intractable neurogenic vesical dysfunction to a situation manageable by use of a urinary collecting bag. Ureterosigmoidostomy is contraindicated since the anal sphincter is likewise incompetent.

Aftercare. For every patent, urinary rehabilitation must be continuously coordinated with general rehabilitation. Because the survival of these patients depends upon conservation of renal function, lifelong and close general medical as well as urologic follow-up is necessary.

Care of patients with other types of neurogenic bladder

The care needed by the patient depends entirely on the part of the process of micturition interrupted, and this varies with each patient. The previous detailed discussion of "cord" bladders, however, covers the management of most problems that will be encountered. The prognosis in each instance is usually dependent on whether the primary neurologic disease is reversible, controllable, or progressive.

The care required by children with neurogenic bladders is basically the same as that needed by adults. Rehabilitation may be more difficult depending on the age of the child, but some children (especially younger ones) adjust remarkably well to their situations and lead relatively happy lives. The parents, of course, must be actively involved in the reeducation program for their child.

QUESTIONS

1. Describe two types of neurogenic bladder.
2. What is the main cause of death in patients with neurogenic bladder?
3. How is sexual function disturbed in males with neurogenic bladder?
4. What is the most frequent cause of severe neurogenic bladder disease?
5. Name some medical diseases that are responsible for neurogenic bladders.
6. What is meant by the Credé maneuver?
7. Name some diagnostic urologic procedures used for assessing the neurogenic bladder.
8. What is a cystometrogram?
9. How long does the acute stage of spinal shock last?
10. What serious complications occur from neurogenic bladder?
11. What are the determining factors as to whether a patient must wear a catheter or not for a neurogenic bladder?
12. List several methods by which a patient with an upper motor neuron bladder may initiate micturition.
13. When all methods fail for utilization of the neurogenic bladder, what other solutions are available?

REFERENCES

Bergstrom, N. I.: Ice applications to induce voiding, Amer. J. Nurs. **69**:283, 1969.

Bors, E., and Comarr, A. E.: Neurological urology, Baltimore, 1971, University Park Press.

Comarr, A. E.: The practical urological management of the patient with spinal cord injury, Brit. J. Urol. **31**:1, 1959.

Comarr, A. E.: Traumatic cord bladder: management and complications, Surg. Clin. N. Amer. **45**:1409, 1965.

Currie, R. J., Bilbisi, A. A., Schiebler, J. C., and Bunts, R. C.: External sphincterotomy in paraplegics: technique and results, J. Urol. **103**:64, 1970.

de Gutierrez-Mahoney, C. G., and Carini, E.: Neurological and neurosurgical nursing, ed. 4, St. Louis, 1965, The C. V. Mosby Co.

Delehanty, L., and Stravino, V.: Achieving bladder control, Amer. J. Nurs. **70**:312, 1970.

Ellenberg, M.: Diabetic neurogenic vesical dysfunction, Arch. Intern. Med. **117**:348, 1966.

Ferguson, D. E., and Geist, R. W.: Pre-school urinary tract diversion for children with neurogenic bladder from myelomeningocele, J. Urol. **105**:133, 1971.

Hoffman, C. A., Jr., and Bunts, R. C.: Present urologic status of World War II paraplegics, J. Urol. **86**:60, 1961.

Martin, A. M.: Nursing care in cervical cord injury, Amer. J. Nurs. **63**:60, 1963.

Trigiano, L. L.: Independence is possible in quadriplegia, Amer. J. Nurs. **70**:2610, 1970.

CHAPTER 13

Other disorders of the urinary system

UROLOGIC DISORDERS AFFECTING WOMEN

Many diseases of the urinary system affect both men and women; these have been discussed elsewhere. Several important disorders of the urinary tract, however, are peculiar to women because of the anatomic proximity and common embryologic origin of the ureter, bladder, urethra, and reproductive organs and because of the high incidence of disease in the reproductive system.

Fistulas

Fistulas draining urine from the bladder, ureter (Fig. 13-1), or urethra into the vagina are not uncommon. Their frequency, however, is being reduced by improved delivery and surgical techniques. Until repair of the fistula can be undertaken, the patient is incontinent of urine. This is an exceedingly demoralizing condition, and the patient needs practical help in managing the situation (Chapter 4) as well as assurance that the medical and nursing personnel understand her problem. Until surgical repair is undertaken, the urinary leakage is managed with absorbent pads or a vaginal rubber diaphragm to which a tubing is attached to collect the urine.

Care of urinary incontinence in women is difficult and time-consuming. Unless great care is taken, odor is a problem. When fistulas persist, married couples have special problems that require patience and understanding. They should be encouraged to plan together a recreational and activity schedule that will help to minimize tensions until normal sexual relations can be resumed.

The results of reconstructive operations for fistulas are not always successful. The patient must sometimes have several operations, and each successive hospitalization increases her anxiety about the outcome of surgery

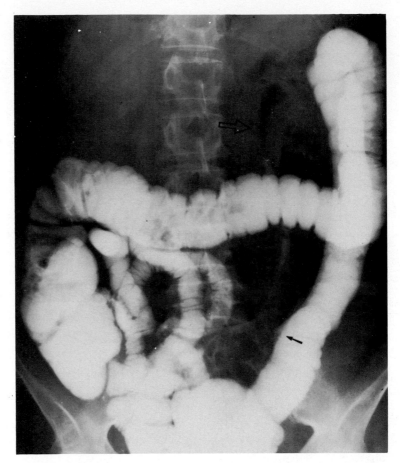

Fig. 13-1. Barium enema reveals ureterocolonic fistula (arrow). Note that some of the contrast agent and colonic gas have entered left upper urinary system, demonstrating a bifid renal pelvis and some of the calyces (large arrow).

and lessens her reserve in accepting the discomforts and inconveniences entailed. All possible nursing measures should be taken to prevent infection and to be certain that free drainage of urine is ensured. Obstruction of drainage tubes may place pressure against the newly repaired vesicovaginal wall and cause healing tissue to break down, resulting in recurrence of the fistula.

Ureterovaginal fistulas. Ureterovaginal fistulas are a complication of gynecologic surgery infrequently. In the treatment of cancer of the cervix, either by irradiation, panhysterectomy (excision of entire uterus, including the cervix), or radical hysterectomy, the blood supply to the ureter sometimes is impaired. The ureteral wall sloughs and a fistula opens from the ureter to the vagina. In other instances iatrogenic trauma to the ureter occurs. This causes a constant drip of urine through the vagina. The excretory urogram may be normal or show evidence of ureteral obstruction.

Certain ureterovaginal fistulas heal spontaneously after a period of time. If healing does not occur, ureteral plastic procedures may be attempted. The ureter may have to be reimplanted into the bladder (ureteroneocystostomy) or be transplanted to the bowel or to the skin through an abdominal opening, or a nephroureterectomy may be performed (Chapter 8).

Occasionally a female child is constantly incontinent of small amounts of urine but otherwise seems to void normally. This is not a true fistula but rather a common sign of an ectopic ureteral opening into the vagina or distal to the urethral sphincter. (See discussion of anomalous ureters in Chapter 2.)

Vesicovaginal fistulas. Vesicovaginal fistulas, or fistulas between the bladder and the vagina, may follow irradiation of the cervix, gynecologic surgery, or trauma during delivery of a baby. It is often possible to repair traumatic fistulas at once if they are recognized. Late recognition makes it impossible to perform surgery to repair the fistula until the inflammation and induration have subsided; this may take 3 to 4 months. An incision for repair is made into the bladder suprapubically or vaginally. The fistula tract is removed and the defect from the bladder to the vagina is closed in three nonopposing layers or with a pedicle graft from the mucosal wall of the bladder or other suitable donor site.

Postoperatively, the patient has a suprapubic tube, a urethral catheter, or both to divert the urine during healing. These tubes are sometimes attached to a suction drainage apparatus to ensure that the bladder is kept empty (Chapter 4). Urinary diversion may be maintained for as long as 3 weeks or more until the wound is completely healed. The catheters should not be irrigated unless it is absolutely necessary, and only very gentle pressure should be used when irrigating them. Signs of urinary drainage from the vagina should be noted. There is normally a small amount of serosanguineous drainage from the vagina for a few days postoperatively. Vaginal douches may be ordered; they should be sterile and given very gently. The patient is restricted to bed rest for several days; then she is usually allowed to sit at the side of the bed. She must remain in her room or beside her bed if suction is being used. Such confinement is tiring since the patient is usually not acutely uncomfortable. Visitors, television, radio, reading materials, and a variety of occupational therapy activities may help fill the time.

Stress incontinence

Urinary incontinence accompanying activity that increases intra-abdominal pressure such as coughing, laughing, walking, or lifting is known as stress incontinence. It is almost exclusively seen in women since the female urethra lacks the interposition of the prostate gland between the internal (smooth muscle) and external (striated muscle) urethral sphincters. Consequently, the two sphincters are intimately associated anatomically, and for adequate function they depend upon the integrity of pelvic supporting structures.

In some instances, obstetric trauma or frequent pregnancy is a factor in the weakening of pelvic supports. In others the cause of stress incontinence is obscure. It can occur in young women as well as in elderly or obese women who have relaxed pelvic musculature. For some patients, sphincter exercises improve the condition (Chapter 4); surgery may be necessary for others. If surgery is indicated, most patients are benefited by reconstruction of the pelvic supports from below (anterior colporrhaphy) combined with sphincteric plication. (See a gynecologic nursing textbook for discussion of care of a patient undergoing this procedure.) If this type of surgery fails, suspension of the urethra and bladder may be carried out via an abdominal approach. This procedure is known as a fascial sling operation or, more often, a vesicourethropexy. The bladder neck is angulated and elevated and the urethra lengthened by this operation. A combined vaginal-abdominal operation may be performed.

Prior to a vesicourethropexy, cystoscopy and cystometry (Chapter 12) may be done to rule out neurogenic bladder and other causes of incontinence. The degree of incontinence may be tested by filling the bladder and then having the patient cough or strain while standing. Then, with the patient in a lithotomy position, the doctor usually fills the bladder with normal saline solution and supports the sides of the bladder neck with ring forceps in the vagina. The ability of the bladder to hold urine under pressure with this support is tested. If the patient can cough and strain down without being incontinent, she is considered a good candidate for the operation. It is done through an incision in the suprapubic area. The bladder is not incised. A small urethral catheter is usually inserted and should be connected to continuous drainage to prevent the pressure of a full bladder on the sutures. If a catheter is not inserted, the nurse should be sure that the patient voids within the time interval specified by the doctor. If the patient does not void, the doctor should be notified. He will usually order catheterization. Mineral oil is frequently ordered to lessen the need to strain for defecation. The patient is usually allowed out of bed, but some physicians order bed rest for several days postoperatively. A vaginal pack is often kept in place several days.

Ureteral obstruction

The most common ureteral obstructions peculiar to women are physiologic hydronephrosis of pregnancy and obstruction of a kidney secondary to accidental ligation of a ureter during gynecologic or pelvic surgery.

Hydronephrosis of pregnancy. Hydronephrosis of pregnancy (Fig.

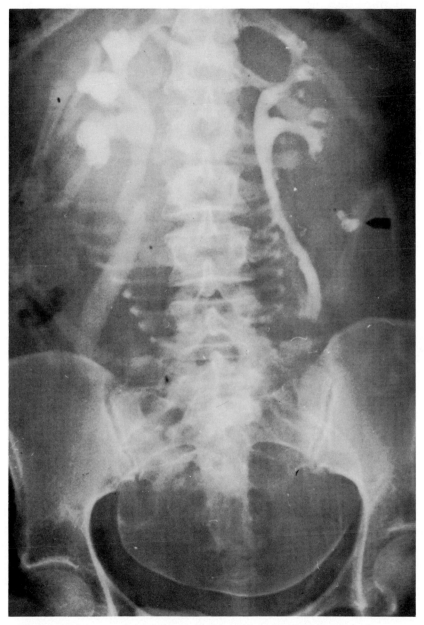

Fig. 13-2. Excretory urogram of woman with near-term pregnancy. Note calcified fetal head in pelvis and ribs and long bones of extremities. Both ureters are dilated, more so on right, with obstruction at junction of mid- and lower thirds. Arrow on right points to calcific densities representing two teeth in dermoid tumor of left ovary, an incidental finding.

13-2) is of special importance because the resulting stasis of urine in the dilated upper urinary tract predisposes to infection. This infection is commonly termed pyelitis of pregnancy but is, in fact, an acute pyelonephritis (Chapter 9).

Ureteral dilatation is first perceptible during the sixth week of pregnancy. There is a decrease in ureteral peristalsis as pregnancy progresses, and ureteral and renal pelvic dilatation increases. In most women, some degree of hydronephrosis is present at term. Regression normally occurs after delivery and is complete within 3 months.

Pressure by the gradually enlarging uterus upon the ureters is a factor in the genesis of physiologic hydronephrosis. However, the relaxant effect of progesterone, a hormone normally secreted during pregnancy, on the ureteral smooth muscle is also an important factor. The reproductive organs and the upper urinary tract have a common embryologic origin and, as a result, the hormonal mechanism intended to relax the uterus appears to have a similar effect on the embryologically related ureters and renal pelves.

Urinary infection during pregnancy seems to be related partly to physiologic hydronephrosis and partly to the incidence of asymptomatic bacteriuria which, for reasons as yet obscure, occurs in more than 5% of pregnant women. Elimination of the bacteriuria seems to lessen the incidence of acute pyelonephritis as a complication of physiologic hydronephrosis and to reduce the incidence of premature delivery, which often occurs in mothers with urinary tract infection.

The treatment of acute pyelonephritis of pregnancy is similar to that for other infections of the kidney (Chapter 9). Chemotherapy may have to be continued for months to ensure that the urine remains sterile until term. Every patient with acute pyelonephritis during pregnancy should have medical follow-up until the ureters have returned to normal. This may be 3 or more months after delivery. Inadequate treatment leads to chronic pyelonephritis and its serious consequences (Chapter 9).

Accidental ligation of ureter. When a ureter is accidentally ligated or compressed during pelvic operations, the patient may have no symptoms. Usually she complains of pain in the kidney region or the flank, or if both ureters are ligated, she may have anuria. Immediate deligation is indicated. When a ureter is completely ligated, function in the respective kidney will often cease. Since the other kidney is functioning, no untoward symptoms may be immediately evidenced. If any function continues in the kidney with its ureter ligated, symptoms of obstruction may ensue (Chapter 8). If performed early, excretory urography reveals the problem.

Late treatment of a patient with a ligated ureter consists of provision for urinary drainage by placing a pyelostomy or nephrostomy tube into the obstructed kidney. This requires a second operation, at which time an attempt to remove the ligature from the ureter may also be made. If removal of the ligature is impossible, resection and anastomosis of the ureter may be attempted. (See Chapter 8 for discussion of this procedure.) If this is impossible, nephrectomy may be necessary, but it must be known that the other kidney is normal. Otherwise the surgeon may elect to perform some diversionary procedure such as ureterosigmoid anastomosis, cutaneous ureterostomy, or construction of an ureteroileal conduit (Chapter 10). If the ligature is removed from the ureter, it is important to watch for urinary drainage from abnormal sites. Such drainage is indicative of fistula formation as the result of ureteral necrosis caused by the accidentally placed ligature and/or subsequent surgery.

URINARY DISORDERS PRIMARILY AFFECTING CHILDREN
Enuresis

According to the 1970 census, there are almost 3 million people with enuresis in the United States. Enuresis is the involuntary nighttime discharge of urine as a result of uncertain pathologic or functional causes. It may also be voluntary, representing a behavior pattern for obtaining attention or pure laziness (for example, inconvenience of outdoor toilet).

The normal infant is born with an automatic bladder, that is, one that, when filled to a certain point, empties reflexly. Voluntary control is a learned function and is not possible until the higher nervous centers have developed fully. Children between the ages of 1 and 2 years usually recognize the imminence of micturition and can prevent voiding for a period of time. Complete day and night control, however, may not occur for several years. Children vary in the rate at which they develop voluntary urinary control just as they vary in other development. However, by the age of 4½ years, 87.8% of all children have complete day and night control. By this age the bladder capacity usually has doubled and is between 200 and 400 ml. Ability to start the urinary stream at will, regardless of the amount of filling, and ability to stop voiding in midstream does not occur until the child is about 5 years of age.

Enuresis needs to be carefully evaluated as to its cause. It has become apparent, however, that a small bladder capacity is a common accompaniment of enuresis. This may improve spontaneously, or the child may learn to compensate for it by drinking small amounts of fluid and emptying his bladder voluntarily at relatively short intervals both in the daytime and during the night.

Uninhibited bladder contractions, urinary tract infection, or other pathologic conditions may cause enuresis. It is important, therefore, that the child with enuresis be given the benefit of a complete urologic examination. A cystometrogram should be obtained and excretory urography and cystoscopy are often advisable. Enuresis may be the only symptom of a disease that is gradually damaging the kidneys and, if uncorrected, may lead to uremia and death.

If enuresis seems to be a behavior symptom, psychiatric help is indicated. Bed-wetting in the absence of pathologic disorders and inconsistently related to fluid intake suggests an insecure child.

Training program to increase bladder capacity. A training program with the objective of increasing the bladder capacity may be attempted for a nocturnal bed wetter and frequent daily voider. A record of both intake and output is kept for a few days prior to initiation of the program; this is used as a comparative record. During the training period, fluids are forced during the day and the child is encouraged to postpone voiding as long as possible. If he is old enough, it is often advantageous to have the child help keep the measurements and the records during the training program; this encourages him to try for larger and larger capacities. The program should be continued until the bladder capacity is at least 250 ml. and preferably 400 ml.; this takes 3 to 6 months. The doctor may also order anticholinergic or ganglionic blocking drugs such as propantheline (Pro-Banthine), nortriptyline (Aventyl), or imipramine hydrochloride (Tofranil).

EXTERNAL TRAUMA TO URINARY TRACT

The urinary tract may be seriously damaged by external trauma. Hematuria following trauma is a cardinal symptom of urinary tract injury; this may be gross or microscopic. Knowledge of the location of the blow or the location of pain following the blow helps to localize the injured part of the tract. Injuries of the upper abdomen or lower thorax often are associated with renal damage. Fifteen percent of patients with fractured pelves have coexistent rupture of the urethra or bladder; injury of the perineum (saddle injury) frequently causes rupture of the urethra. A mass may develop as a result of extravasation of blood or urine into the tissues, or if the wound is open, urine may leak from it. Inability to void is an important symptom that may indicate traumatic renal shutdown, loss of continuity of the ureters or urethra, or obstruction of the ureters or urethra by clot formation. Falling blood pressure, rising pulse rate, and appearance of shock indicate internal bleeding that may be from the urinary tract or other injured internal organs. The spleen is the most commonly injured abdominal organ.

The emergency management of genitourinary injuries is that of injuries generally. Adequate oxygenation must be ensured; hemorrhage and shock must be combated with fluid therapy. (See a medical-surgical nursing textbook for details.) Definitive treatment of the injury is rarely indicated until shock has been adequately treated and definitive inves-

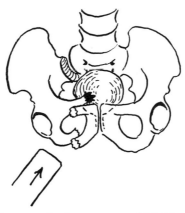

Fig. 13-3. Fracture of pelvis may lead to rupture of bladder. (Unpublished illustration of Dr. B. G. Clarke and Dr. L. Del Guercio.)

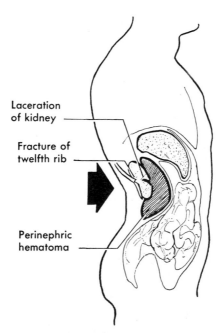

Fig. 13-4. Fractured rib may lacerate kidney. Note hematoma resulting from hemorrhage from kidney into adjacent tissue. (Adapted from unpublished illustration of Dr. B. G. Clarke and Dr. L. Del Guercio.)

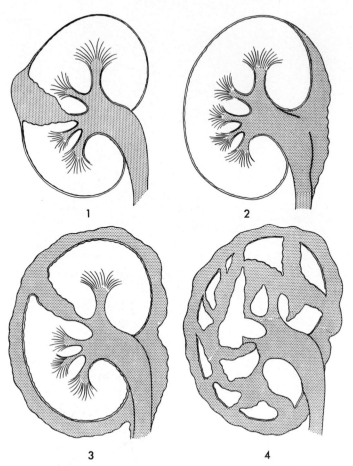

Fig. 13-5. Four degrees of renal trauma. **1,** Urine is extravasating from split in renal parenchyma but confined under renal capsule. **2,** Urine is extravasating through tear in renal pelvis. **3,** Urine is extravasating through rent in kidney and capsule and surrounds kidney and renal pelvis. **4,** Kidney is shattered and urine is extravasating in all areas.

tigative procedures, including radiographic studies, can be completed. Persistent bleeding or urinary extravasation require prompt operative treatment.

When the bladder or urethra has been damaged (Fig. 13-3), provision must be made at once for urinary drainage. A cystostomy frequently is performed, but nephrostomies may be necessary. Reparative surgery is undertaken as soon as the patient's condition warrants it. The care is similar to that for a patient having reconstructive surgery of the bladder and urethra for other reasons (Chapter 8), except that it must be adapted as required by coexisting problems caused by the trauma.

The kidney may be contused, torn, or completely ruptured by an external blow (Figs. 13-4 and 13-5). Since spontaneous healing may occur, the patient may be observed closely and surgical intervention undertaken only if the kidney has been ruptured or hemorrhage continues. Whenever possible, the kidney is preserved, and surgery is never undertaken before the presence of a functioning contralateral kidney is ascertained. The care is the same as that of any patient having renal surgery (Chapters 10 and 11).

QUESTIONS

1. List some causes of vesicovaginal and ureterovaginal fistulas.
2. List some causes of urinary stress incontinence in the female.
3. List some procedures to correct urinary stress incontinence in the female.
4. What is meant by hydronephrosis of pregnancy and what are two causes?
5. Is enuresis a common problem?
6. What tests may be performed in evaluating enuresis?
7. What drugs are used for enuresis?
8. When the spleen is injured by trauma, what urinary organ may also be injured?
9. When the liver is injured by trauma, what urinary organ may also be involved?
10. What urinary tract trauma accompanies a fractured pelvis?

REFERENCES

Alexander, L.: Tackling the problem of enuresis, RN **29**:46, 1966.
Berry, J. L., and Dahlen, C. P.: Evaluation of procedure for correction of urinary incontinence in men, J. Urol. **105**:105, 1971.
Carlton, C. E., Jr., Scott, R., Jr., and Guthrie, A. G.: Initial management of ureteral injuries: report of 78 cases, J. Urol. **105**:335, 1971.
Celano, P. J.: Vaginal fistulas, Amer. J. Nurs. **70**:2131, 1971.
Gabriel, H. S.: You can help the elderly incontinent, RN **29**:52, 1966.
Kelso, J. W., and Funnell, J. W.: Management of gynecologic-urologic complications, Amer. J. Obstet. Gynec. **79**:856, 1960.
Muellner, S. R.: Development of urinary control in children, J.A.M.A. **172**:1256, 1960.
Reid, R. E., and Herman, J. R.: Rupture of the bladder and urethra: diagnosis and treatment, New York J. Med. **65**:2685, 1965.
Rose, J. F.: Management of the patient with trauma to the urinary tract, Med. Clin. N. Amer. **48**:1633, 1964.
Troup, C. W., and Hodgson, N. B.: Nocturnal functional bladder capacity in enuretic children, J. Urol. **105**:129, 1971.
Valk, W. L., and Foret, J. D.: The problem of vesicovaginal and ureterovaginal fistulas, Med. Clin. N. Amer. **43**:1769, 1959.
Walker, J. A.: Injuries of ureter due to external violence, J. Urol. **102**:410, 1969.
Werry, J. S., and Cohrssen, J.: Enuresis—an etiologic and therapeutic study, J. Pediat. **67**:423, 1965.
Wharton, L. R., Jr., and TeLinde, R. W.: An evaluation of fascial sling operation for urinary incontinence in female patients, J. Urol. **82**:76, 1959.

CHAPTER 14

The adrenals

The paired adrenal glands are really composed of two structures with entirely unrelated functions. The cortex secretes a variety of glucose-regulating, mineral-regulating, and sex hormones, while the medulla is concerned with vasoconstriction. The glands normally lie superior and medial to each kidney and in direct proximity. The right adrenal is triangular in shape and hugs the vena cava. It is recessed behind the liver. Its length is approximately 3 cm. and it weighs between 5 and 7 grams. It is heavier in the male. It is supplied by many small arteries that arise from the renal and aortic vessels. Its blood is discharged through several veins, the chief of which is the middle vein emptying into the vena cava or renal vein. The exact vascular distribution varies in different people. Lymphatic drainage occurs but no special significance for this has been determined. The celiac and renal nerve plexuses supply this endocrine organ. The left adrenal differs only in its location in proximity to the aorta instead of the vena cava and a slightly different shape.

The normal adrenals are largely under the control of the anterior pituitary hormone, corticotropin (ACTH). Adrenal products, in turn, have a feedback inhibitory effect on the pituitary.

ADRENAL MEDULLA

Anatomically, the central portion of the adrenal is known as the medulla and it secretes epinephrine and norepinephrine, both powerful vaso-constricting substances. They are produced in excess during stress or in the presence of a pheochromocytoma or neuroblastoma. The tissue is reddish brown in color and stains brown with the application of chromic acid. Thus the term "chromaffin cells" is applied to this tissue of ectoder-

346

mal origin. Ectopic medullary tissue may occur in the kidney, along the great abdominal vessels, next to the bladder or vagina, or anywhere sympathetic nerve tissue is found.

Pheochromocytoma is a rare, familial tumor that occurs bilaterally in 10% of its victims and that is malignant in the same percentage. It involves children and young adults most often. The patient is subject to bouts of nervousness, headache, sweating, flushing, tachycardia, fever, and intermittent hypertension, or the blood pressure may be constantly elevated. The urine is collected for 12 or 24 hours and the vanillylmandelic acid (VMA) content measured. This is a metabolic product of epinephrine and norepinephrine. The test is the most accurate means of diagnosis but must be carried out when the tumor is exhibiting the signs mentioned. The majority of patients with hypertension will show a blood pressure drop when phentolamine methanesulfonate (Regitine) is given intravenously. This is used both as a test and for medical management. The histamine stimulation test is not reliable and occasionally is hazardous. The tumor is difficult to demonstrate, but retroperitoneal pneumography with or without transfemoral aortography is often rewarding. The catheter tip should be well away from the adrenal arteries; the translumbar puncture method would be dangerous and is contraindicated. The excretory urogram may show downward and outward displacement of the kidney, but it is often normal. The transabdominal surgical approach is the best way to search for and remove the tumor(s).

During and after such surgery the patient is subject to marked fluctuation in blood pressure and pulse, and constant nursing attention to these vital signs is paramount. The physician may have to help regulate the intravenous drip of phentolamine or phenylephrine, which may be needed for many hours. The patient should be in the intensive care unit until the vital signs are well stabilized without drugs. In the later postoperative period the patient may be weak and will need assistance in ambulation and personal needs.

Neuroblastomas occur up to middle age and in either sex but most often in young children. Besides the adrenal site, the malignancy may occur elsewhere in the retroperitoneal or mediastinal areas. Local and distant metastases to the bones, lymph nodes, lungs, and liver are frequent. They grow to a large size, and in addition to causing signs and symptoms from their expansion, they may cause fever, pain, and general malaise. In the adrenal area they push the kidney down and out and often contain calcifications. Excretory urography shows the kidney is functioning and is less distorted than when involved with hydronephrosis or Wilms' tumor, the chief entities to be distinguished. The vena cavogram may show obstruction. Treatment is usually surgical excision followed by irradiation and chemotherapy. The prognosis is poor since the diagnosis is often made late. The nursing care is similar to that after removal of Wilms' tumor.

ADRENAL CORTEX

The outer portion of the adrenal gland is called the cortex. It comprises 80% of the gland's size and is yellow in appearance. It is divided into several zones, each secreting its own endocrine substance. The outer zona glomerulosa secretes aldosterone, a mineralocorticoid capable of altering the fluid and electrolyte balance of the body through interaction with the kidneys (see discussion of renovascular hypertension in Chapter 7).

The zona fasciculata and zona reticularis form glucocorticoids, 17-ketosteroids (androgens), and estrogens and progesteroids. Since sex hormones are secreted by the adrenal gland as well as by the gonads, their precise balance is necessary for normal sexual development and function. More than fifty steroids that arise from the cortex have been isolated. Drugs taken by the pregnant female or oversecretion from her own endocrine organs may affect the fetus, producing an abnormal offspring.

Cushing's syndrome

Cushing's syndrome is an extremely hyperglucocorticoid state; that is, excess amounts of glucocorticoid hormones (those controlling carbohydrate metabolism) are secreted by the adrenal cortex. It may be caused by benign hyperplasia or neoplasm of the adrenal cortex. The patient is obese and there is a prominence referred to as "buffalo hump" just below the posterior portion of the neck (Fig. 14-1). Hypertension, diabetes mellitus, brawny edema (especially of the sacral area), muscle wasting, and generalized weakness occur. A rounded moon face and a plethoric, reddened countenance are typical. Females have amenorrhea. Personality changes, usually of the depressive type, are common. Osteoporosis is also common and may lead to fractures. Some patients exhibit hirsutism (excessive hairiness), especially of the face. The skin is thin, with a reduction in subcutaneous tissue. This is in contrast to obese hirsutes who are not suffering from Cushing's syndrome; they have thick skin. Laboratory studies often reveal hyperglycemia (a diabetic glucose tolerance curve), glucosuria, erythrocytosis, leukocytosis, lymphopenia, eosinopenia, decreased levels of serum chloride and potassium, an increased urinary corticoid excretion, and normal or elevated 17-ketosteroid excretion. If carcinoma rather than benign hyperplasia causes the syndrome, excretion of both corticoids and 17-ketosteroids is markedly increased. Without treatment the patient with Cushing's syndrome most often dies relatively early in life, either from complications of diabetes mellitus or from a vascular accident. If 1 mg. of dexamethasone is given at midnight and the 8 A.M. plasma cortisol level is 12 μg% or higher,

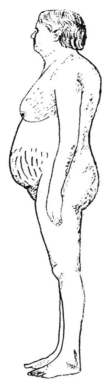

Fig. 14-1. Cushinoid patient shows "moon" face, "buffalo hump" of shoulder region, and marked obesity of trunk with relative thinness of the extremities. Some patients have hirsutism.

further refined tests of the pituitary-adrenal function are in order since it is likely that Cushing's syndrome is present. The nurse's support of the emotionally unstable patient is her chief role in this case.

Adrenogenital syndrome

A state of virilism due to hyperplasia or tumor of the adrenal cortex is known as the adrenogenital syndrome. Congenital adrenal hyperplasia in females results in pseudohermaphroditism. The chief manifestation in female infants is hypertrophy of the clitoris, which requires clitorectomy. If recognized early, the disease can be treated successfully by administration of cortisone to suppress the pituitary hyperexcretion of ACTH, thereby decreasing the adrenal excretion of androgen. In the preadolescent male, precocious puberty is the principal manifestation of the syndrome. In the preadolescent or adult female, virilization (masculinization) and signs of protein conservation such as excessive muscle development appear. The majority of cases of adrenogenital syndrome appearing at puberty or later are caused by neoplasms.

In patients with hyperplasia of the adrenal cortex there is a marked endocrine response (an increase in urinary excretion of corticoid hormones and eosinopenia) when adrenocorticotropic hormone (ACTH) is administered. If there is carcinomatous glandular involvement, little or no endocrine response is obtained by the administration of the ACTH.

Other test agents used to differentiate the various hypercorticism states according to output of corticoids and 17-ketosteroids include metyrapone (inhibits the final step in cortisol biosynthesis) and dexamethasone. (Interested nurses should consult a textbook on endocrinology.)

Surgically, the adrenal glands may be approached anteriorly through the peritoneal space, by incision through the thorax and diaphragm, or quite readily through a posterior incision. Since they are recessed deep within the body, difficulty in their exposure and dissection is often encountered, especially in the obese subject. The frequency of involvement of both glands by tumors or hypertrophy requires exploration of both sides. The cushinoid patient, because of huge abdominal apron, presents a special problem in surgical positioning and approach. Two operating tables may be required, with the patient's abdomen drooping between them. Both adrenals are approached posteriorly and both glands or all of one gland and four fifths of the other gland may need to be excised.

Adrenal cortical tumors

Adrenal cortical tumors are usually benign adenomas (functional or nonfunctional) but may be malignant and excrete large amounts of steroids.

The aldosterone-secreting tumor of the cortex is small and often multiple and bilateral. Its diagnosis therefore is made by detection of blood chemistry abnormalities. The serum potassium level is characteristically low and the CO_2 elevated. The patient exhibits weakness, polydipsia, polyuria, and, infrequently, paresthesias or tetany. Although the patient's elevated blood pressure makes the physician suspect this possibility, it is difficult to distinguish this cause of hypertension from the essential or the renovascular form. The latter may exhibit the same blood chemistry findings (secondary hyperaldosteronism). The chief distinction is found in the bioassay of angiotensin in the peripheral venous blood. This is elevated or increased in renovascular hypertension after a low-salt diet and exercising, but primary aldosteronism does not show such activation of the renin system. Since the tumor(s) is invariably located within the adrenals, a posterior bilateral adrenal exposure is made. If no definite tumor is seen, the left adrenal is removed and sectioned since three out of four occur on this side. If a tumor is not found by this maneuver, four fifths of the right adrenal is removed. The residual tissue is usually sufficient to prevent hypocorticism. Most patients are cured by removal of a functioning adenoma.

Total adrenalectomy. After bilateral total adrenalectomy the patient no longer produces the adrenal steroids essential for the maintenance of life. Fortunately, it is now possible to replace this loss by giving hormones.

During the period when the appropriate replacement necessary for maintaining the patient in reasonably good health is being determined, the chemical analyses of blood (usually serum sodium, potassium, and chloride) and the blood pressure are carefully and frequently checked; drugs and dosages are varied accordingly. Each patient requires individual prescriptions according to his physiologic needs.

The hormones most frequently used in the past for replacement therapy were cortisone and hydrocortisone. Cortisone may be administered intravenously or orally; hydrocortisone is the parenteral preparation. Both of these drugs exert a regulatory effect on carbohydrate metabolism and have an adverse effect on regulation of electrolyte balance. Sodium is retained and potassium is excreted. These effects on the two electrolytes are reduced by the administration of the newer synthetic steroids, prednisone and prednisone. They are many more times potent than hydrocortisone.

Nursing care of patient having adrenal surgery

Nursing care of the patient with adrenal malfunction must be individualized according to his particular needs (Table 6). Attempts are made to prevent, insofar as possible, extra outpouring of hormones in patients with hyperfunction of the adrenal glands and to decrease the need for excessive hormones in patients with hypofunctioning adrenal glands.

Preoperative period. During the preoperative period the nurse assists in diagnostic procedures and in the maintenance or reestablishment of optimum physical and mental status. Since any stressful situation tends to increase the hormonal imbalance in patients with either cortical or medullary adrenal disease, the nurse should take special care to explain all anticipated procedures to the patient and to assure their smooth execution. She needs to listen to the patient's problems and complaints and should make sincere attempts to alleviate them so as to provide a restful, relaxed situation.

Adrenocortical hyperfunction

The patient with hyperadrenocorticism is likely to be quite emotionally labile; he is commonly negativistic. Consequently, the nurse must be tactful in handling situations. Since these patients are frequently abnormal in appearance (Cushing's syndrome and adrenogenital syndrome), privacy needs to be maintained. Sensitiveness about their appearance plus the depression that is of physiologic origin and is a result of the disease make these patients suicidal risks. They require close observation, and

Table 6. Synopsis of physiology and pathophysiology of adrenal cortex*

Adrenal cortical hormones	Functions	Manifestations of underproduction	Manifestations of overproduction
I. Mineralo-corticoids (aldosterone and deoxy-corticosterone)	Proinflammatory effect		
	Electrolytic effect—inhibits renal tubular resorption of potassium and enhances resorption of sodium	Hyperkalemia; hyponatremia (dehydration, decreased blood volume, circulatory collapse, shock, increased capillary permeability)	Hypokalemia (muscle weakness, cardiac arrhythmias etc.); hypernatremia (water retention, increase in blood volume, increase in blood pressure, cardiac involvement)
II. Glucocorti-coids (cortisone and hydrocortisone)	Metabolic effect (a) Gluconeogenesis —conversion of protein to glucose (protein catabolic effect)	Hypoglycemia; decrease in liver glycogen	Hyperglycemia; negative nitrogen balance; osteoporosis
	(b) Insulin antagonism	Hypersensitivity to insulin administration	Delayed wound healing
	Electrolytic effect—same as mineralocorticoids, though to lesser degree	See mineralocorticoids	
	Anti-inflammatory effect—opposes inflammatory process (chief clinical use of glucocorticoids in addition to replacement therapy)		Vulnerability to infection—depression of inflammatory response, a body defense mechanism
	Enable body to withstand stress situations (essential for life—exact mechanism unknown)	Vulnerability to minor stress (emotional and physical)	
	Depression of lymphoid tissue, fibroblasts, and eosinophils	Eosinophilia; lymphocytosis	Eosinopenia; lymphopenia; delayed wound healing

*From Reich, B. H., and Ault, L. P.: Nursing care of the patient with Addison's disease, Amer. J. Nurs. 60:1253, 1960.

Table 6. Synopsis of physiology and pathophysiology of adrenal cortex
—cont'd

Adrenal cortical hormones	Functions	Manifestations of underproduction	Manifestations of overproduction
III. Gonadlike hormones— androgens (testosterone)	Masculinizing effect	Loss of body hair; decrease in muscle mass	Masculinization
	Protein anabolic effect	Weakness	Increased strength, muscle mass, and libido; sense of well-being
Estrogens (estrogen)	Feminizing effect		Feminization

protective measures to prevent self-destruction should be taken when indicated.

Peptic ulcer is likely to occur, and any epigastric distress calls for a consideration of this possibility. Antacids are frequently administered.

If osteoporosis is present, care must be taken to prevent falls, which may readily cause fractures. Siderails or low beds are indicated. Since muscular weakness is frequently present, the patient should be assisted in ambulation as necessary.

Patients with abnormal fat deposits and thin skin such as occur in Cushing's syndrome bruise easily and are prone to decubitus ulcer formation, as are those in whom paralysis is a symptom (primary aldosteronism). Alternating air pressure mattresses should be used, and the bedridden patient should be turned at least every 2 hours. Careful skin care over pressure points is essential.

Increased output of cortisone predisposes the patient to infection. Catheterization should be avoided, if possible, and strict asepsis used in any procedures requiring entrance into a closed body cavity or breakage of skin. No one with known upper respiratory, staphylococcal, or other infections should be allowed to come into contact with the patient.

Food and fluid intake may need to be carefully recorded to ensure adequate diet control. Diets low in sodium and high in potassium are frequently ordered preoperatively. Potassium intake may be supplemented by the administration of enteric-coated potassium tablets or potassium cocktails. Insulin and/or diets similar to those used for patients with diabetes mellitus may be ordered for patients with excessive hyperglycemia. (See a medical nursing textbook for a discussion of the care of a patient with diabetes mellitus.)

Urinary output should be recorded as to the time and amount of each voiding. If serious polyuria develops (see discussion of fluid intake and output in Chapter 4), vasopressin (Pitressin) may be ordered to prevent dehydration.

The patient's mouth is often very dry, and frequent mouth care should be given. Cold drinks at intervals may also help to relieve the discomfort, but special care must be taken that the fluids offered are not restricted on the prescribed diet.

Postoperative period. Regardless of removal of the diseased tissue and hormonal replacement, preoperative symptoms usually do not subside for several weeks postoperatively. The general care required during the preoperative period must therefore be continued.

Since the hormonal replacement is delicately regulated on the basis of continuous observations of electrolytic, metabolic, and blood pressure balances, the patient who has had adrenal surgery needs to be given constant nursing attention until hormonal stability is regained or a maintenance regimen is established.

The operative incision is often close to the diaphragm and therefore special care should be taken to have the patient turned frequently. He should be encouraged to breathe deeply and to cough. Since the incision is painful, it should be firmly supported during coughing and turning. Dyspnea or sudden chest pain should be reported at once because a spontaneous pneumothorax may occur.

The patient usually returns from the operating room with a gastric tube in place since the surgery may require entrance into the peritoneal cavity and considerable manipulation of abdominal organs. This tube should be attached to the prescribed drainage. Special mouth care should be given to prevent stomatitis and parotitis.

The patient is usually kept in bed for 1 to 2 days postoperatively. Because the vascular system is quite unstable, he is usually kept flat during at least the first 24 hours; this does not preclude turning from side to side. When the patient is permitted to be out of bed, most doctors order elastic bandages applied to both legs. The first time the patient gets up he should sit in a chair and his blood pressure should be checked frequently. If hypotension occurs, he should be returned to bed. Specific orders for the type, amount, and progression of ambulation should be obtained from the doctor.

Adrenocortical resection

Hormonal balance is exceedingly labile during the first several days after all or part of the adrenocortical tissue or a tumor of it is removed. Intravenous or intramuscular replacement of hormones therefore must be constantly adjusted. Hydrocortisone may be given continuously by intravenous drip, and drugs to raise the blood pressure are often given intravenously. The rate of infusions containing pressor drugs are regulated in accordance with frequent blood pressure readings (usually every 15 minutes). The nurse is responsible for making accurate blood pressure recordings and for adjusting the rate of flow of the infusion containing pressor drugs according to the doctor's orders. The doctor usually leaves an order for the rate of flow to be increased if the pressure drops below a specified level; there is usually an order to decrease the rate if the pressure rises. If there is no order, the doctor must be notified of changes in blood pressure. When the blood pressure does not respond appropriately to the prescribed rate of infusion flow, the doctor should also be notified.

When a patient has had adrenocortical resection, the nurse should observe him carefully for signs of hypoglycemia. These are headache, weakness, perspiration, trembling, emotional instability, visual disturbances, and apprehension.

When the patient is able to eat, the nurse should check to see that he has eaten the food served. The diet is prescribed to meet the patient's physiologic needs, and if it is not eaten, the doctor should be notified so that replacement can be given as necessary. The patient on regular meals should be watched especially closely for hypoglycemic reactions between 5 and 6 A.M. Hypoglycemic reactions also often follow any mentally or physically stressful activity. If a meal must be delayed or omitted for any reason, the fasting period should be kept at a minimum and the patient's activities curtailed during the fast since any physical exercise stimulates carbohydrate metabolism. If a hypoglycemic reaction occurs, the doctor usually orders glucose given by mouth or intravenously. He should be notified as soon as this condition is suspected because the patient may quickly lapse into coma.

The nurse should also be alert for symptoms of addisonian crisis. Shock with extremely low blood pressure, cyanosis, nausea and vomiting, and severe abdominal pain occurs in patients with this condition. The patient is extremely weak and hard to arouse. This complication also requires immediate treatment. The doctor will probably order increased amounts of hydrocortisone; saline solutions and DOCA are also usually ordered. Absolute bed rest may be ordered to decrease physical stress. Markedly increased urinary output indicates the need for vasopressin to control excessive diuresis. This symptom should be treated promptly, too, to prevent dehydration and electrolyte embalance.

Rehabilitative period

Permanent replacement therapy. The patient who requires hormonal substitution for the remainder of his life presents a serious rehabilitative problem. Prognosis depends on his acceptance of the situation and his understanding of his limitations and therapy. It is important for the patient to have the support of family members and for them to understand the management and be willing to assume the responsibility for his therapy if he is unable to do so himself. The patient must know that his therapy cannot be discontinued for a single day and that it does not provide leeway for the excessive hormonal needs engendered by unusually stressful situations, either physical or mental. Because of this, he must learn to recognize and avoid stress-producing situations such as job tensions, family quarrels, and excessive exercise. Fasting, extremes of temperature, and fatigue should also be avoided.

If symptoms of inadequate hormones occur, medical advice should be sought at once. The symptoms are similar to those of waning effectiveness of corticosteroid therapy or, in extreme situations, those of addisonian crisis. If any infection, no matter how minor, or any other physical symptoms such as vomiting, diarrhea, or injury occur, the person should seek medical advice. Since pregnancy is a stress, the physician should be consulted about family planning. Additional hormones may be needed by the woman during the period of gestation and delivery.

Because sudden, unexpected stressful situations such as accidents or incapacitating illness may occur, the patient should always carry an identification card on which is noted his name, address, and telephone number; his doctor's name, address, and telephone number; and the prescribed corticoid therapy with the dosage to be used in event of an emergency. Patients on prolonged cortisone therapy have a predisposition to dental caries. Therefore good dental hygiene and regular visits to the dentist are important for maintenance of general health. Although replacement therapy may seem to restrict the usual life pattern markedly, the person who has been helped to accept his limitations and live with them is able to have a relatively normal life. (President John F. Kennedy was an example.) It is important to remember that the patient is far less restricted than he was with a diseased adrenal cortex.

Temporary replacement therapy. The patient requiring only temporary replacement of either adrenal cortical or medullary hormones is gradually removed from drug therapy. During this period he should be observed for the same untoward symptoms as a person on permanent replacement therapy. Drugs are often discontinued before the patient is discharged from the hospital. If they have not been discontinued, the patient must be taught the importance of taking them regularly. Regardless of whether he is on drug therapy or not, the patient and his family should know the untoward symptoms of hormonal deficiency and the need to seek immediate medical attention if these symptoms occur. The doctor usually wishes the patient to be encouraged to lead a less stressful life than usual for several months. Regular medical follow-up should be continued until the doctor determines it is no longer necessary.

QUESTIONS

1. Name the two main sections of the adrenal gland.
2. Name some tumors arising in the adrenal medulla.
3. Name some diseases of the adrenal cortex.
4. What are the three types of hormones secreted by the adrenal cortex?
5. What type of secretion arises in the adrenal medulla?
6. What is meant by the adrenogenital syndrome?
7. What medication is necessary after total adrenalectomy?
8. Which adrenal tumor tends to occur in other members of the family?
9. Patients with insufficient adrenal cortical secretion suffer from what disease?
10. What are the symptoms of this disease?
11. What is meant by virilism?

REFERENCES

Biglieri, E. G., Hane, S., Slaton, P. E., Forsham, P. H., Herron, M. A., and Horita, S.: Steroid secretion in adrenal disease, J. Clin. Invest. **42:**516, 1963.

Bradley, J. E., Young, J. D., Jr., and Lentz, G.: Polycythemia secondary to pheochromocytoma, J. Urol. **86:**1, 1961.

Cerny, J. D., Nesbit, R. M., Conn, J. W., Bookstein, J. J., Rovner, D. R., Cohen, E. L., Lucas, C. P., Warshawsky, A., and Southwell, T.: Preoperative tumor localization by adrenal venography in patient with primary aldosteronism: comparison with operative findings, J. Urol. **103:**521, 1970.

Conn, J. W., Knopf, R. F., and Nesbit, R. M.: Clinical characteristics of primary aldosteronism from an analysis of 145 cases, Amer. J. Surg. **107:**159, 1964.

Cox, R.: Bilateral adrenalectomy: a case report, J. Amer. Ass. Nurs. Anesth. **34:**48, 1966.

Frohman, I. P.: The adrenocorticosteroids, Amer. J. Nurs. **64:**120, 1964.

Konnak, J. W., and Cerny, J. C.: Surgical treatment of Cushing's syndrome, J. Urol. **102:**653, 1969.

Pickett, L. K., and Voorhess, M. L.: Neuroblastoma in childhood, Surg. Clin. N. Amer. **44:**1469, 1964.

Shea, K. M., O'Connor, C. P., Karoflis, E. G., Thorn, G. W., and Kozak, G. P.: What and how to teach a patient with adrenal insufficiency, Amer. J. Nurs. **65:**80, 1965.

Weinberg, M. A.: Pheochromocytoma, Arch. Intern. Med. **112:**677, 1963.

Winter, C. C.: Correctable renal and adrenal hypertension. In Tice's practice of medicine, Hagerstown, Md., 1968, Hoeber Medical Division, Harper & Row.

Index

359